REHABILITATION IN CANCER CARE

REHABILITATION IN CANCER CARE

Edited by

Jane Rankin
MSc, BSc (Hons), MCSP, SRP

Karen Robb
PhD, BSc, PGCAP, MCSP, SRP

Nicola Murtagh
MBA, DipM, Grad Dip Phys, MCSP, SRP

Jill Cooper
MSc, P Dip, Dip M, DipCOT, SROT

Sian Lewis
BSc (Hons), PG Dip, RD

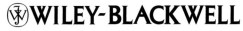

WILEY-BLACKWELL

A John Wiley & Sons, Ltd., Publication

This edition first published 2008
© 2008 Blackwell Publishing Ltd

Blackwell Publishing was acquired by John Wiley & Sons in February 2007. Blackwell's publishing programme has been merged with Wiley's global Scientific, Technical and Medical business to form Wiley-Blackwell.

Registered office
John Wiley & Sons Ltd, The Atrium, Southern Gate, Chichester, West Sussex, PO19 8SQ, United Kingdom

Editorial offices
9600 Garsington Road, Oxford, OX4 2DQ, United Kingdom
2121 State Avenue, Ames, Iowa 50014-8300, USA

For details of our global editorial offices, for customer services and for information about how to apply for permission to reuse the copyright material in this book please see our website at www.wiley.com/wiley-blackwell.

Library of Congress Cataloging-in-Publication Data

Rehabilitation in cancer care / edited by Jane Rankin . . . [et al.].
      p.   ;   cm.
   Includes bibliographical references and index.
   ISBN-13: 978-1-4051-5997-5 (pbk. : alk. paper)
   ISBN-10: 1-4051-5997-9 (pbk. : alk. paper)   1. Cancer—Palliative treatment.
   2. Cancer—Patients—Rehabilitation.   I. Rankin, Jane, 1964–
   [DNLM: 1. Neoplasms—rehabilitation—Great Britain.   2. Allied Health Personnel—Great Britain.   3. Palliative Care—methods—Great Britain.   4. Patient Care Team—Great Britain.
   QZ 266 R345 2008]
   RC271.P33.R44   2008
   616.99′4029—dc22

                                                                                2008006137

A catalogue record for this book is available from the British Library.

Set in 10/12.5 pt Sabon by Aptara Inc., New Delhi, India
Printed in Singapore by Markono Print Media Pte Ltd

1   2008

CONTENTS

SECTION 3: SYMPTOM MANAGEMENT

CONTRIBUTORS

Editors

Jill Cooper
Head Occupational Therapist, Royal Marsden NHS Foundation Trust, London

Sian Lewis
Clinical Head Dietitian, Velindre Cancer Centre, Wales

Nicola Murtagh
Head of Therapies, Royal Marsden NHS Foundation Trust, London

Jane Rankin
Lead Cancer Physiotherapist, Cancer Centre, Belfast City Hospital, Belfast Health and Social Care Trust, Belfast, Northern Ireland

Dr Karen Robb
Consultant Oncology Physiotherapist, Physiotherapy Department, St Bartholomew's Hospital, London

Contributors

Lorraine Ashcroft
Senior Oncology Head and Neck Cancer Physiotherapist, Cancer Centre, Belfast City Hospital, Belfast Health and Social Care Trust, Belfast, Northern Ireland

Tessa Aston
Macmillan Specialist Dietitian, Palliative Care Team, The Rutson Hospital, Northallerton, North Yorkshire

Rachel Barrett
Highly Specialist Haematology Dietitian, Department of Nutrition & Dietetics, Guy's and St Thomas' NHS Foundation Trust, Guy's Hospital, London

Philomena Canning
Senior Occupational Therapist, Royal Marsden NHS Foundation Trust, Sutton, Surrey

Joanne Carr
Senior Oncology Physiotherapist, Beaumont Hospital, Dublin, Ireland

Karen Chambers
Senior Occupational Therapist, Cancer Centre, Belfast City Hospital, Belfast
Health and Social Care Trust, Belfast, Northern Ireland

Professor Robin Davidson
Clinical Psychology Department, Belfast City Hospital, Belfast Health and Social
Care Trust, Belfast, Northern Ireland

Iona Davies
Macmillan Lymphoedema Physiotherapist, Lymphoedema Clinic, Singleton
Hospital, Swansea

Rhian Davies
Specialist Lymphoedema Physiotherapist, Bromyard, Herefordshire

Merian Denning
Senior Physiotherapist, Water Lane Physiotherapy Clinic, Wilmslow, Cheshire

Sue Desborough
Lymphoedema Therapist, Lymphoedema Clinic, St Giles Hospice, Lichfield,
Staffordshire

Nicola Evans
Head Occupational Therapist, Cancer Centre, Belfast City Hospital, Belfast Health
and Social Care Trust, Belfast, Northern Ireland

Charlie Ewer-Smith
Macmillan Occupational Therapist, Occupational Therapy, Bristol Haematology
and Oncology Centre, Bristol

Dr Paul A. Fenton
Specialist Registrar in Clinical Oncology, Wessex Rotation, Southampton General
Hospital, Southampton

Paula Finlay
Senior Neuro-oncology Physiotherapist, Cancer Centre, Belfast City Hospital,
Belfast Health and Social Care Trust, Belfast, Northern Ireland

Sarah Fisher
Clinical Director, The Beacon Specialist Community Cancer and Palliative Care
Service, Guildford, Surrey

Dr Jacqueline Gracey
Faculty of Life and Health Sciences (Physiotherapy), University of Ulster at
Jordanstown, Newtownabbey, Northern Ireland

Mandy Hamilton
Senior Specialist Oncology Dietitian, Cancer Centre, Belfast City Hospital, Belfast
Health and Social Care Trust, Belfast, Northern Ireland

Melanie Lewis
Lead Macmillan Lymphoedema Physiotherapist, Lymphoedema Clinic, Singleton Hospital, Swansea

Gemma Lindsell
Senior Occupational Therapist, Royal Marsden NHS Foundation Trust, Sutton, Surrey

Karen Livingstone
Senior Physiotherapist, Neil Cliffe Cancer Care Centre, Wythenshawe Hospital, Manchester

Daniel Lowrie
Senior Occupational Therapist, Royal Marsden NHS Trust, London

Gillian Lusty
Specialist Speech and Language Therapist (Oncology), Cancer Centre, Belfast City Hospital, Belfast Health and Social Care Trust, Belfast, Northern Ireland

Pippa McCabe
Senior Gynae-oncology Physiotherapist, Cancer Centre, Belfast City Hospital, Belfast Health and Social Care Trust, Belfast, Northern Ireland

Dr Doreen McClurg
Clinical Specialist Physiotherapist, Belfast City Hospital, Belfast Health and Social Care Trust, Belfast, Northern Ireland

Debbie McKinney
Senior Lung Cancer Physiotherapist, Cancer Centre, Belfast Health and Social Care Trust, Belfast, Northern Ireland

Sallyanne McKinney
Upper Gastrointestinal Cancer Specialist Dietitian, Nutrition and Dietetic Department, The James Cook University Hospital, Middlesbrough

Jennifer Miller
Senior Occupational Therapist, Royal Marsden NHS Foundation Trust, Sutton, Surrey

Brenda Nugent
Senior Oncology Dietitian, Cancer Centre, Belfast City Hospital, Belfast Health and Social Care Trust, Belfast, Northern Ireland

Catriona Ogilvy
Senior Occupational Therapist, Royal Marsden NHS Foundation Trust, London

Debbie Pearson
Macmillan Occupational Therapist, Palliative Care Team, The Rutson Hospital, Northallerton, North Yorkshire

Dr Gillian Prue
Health and Rehabilitation Science Research Institute, University of Ulster at Jordanstown, Newtownabbey, Northern Ireland

Lena Richards
Senior Physiotherapist (Sarcoma), Christie Hospital, Withington, Manchester

Dr Geoff Sharpe
Consultant Clinical Oncologist, Southampton General Hospital, Southampton

Sarah Taggart
Senior Haematology Physiotherapist, Belfast City Hospital, Belfast Health and Social Care Trust, Belfast, Northern Ireland

Kathy Thompson
Macmillan Occupational Therapy, Specialist for Neuro-oncology, Cookridge Hospital, Leeds, West Yorkshire

Helen White
Speech and Language Therapy Team Leader, Royal Marsden NHS Foundation Trust, Sutton, Surrey

Heidi Williams
Senior Upper Gastrointestinal/ENT Physiotherapist, Rehabilitation Centre, The James Cook University Hospital, Middlesbrough

Val Young
Physiotherapy Superintendent in Oncology, Physiotherapy Department, Southampton General Hospital, Southampton

FOREWORD

Gone are the days when cancer was an inevitable pathway to death. Many cancers now respond to the new treatments and some, such as breast cancer, have become much more of a chronic disease state than a terminal illness. It is therefore increasingly important that patients do have the support they need to rehabilitate back to an active and enjoyable lifestyle, despite the limitations that their disease and its treatments may have imposed.

The National Council for Palliative Care has defined supportive care as a process which 'helps the patient and their family to cope with cancer and treatment of it, from pre-diagnosis, through the process of diagnosis and treatment, to cure, continuing illness or death and into bereavement. It helps the patient to maximise the benefits of treatment and to live as well as possible with the affect of the disease. It is given equal priority alongside diagnosis and treatment'.

Rehabilitation is an essential core component to cancer care and much rehabilitation depends on those professions such as physiotherapy, occupational therapy, dietetics, speech and language therapy and podiatry. As rehabilitation occurs, the professions of medicine and nursing tend to take a back seat, having had a major role in aspects of disease management and control, but a lesser role in rehabilitation.

This book is an important introduction for those who are looking after patients with cancer. It helps them understand why people with cancer and even those receiving palliative or terminal care can benefit greatly from rehabilitation and rehabilitation techniques. It also provides the reader with an understanding of tumour growth and the way the different cancers behave, their responses to treatment and how this impacts on the patient.

Although the more common forms of cancer, the symptoms and the side effects of treatment may be well known, they may often need the specialist intervention of an allied health professional to ensure that patients can cope with the situation they are faced with. All interventions and rehabilitation need to be evaluated and this book provides an evidence base for such interventions, thereby providing an important resource to those professionals working within rehabilitation or who are training up in rehabilitation in cancer.

Multi-professional working must have patients and their family at the heart of decision making. It is only by addressing all aspects of patient care in a holistic way that a patient's needs can be met. It is so often the smaller detail of daily living that can grind patients down, destroy their morale, their self-confidence and their self-esteem. Attention to detail is crucial if patients are to be adequately supported. Thus the chapters on multi-professional management of patients are particularly important. They cover all of those broad areas and address the types of questions that patients themselves ask, such as "is there anything I should not eat?" or "what should I avoid doing?" By helping patients venture towards the boundaries of their ability, they are able to push those boundaries further and further and achieve more. It is the rehabilitative services that allow patients to live independently, to return home from hospital and to cope within the restrictions of disease and treatment. This book is one to be taken off the shelf to refer to time and time again.

Professor the Baroness Finlay of Llandaff
September 2007

ACKNOWLEDGEMENTS

The inspiration for planning this book was created at an executive meeting of the Association of Chartered Physiotherapists in Oncology and Palliative Care (ACPOPC) when it was planned to propose a physiotherapy-specific cancer rehabilitation book. The need for such a publication had been highlighted for some years by the group's membership. After initial discussion, it was realised that an allied health profession (AHP) book would promote interdisciplinary working and be of more benefit to clinicians, managers, educators, students and patients. As such, the other professions such as occupational therapy, dietetics, speech and language therapy and podiatry were contacted. On behalf of ACPOPC, I thank the link professional leads (Jill Cooper, Tricia Knox, Chris Timney and David McKeown) for their support and enthusiasm, for recruiting their chapter contributors and additional members for the editorial panel and for being available for professional advice. Without their networking and persuasive skills, the book would never have been published in its AHP team format.

On behalf of the editorial committee, I also thank the 44 multi-professional health care staff from all areas of care provision and education that contributed to this book. It has been refreshing to see such dedication and professionalism in everyone's approach to the project. More so, the support and respect shown by and to all professions has been inspiring.

I also thank Val Young for her continued back up regarding interprofessional communication and manuscript completion. As always, Val was happily behind the editorial committee ensuring timely progress.

Jane Rankin
Editor

SECTION 1

INTRODUCTION TO ONCOLOGY AND PALLIATIVE CARE

Chapter 1

CANCER AND ITS MANAGEMENT – AN INTRODUCTION

Dr Geoff Sharpe and Dr Paul A. Fenton

Cancer is a major public health issue and impacts on everyone's life, either directly or indirectly. It can occur at all ages, may affect the rich or the poor and represents a huge burden not only for individuals but also for their families and their societies. It remains one of the leading causes of death in the world, particularly in developing countries.

The World Health Organization (WHO) reports 7.6 million people dying from cancer in 2005, with more than 70% occurring in low- and middle-income countries where resources for prevention, diagnosis and treatment of cancer are limited or non-existent. Based on conservative projections, cancer deaths worldwide will continue to rise with an estimated 9 million people dying in 2015, rising to 11.4 million by 2030 (World Health Organization, 2006a).

It is thought that many of these deaths are avoidable, with at least one-third of cancers being preventable and others detected early and cured with appropriate treatment. Even patients with advanced, recurrent or incurable cancer may still benefit from life-extending or palliative treatment and supportive care.

Cancer in the UK

Incidence

In the UK, 233 621 persons were diagnosed with cancer (excluding non-melanoma skin cancer, NMSC) during 2004, with four types – breast, lung, colorectal and prostate – accounting for over half of all new cases (Figure 1.1) (Office for National Statistics, 2006). Breast cancer remains the most common cancer in the UK despite the fact that it is rare in men, whilst lung cancer is the most common cause of cancer death. Overall, cancer is responsible for around one quarter of all deaths in the UK.

The overall incidence of cancer over the preceding decade had remained fairly constant but this masks large changes in reported incidence trends for individual cancers, with large decreases in invasive bladder and stomach cancers and large increases in melanoma, uterine, oral and kidney cancers.

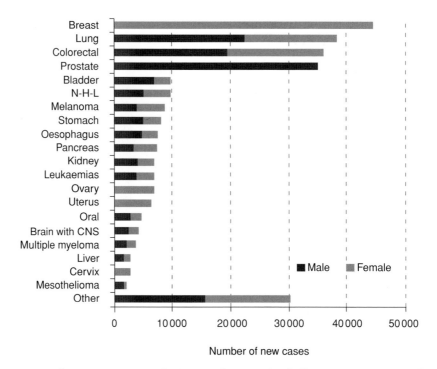

Figure 1.1 The 20 most commonly diagnosed cancers (excluding NMSC), UK, 2004. [Office for National Statistics (www.statistics.gov.uk). Crown Copyright. Reproduced under the terms of the Click-Use Licence.]

Age

In the UK, cancer remains predominantly a disease of older persons, with the majority being diagnosed after the age of retirement (Figure 1.2).

Cancer in children (0–14 years) and young adults (15–24 years) is uncommon and together represents just over 1% of all cases. Many of the types of cancer seen in children are rarely seen in adults and, conversely, the common adult cancers are rare in children. The commonest cancers in childhood are haematological (leukaemia/lymphoma) followed by tumours of the central nervous system. The most common cancers in teenagers and young adults include lymphoma, testicular cancer, melanoma, leukaemia and bone and connective tissue tumours.

Cancer and its management

The WHO Cancer Control Series (2006b) identifies the four main components of cancer control as:

- Prevention
- Early detection

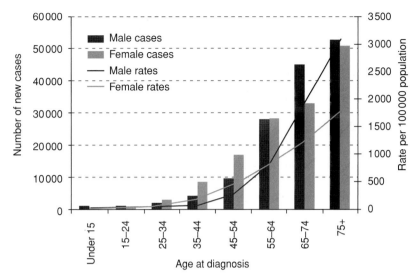

Figure 1.2 Number of new cases and rates by age and sex (excluding NMSC), UK, 2004. [Office for National Statistics (www.statistics.gov.uk). Crown Copyright. Reproduced under the terms of the Click-Use Licence.]

- Diagnosis and treatment
- Palliative care

Cancer may be defined as the uncontrolled growth and spread of abnormal cells, which, if left unchecked, leads to ill health and death. It is not a single condition but rather a collection of over 200 diseases arising from such uncontrolled growth amongst different cell types and organs.

The mechanisms involved in the causation and development of many of these cancers are not fully understood and these involve complex interactions between genetic, lifestyle and environmental factors, i.e. 'nature and nurture'. This is reflected in the epidemiology of cancer, which shows marked variations in both the type and the frequency of cancers between and within different populations.

An understanding of the factors involved in the causation and progression of cancer is essential to prevent, detect and successfully treat the disease.

Prevention of cancer

Lifestyle choices

It is estimated that around half of all cancers diagnosed in the UK could be avoided if people made appropriate lifestyle choices (Cancer Research UK, 2005):

- Smoking – The links between cancer and smoking are now well proved. It is reported to be the single biggest cause of cancer in the world and accounts for one in four cancer deaths in the UK, mainly due to lung cancer. Stopping smoking can greatly reduce the risk of smoking-related cancers, with the risk of lung cancer falling to about half of that of a smoker within 10 years.

- Obesity – Studies of obesity in adults have revealed a relationship between excess body weight and cancer, especially kidney, uterus and colon cancers as well as breast cancer in post-menopausal women.
- Diet – It is not currently possible to identify and quantify all risk factors and protective factors in the diet, but there is agreement that diet may be an important component of cancer risk. There is clear association between alcohol intake and some cancers of the upper aerodigestive tract.
- Physical activity – There is growing evidence for a direct link between physical inactivity and cancer, particularly of the colon, which is independent of body weight.
- Exposure to sunlight – Ultraviolet exposure has increased in recent decades in the UK population due to holidays abroad and the use of sunbeds and sunlamps. During this period there has been parallel increase in all skin cancers, including a three- to fourfold increase in melanoma. It remains an occupational risk for outdoor workers.
- Occupation – Historically, a large number of occupations were hazardous to health, including exposure to carcinogens (substances associated with the development of cancer). Such exposure is now banned or regulated in the UK and the majority of occupation-associated cancers seen today are the result of exposure many years ago. Much of this exposure occurred in small numbers of workers in specific occupations, but large numbers of people may have been affected by occupational exposure to asbestos. This is known to be associated with a long latency period leading to mesothelioma and lung cancer in later life. It is estimated that the mesothelioma death rates in the UK will not peak until 2013.
- Infections – Cancer itself is not infectious, but there are a number of infective agents that can be implicated in the development of cancer. These include human immunodeficiency virus (Kaposi's sarcoma, lymphoma and other cancers), hepatitis B and C (liver cancer), *Helicobacter pylori* (stomach cancer), human papilloma virus (HPV; cervix and other anogenital cancers) and Epstein–Barr virus (some nasopharyngeal cancers and lymphomas).

Vaccines against the HPVs are being introduced in a national vaccination programme in the UK. They have been found to be effective against the main strains of HPV linked to cervical cancer and it is estimated that vaccinating girls at around the age of 12 years has the potential to prevent many, but not all, of the 3000 cervical cancers currently diagnosed each year.

Inherited/familial cancer

Cancer is common and many people diagnosed with cancer may have a relative who has also been affected, either due to chance or due to environmental reasons. True family cancer syndromes are uncommon and account for only around 5% of all cancers. They are due to inherited genetic mutations that increase an individual's risk of developing the disease. There are many such syndromes, each one associated with different genetic changes and characteristic tumour types and presentations.

Features suggestive of a family cancer syndrome include:

- Many cancers diagnosed within one side of a family
- Two or more close blood relatives diagnosed with the same cancer
- Cancer diagnosed at an earlier age than usual
- Individuals developing more than one type of cancer
- Cancers occurring in individuals with other unusual physical features, including birth defects

Some syndromes, but not all, are associated with specific mutations that can be identified in the laboratory. Such genetic testing needs careful consideration because:

- Inheritance of such a mutation does not always mean that individual will necessarily develop cancer
- Absence of such a mutation does not mean that individual will not develop cancer.
- At what age should the test be done?
- Does knowledge of the test result alter that individual's medical management?
- The impact on the family
- The impact on the individual

Consequently, referral to specialist cancer genetics teams for assessment and counselling regarding the risks, benefits and consequences of such testing is essential.

Immunodeficiency

This can be either primary (inherited) or secondary (acquired) usually as a consequence of immunosuppressive therapy, e.g. following organ transplantation or human immunodeficiency virus (HIV)/acquired immunodeficiency syndrome (AIDS). Such individuals are predominantly at risk of lymphoma, skin tumours and some solid tumours.

Detecting cancer early

If cancer cannot be prevented, the next best thing is to detect it early, for at this stage many cancers may still be cured. This is the rationale for screening and self-examination programmes.

Screening

This is the presumptive identification of cancers (or pre-cancer) by means of tests, examinations or other procedures that can be applied rapidly.

The success of cancer screening programmes depends on a number of fundamental principles:

- The target disease should be a common cancer with a known natural history and with high associated morbidity or mortality
- Effective treatment capable of reducing this morbidity or mortality should be available
- Test procedures should be acceptable, safe, inexpensive and have high sensitivity and specificity

Such organised screening programmes include:

- NHS Breast Cancer Screening Programme – It is based on mammography every 3 years for patients aged 50–70 years and is estimated to save around 1400 lives per year in England alone. Patient acceptance rates are relatively high at around 75%.
- NHS Cervical Cancer Screening Programme – It involves a cervical smear performed every 3–5 years (age dependant) on women aged 25–64. This may detect and facilitate treatment for conditions that might otherwise develop into invasive cancer.

  The uptake is high at around 80% and may prevent up to 5000 deaths per year. Despite this, almost half of all cases of cervical cancer in the UK have never had a cervical screening.
- NHS Bowel Cancer Screening Programme – It is currently being introduced across the UK and will be fully operational by 2009. It uses faecal occult blood testing as an initial 2-yearly screening in men and women aged 60–90 years. A positive test leads to further investigations (usually colonoscopy). Around 50% of colonoscopies will prove to be normal, 40% may demonstrate polyps that can be removed before they undergo any malignant change and 10% will be found to have a cancer, hopefully still in the early stages where treatment may be curative.

Self-examination

Some cancers can be usefully detected by self-examination, e.g. melanoma (where early diagnosis may reduce death rates by up to 63%) and perhaps testicular cancers.

There is no evidence to support taught systematic breast self-examination and this has been largely replaced by a more relaxed breast awareness campaign.

Cancer – diagnosis and treatment

Diagnosis

Patients with cancer may present in a variety of manners, both acute and chronic. The initial presumptive diagnosis of cancer is usually made by clinical history and physical examination, supported by appropriate investigations including imaging studies (X-rays, computed tomography (CT) scans, magnetic resonance (MR) imaging and positron emission tomography (PET)), and laboratory tests, including tumour markers and cytology. The definitive pathological diagnosis is usually made following a biopsy.

Staging

This is the term used to define the size and degree of spread (both local and distant) of a cancer with respect to treatment planning and prognosis. The staging may also include other features of specific prognostic value to that particular cancer, e.g. pathological grade or degree of necrosis. There is not a single staging system for all cancers, but the most commonly used one is the American Joint Committee on Cancer (AJCC) TNM classification (Greene *et al.*, 2002), with individual cancers defined according to TNM criteria, where:

T stands for tumour. (This defines the extent of local spread.)
N stands for regional lymph node involvement.
M stands for the presence of metastases; i.e. the cancer has spread to other parts of the body.

A number is added to each letter to indicate specific category grouping and in some cancer types further internationally agreed subgroupings are used. For example, a 4-cm breast cancer with a metastasis in a mobile axillary lymph node on the same side and with no evidence of metastases elsewhere would be classified as:

T2 – Tumour greater than 2 cm but not larger than 5 cm in greatest dimension
N1 – Metastasis to movable ipsilateral lymph node(s)
M0 – No distant metastases

The TNM combinations typically correspond with one of the defined stage groupings (I–IV) for that specific cancer. In the example above, this TNM combination would be in AJCC Stage IIB. Staging is predominantly clinical and is based on physical examination, imaging and biopsy. Pathological staging can only be assigned following surgery to remove or explore the extent of the cancer and combines the results of both the clinical staging and the surgical findings. The TNM category is then modified by the prefix 'p', e.g. pT2.

The formal stage of a cancer does not change over time even if the cancer progresses. It is defined as the stage it was given when it was first diagnosed. It is uncommon for cancers to be restaged, but if they are, they are defined by the prefix 'r'. Precise use of staging is important as it provides a common language by which clinicians can discuss a specific case and is used to identify appropriate clinical trials.

Treatment

Surgery

This is the oldest form of cancer treatment and probably still remains the most important modality today. It offers the greatest chance of cure for many patients, particularly when the cancer is localised. Most patients will have some form of surgery at some point during their cancer journey.

- Preventative surgery – This is the prophylactic removal of non-cancerous tissue that has a high subsequent risk of becoming malignant. Examples would include the removal of pre-cancerous polyps from the colon and even bilateral mastectomy in a patient with a known inherited mutation of specific genes (*BRCA1* or *BRCA2*) where the risk of developing breast cancer is very high.
- Diagnostic surgery – It is performed to confirm the diagnosis of cancer, as well as to give information about type, grade and stage.

  A biopsy is a procedure to remove a small tissue sample for histopathological examination in the laboratory. It may be obtained at open surgery either as an excisional biopsy (whole tumour removed from that site) or as an incisional biopsy (small part of a larger tumour is removed). A tissue biopsy can also be obtained at endoscopy or by needle biopsy of palpable tumours or of deeper lesions using radiological image guidance.

  Fine-needle aspiration of a suspected cancer is a minimally invasive technique that uses a fine needle attached to a syringe. The aspirated cells are assessed by a cytologist who may be able to rapidly confirm the presence of cancer, but since the cells are assessed in the absence of histological architecture, it does require expertise to interpret.
- Radical surgery – It is surgery performed with curative intent. It is normally indicated by only when a cancer appears to be confined to a defined area and is likely to be technically resectable. It may be performed as the initial or only treatment, or as a planned procedure after primary radiotherapy and/or chemotherapy designed to improve the surgical outcome. In larger operations it may be combined with reconstructive surgery.
- Cytoreductive surgery – This surgery is performed to electively debulk the tumour to improve the outcome following subsequent non-surgical treatment. It is typically indicated either where it is technically not possible to remove all the cancer or where radical surgery would be associated with unacceptable effects on the patient.
- Palliative surgery – It is used to treat complications of advanced cancers such as relief of bowel obstruction, orthopaedic intervention for pathological bone fractures or urological management of kidney obstruction. It may also be used to relieve pain unresponsive to other modalities.

Despite continued advances in anaesthesia and surgical techniques, many patients cannot be cured by surgery alone and the use of combined modality treatment is increasingly becoming commonplace for many cancer types. This typically involves the use of post-operative adjuvant radiotherapy, chemotherapy and/or hormone therapy. Such therapy may also be given pre-operatively (neoadjuvant) or, less commonly, perioperatively.

In patients where surgery has little or no role, the non-surgical treatment may be given with curative or palliative intent, depending on the tumour type or stage.

Radiotherapy

Radiation in its various forms has been used to treat cancer almost since its discovery in the late nineteenth century. Modern radiotherapy utilises radiation in two main ways: external beam radiotherapy (teletherapy) and brachytherapy.

External beam radiotherapy.   This comprises the vast majority of radiotherapy techniques. A variety of beams may be used, but most commonly high-energy X-rays (photons) produced by a linear accelerator.

A linear accelerator works by producing electrons, which are accelerated to very high speeds and forced to collide with a metal target thick enough to stop them. Part of the energy loss from this collision results in the production of X-rays, which can be filtered to produce a uniform beam of appropriate quality for therapy. If the target is replaced by a scattering foil, the linear accelerator can produce electron beams suitable for treatment, i.e. a dual modality unit.

Older units based on cobalt-60 deliver gamma rays and can be considered to be equivalent to a low-energy linear accelerator.

Radiation causes damage to the DNA in cells either by a 'direct hit' or, more commonly, by producing free radicals through interactions with cellular molecules (Figure 1.3). A sufficient level of DNA damage will cause cell death through apoptosis (programmed cell death) or when the cell attempts to divide (mitotic cell death); lesser

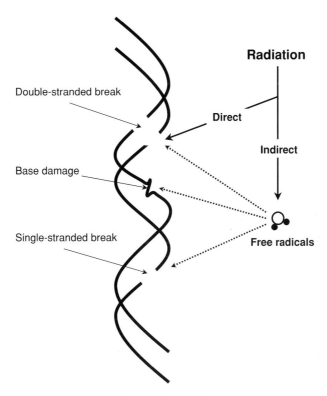

Figure 1.3   Direct and indirect DNA damage from radiation.

amounts of damage can be repaired and may not cause cell death. Double-stranded DNA breaks are the most lethal type of damage.

The effect of radiation on a cancer is determined by the 'five Rs' of radiobiology (Steel, 2002):

- Repair (the ability of the cancer cell to repair DNA damage)
- Repopulation (the speed at which the cancer replaces killed cells)
- Reoxygenation (the level of oxygenation is important in free-radical formation)
- Redistribution (the return of cells to a more even assortment through the cell cycle after killing of cells during its more sensitive phases)
- Radiosensitivity (the inherent susceptibility to radiation damage which varies between cancer types)

Radiation treatments are commonly fractionated – a total dose divided into a number of treatments (fractions) given over a set period of time. The details of fractionation – fraction size, frequency and number – depend on the goals of treatment and the radiobiology of the cancer and normal tissues involved. Fractionation is aimed at optimising the 'therapeutic ratio' – the balance between tumour response and normal tissue toxicity.

Conventional fractionation usually involves giving daily treatments of 2 gray (Gy) (unit of absorbed dose: 1 Gy = 1 J/kg) per fraction, 5 days per week, for up to 7 weeks – e.g. for a radical treatment, 60–70 Gy in 30–35 fractions over 6–7 weeks.

Hypofractionation is commonly employed for palliative treatments; a small number (1–10) of large fractions (greater than 2 Gy per fraction) are given. Symptom and cancer response are satisfactory and treatment takes much less time, but late unwanted side effects may be worse (compared to equivalent conventionally fractionated treatment); this is often less relevant for palliative patients.

Hyperfractionation is treatment with an increased number of smaller fractions (less than 2 Gy per fraction) over the same time period (e.g. twice daily and/or weekends). This may reduce late side effects in some tissues (improving the therapeutic ratio), which in turn may allow a higher total dose to be given.

Accelerated fractionation is treatment with the same size and number of fractions over a shorter period of time (e.g. twice daily and/or including weekends). This has the advantage of reducing the repopulation of tumour cells by limiting the time between fractions (a minimum gap of 6 h between treatments is necessary to allow normal tissue recovery) and can be more effective in rapidly growing tumours.

Hyperfractionation and acceleration can be utilised together (HART) to give a higher total dose in a larger number of fractions and so combine the improved therapeutic ratio of hyperfractionation and the reduced repopulation effect of acceleration. If this is given on a continuous basis, 7 days per week, this is termed CHART.

Radiotherapy planning involves ensuring that the patient can be accurately and reproducibly positioned and that the target can be effectively treated while minimising the normal tissue toxicity. Patients are aligned on the treatment couch with lasers and, if necessary, reference tattoos over anatomical landmarks. Immobilisation devices such as shells for the head and neck, armrests and vacuum bags may be used to ensure reproducibility of body position. Factors such as bladder and bowel filling can have a profound effect on the position of abdominal organs and patients may therefore be asked to have them empty or full depending on the treatment situation.

The target is identified through clinical examination, plain X-rays, CT and MR imaging (with occasional use of nuclear medicine and PET techniques). In conventional planning the patient is then positioned in a simulator – a diagnostic X-ray machine mounted on a radiotherapy gantry that can reproduce treatment conditions – and treatment fields are planned in relation to bony landmarks to cover the target volume (including a margin for microscopic spread of cancer and variations in set-up and patient parameters).

For CT planning, a dedicated scanning is performed in the reproducible treatment position. Using planning software the clinician draws the target volume on the CT images, which can be fused with other images, e.g. MR, from which a treatment plan is designed. The standard rectangular treatment field can be shaped by leaves in the machine treatment head (multi-leaf collimators, MLC) or individual lead-alloy blocks to conform the high-dose region more closely to the target volume, so-called conformal therapy. Most modern radical treatments implement conformal techniques and many palliative treatments are now being CT planned because it reduces appointment times for patients and allows clinicians greater flexibility.

During radiotherapy treatment it is possible to image the target volume being treated to ensure accuracy of delivery. This is achieved either by X-ray or by CT images taken on the treatment unit and can be used to adapt treatment to any changes in set-up or patient/cancer characteristics. This is the basis of image-guided or 'adaptive' radiotherapy.

The side effects of radiotherapy can be divided into early and late effects and are related to the area receiving treatment and the dose of radiation (Figure 1.4). Early effects are usually reversible and most recover within several weeks of finishing radiotherapy. Late effects occur months to years after radiotherapy and are usually permanent. It is predominantly the potential late effects in tissues adjacent to the cancer that limit the dose of radiation that can be given. Knowledge of the radiation tolerance of normal tissues is essential for successful radiotherapy planning.

Radiotherapy in children is a specialist area and is limited to 14 centres in the UK. Children may require careful preparation in order to comply with treatment planning and delivery, with some very young children needing anaesthesia at each appointment. Planning takes on an extra dimension as the effect of treatment on growth, development and education can be profound, particularly in the younger child.

Intensity-modulated radiotherapy (IMRT) is a three-dimensional technique that utilises the MLC of the modern linear accelerator to vary the intensity of radiation delivered across a treatment beam and so create a further dimension of conformality. It is particularly useful when trying to conform radiotherapy to a target volume which has significant concavity and convexity, e.g. treatment of a cancer wrapped around the spinal cord, but where the dose to the cord itself must be kept low. It utilises a different 'inverse' approach to planning, in which the dose constraints to

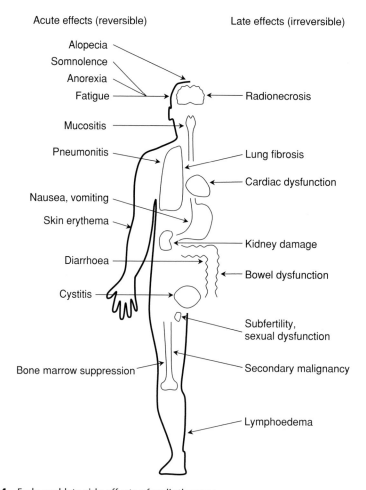

Acute effects (reversible) Late effects (irreversible)

Alopecia
Somnolence
Anorexia
Fatigue — Radionecrosis

Mucositis

Pneumonitis — Lung fibrosis

Cardiac dysfunction

Nausea, vomiting
Skin erythema

Kidney damage

Diarrhoea
Bowel dysfunction

Cystitis

Subfertility,
sexual dysfunction

Bone marrow suppression — Secondary malignancy

Lymphoedema

Figure 1.4 Early and late side effects of radiotherapy.

normal tissues and structures are applied first and the planning system then defines the maximum dose that can be delivered to the cancer within those constraints.

Stereotactic radiosurgery (SRS) is a specialised form of radiotherapy delivered with great accuracy and traditionally as a single large fraction of radiation. It was developed for use in the management of small spherical intracranial lesions such as metastases, small primary tumours and other pathologies including vascular mal-formations. It has evolved to include extracranial lesions and may involve several fractions rather than a single one. It can be delivered on dedicated units such as the 'Gamma-knife' or on modified linear accelerators.

Stereotactic radiotherapy (SRT) combines the accuracy of SRS with the physical and biological benefits of fractionated conformal radiotherapy and has a role in larger, more irregular lesions.

Deep and superficial X-ray therapy units operate at a much lower potentials than linear accelerators, i.e. 50–150 kV for superficial X-rays and 150–500 kV for

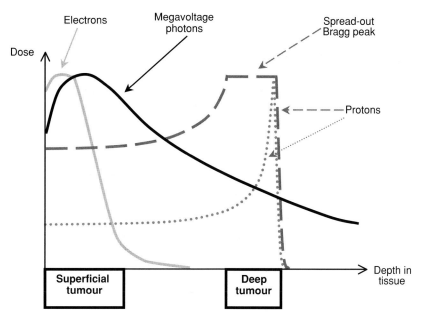

Figure 1.5 Depth-dose properties of electron, megavoltage photon and proton beams.

orthovoltage X-rays. The main use of superficial X-ray treatment is for the treatment of skin cancers. Orthovoltage units produce more penetrating beams and can be used for a variety of treatments but are particularly useful in the palliation of superficial bone metastases, e.g. ribs.

Electron beams have physical characteristics that are useful in the management of more superficial cancers (<5 cm deep) as the dose to tissues falls off rapidly beyond the target volume (Figure 1.5). They are principally used in the treatment of skin cancer, chest wall irradiation in breast cancer and in treating lymph nodes, especially in head and neck cancers. They have a relative biological effectiveness (RBE) similar to photons.

Photons and electrons are not the only options available, particularly for the treatment of deep-seated cancers. Hadron therapy includes the use of heavy particle beams, such as protons and neutrons.

Proton beams are typically produced from a cyclotron and differ from standard photon therapy by delivering their peak energy at the end of their trajectory, i.e. the Bragg peak (Figure 1.5). This means that tissue beyond this target point remains largely unaffected and tissue in front gets relatively little dose. The Bragg peak is too narrow to be used to treat a clinically relevant volume and so several beams of different energies can be superimposed to create a uniform dose region over a larger and clinically relevant target. This region is known as the (SOBP) 'spread-out Bragg peak'. Protons have a similar biological effectiveness to photon therapy but have advantages in reducing dose to surrounding normal tissue (the integral dose) and so may improve the therapeutic ratio.

Neutrons can be produced by proton bombardment of a beryllium target. They are intensely ionising and cause more damage to DNA. The double-stranded DNA damage is difficult for the cell to repair and is more likely to lead to cell death. The RBE of fast neutron therapy is several-fold higher than that of photons, both in cancer and in normal tissue.

The treatment of cancers by proton or neutron therapy is limited to a small number of centres throughout the world, mainly due to the enormous cost. They may be used as single-modality treatment or as a 'boost' in combination with more conventional photon therapy.

Brachytherapy. Brachytherapy involves using a radioactive source that emits its radiation over a short distance. This requires the source to be intimately associated with the cancer and allows the absorbed radiation dose to be delivered more effectively whilst minimising unwanted effects on surrounding normal tissues. It may be delivered in three main ways:

- Interstitial therapy – This involves the implantation of radiation sources into a cancer or the placing of such sources directly onto a superficial cancer.

  The cancer may be implanted directly using radioactive wires or indirectly by the placing of guide tubes within the cancer and subsequent after-loading with radioactive wires, which can be done manually or preferably by remote techniques. Historically, sealed radium sources were used for the majority of brachytherapy treatments but have been totally replaced by other radionuclides of which iridium-192 is most commonly used.

  Such treatments are usually completed quickly, typically 3–5 days, but do require the patient to be in hospital with appropriate radiation protection measures.

  It may be indicated in the primary treatment of some small cancers, including head and neck, skin, anogenital and breast, or as part of salvage therapy for recurrent cancers. It is rarely used in the UK and expertise is limited to a few centres.

- Intracavitary therapy – It is the insertion of sealed radioactive sources into body cavities and has been largely confined to the treatment of gynaecological cancers, although the development of small fine-bore after-loading systems has allowed it to be explored in other anatomical sites.

  For gynaecological use, a variety of applicators have been developed, including intrauterine tubes, ovoids for use in the lateral fornix and vaginal tubes. Most modern systems involve after-loading, either using low-/medium-dose-rate systems based on caesium-137 or high-dose-rate (HDR) systems utilising iridium-192 or cobalt-60. HDR systems allow fractionated outpatient therapy. The main indications are in the treatment of cancers of the cervix, endometrium or vagina and may be combined with external beam therapy.

  A type of intracavitary treatment using low-energy X-ray therapy is 'contact therapy' in which the treatment can be delivered directly to tumours within a cavity, much as for skin cancers. It has limited use and but has found some popularity in the management of anal and low rectal cancers.

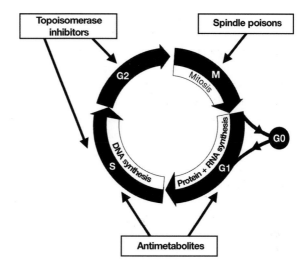

Figure 1.6 Cell-cycle-specific chemotherapy drugs.

• Targeted radiotherapy – This may use elemental unsealed radionuclides, e.g. iodine-131 or strontium-89. The largest experience is with ^{131}I in thyroid cancer, where it is taken up into the gland and concentrated via the normal physiological mechanism.

Radionuclides can also be attached to metabolic agents, e.g. *m*IBG which concentrates in neuroectodermal tumours such as neuroblastoma.

They can also be attached to antibodies, such as in the treatment of lymphoma, to colloids, which may be given directly into body cavities, such as peritoneal or pleural spaces, or to bone-seeking chelates.

Chemotherapy

The origins of chemotherapy can be traced to World War I, when the British and German armies experimented with chemical warfare, using mustard gas to cause blistering of the skin, irritation of the lungs, nausea, fatigue and at times death. It was also noted to cause low white blood cell counts and this is what led to the nitrogen mustards being used in the treatment of leukaemia and lymphoma.

The uncontrolled proliferation of cancer cells involves rapid procession through the 'cell cycle', the sequence of cellular processes that allows replication of DNA and division into daughter cells. If this cycle is disrupted, the cell cannot divide and will become inactive or die. The effect of most chemotherapy is to interfere with this cycle, especially by interfering with the replication, structure and function of DNA.

Some chemotherapy drugs act at specific phases in the cell cycle (Figure 1.6): the *antimetabolites*, such as 5-fluorouracil (5-FU) and methotrexate, interfere with the production and use of the building blocks of DNA and therefore have their greatest activity in G1 and S phases. *Topisomerase inhibitors*, such as irinotecan and etoposide, interfere with a group of enzymes that help to regulate the structure of supercoiled DNA which are particularly active during S and G2 phases leading to DNA and chromosome damage and failure to enter mitosis. *Spindle poisons*, which include the naturally derived vinca alkaloids (from the periwinkle shrub, such as vincristine and vinorelbine) and taxanes (from the yew, such as paclitaxel and docetaxel), alter the structure and function of the microtubules within the mitotic spindle and are therefore most active during M phase.

In contrast, many chemotherapy drugs can cause damage at any point in the cycle. The *alkylating agents*, which include the original nitrogen mustard ('mustard gas') compounds and their derivatives (such as chlorambucil and cyclophosphamide), nitrosureas (such as carmustine and lomustine) and heavy-metal alkylators (such as cisplatin and carboplatin), act through binding to cellular molecules including DNA and disrupting their structure and function. This causes damage to the DNA template, obstructs DNA replication and also causes the breakage of DNA strands leading to cell death.

The *antitumour antibiotics*, derived from micro-organisms, have the ability to kill cells that are not actively dividing as well as those proceeding through the cell cycle; anthracyclines, such as epirubicin and doxorubicin, alter DNA and enzyme structure and function, directly inducing cell death.

Normal body tissues have advantages that allow them to withstand and recover from the assault of chemotherapy better than cancer (intact cellular and DNA repair mechanisms and lower proportion of actively proliferating cells), but toxic effects remain common.

The normal tissues with the highest proliferation rates are the most sensitive to chemotherapy: mucous membranes in the mouth and bowel (mucositis, nausea, vomiting and diarrhoea), hair follicles (alopecia) and bone marrow (anaemia, reduced platelet and white blood cell counts) all exhibit acute toxicity with a wide variety of chemotherapy agents. Each chemotherapy drug has a different spectrum of toxicity; the most common are shown in Figure 1.7.

The dosage and schedule of a chemotherapy drug are clearly important in determining its toxicity and outcome. Early trials of a drug are aimed at determining the maximum tolerated dose and frequency (time to recover from toxicity, e.g. when bone marrow suppression has recovered sufficiently). With most drugs this equates to cycles of chemotherapy given once every 3–4 weeks.

The pharmacokinetic properties of a chemotherapy drug (how it is absorbed, distributed and eliminated from the body) are important factors in its administration, dosage and schedule. Drugs taken orally are absorbed from the gut and pass through the liver before entering the bloodstream, processes which, for many drugs, can cause large and unpredictable variations in the plasma concentration at different times and between patients. Intravenous administration avoids these variations and is the most common method in use. The exposure of the body to a drug is limited by its metabolism and elimination by cellular enzymes and organs (principally the liver and kidneys). For some drugs this occurs within minutes, such as 5-FU which is often given by continuous intravenous infusion over a number of days to account for this. Others take much longer to be eliminated and can therefore be given as a single intravenous infusion over minutes or hours.

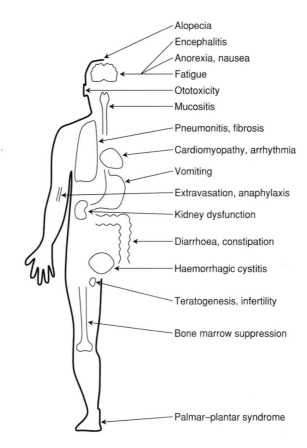

Figure 1.7 Side effects of chemotherapy.

Alternate routes of administration can produce much higher drug concentrations in the vicinity of the tumour than is possible intravenously: intrathecal chemotherapy (into cerebrospinal fluid), intravesical chemotherapy (into the bladder) and intraperitoneal chemotherapy (into the abdominal cavity). These routes have the advantage of avoiding excessive systemic toxicity, but doses remain limited by local toxicity.

Over time, cancer cells develop resistance to chemotherapy; new genetic mutations mean that some cells are able to withstand or recover from chemotherapy better; these survive and reproduce, whilst the others are killed by chemotherapy, leaving a residual population of cells or 'clones' resistant to the drug. Combining chemotherapy drugs can reduce this effect and also has the advantage of attacking different targets within the cancer, therefore enhancing cell kill; the disadvantage is the additional toxicity and this may require reductions in drug dosage to accommodate the combination.

Chemotherapy may have a profound effect on patients with cancer: in some cases cure (e.g. lymphoma and germ cell tumours), while in others disease control with prolongation of life or enhancement of quality of life. The art of its use is the balance between this and the associated toxicity; the ongoing goal is the development of less toxic agents that are increasingly specific for and effective against cancer cells.

Chemoradiation, i.e. the use of concurrent chemotherapy during radical radiotherapy, has now become the standard of care for many solid tumours, based on improvements in response rates, local control and survival.

Other treatments

Hormone therapy is an important and effective treatment in several cancers, where the growth of the cancer is hormone dependent, e.g. some prostate and breast cancers. It works either by stopping hormone production or by blocking the hormone reaching the cancer cell. Examples of such drugs would be goserelin (Zoladex) for prostate cancer that downregulates the production of testosterone and tamoxifen for breast cancer that acts as an anti-oestrogen, blocking the oestrogen receptor on the surface of a breast cancer cell.

Angiogenesis or the formation of new blood vessels has a very important role in the growth and spread of many cancers. It is hoped that the use of natural or synthetic angiogenesis inhibitors will prevent the formation of new vessels, causing cancers to shrink or die. One such drug is bevacizumab (Avastin), a monoclonal antibody directed against vascular endothelial growth factor (VEGF) that prevents angiogenesis in bowel cancer and may have a role in other cancer types.

Other biological treatment strategies are aimed at stimulating the immune system to fight cancer (immunotherapy) and include BCG (bacillus Calmette-Guérin), interferon alpha, other monoclonal antibodies (such as trastuzumab (Herceptin)) and cancer vaccines.

Gene therapies remain experimental treatments that involve the introduction of genetic material (DNA or RNA) into an individual's cells to treat cancer. There are several strategies, including:

- Direct replacement of missing or defective genes with healthy ones
- Manipulation of the immune response genes
- Making cancer cells more sensitive to chemotherapy/radiotherapy
- Making normal tissues more resistant to the side effects of high-dose chemotherapy
- Manipulation of angiogenesis genes

Palliative and supportive care

People dealing with cancer need supportive care, which has been defined by the National Council for Hospice and Specialist Palliative Care Services (2002) as the help that the patient and their family may need to 'cope with cancer and the treatment of it – from pre-diagnosis, through the process of diagnosis and treatment, to cure, continuing illness or death and into bereavement'. It helps the patient to maximise the benefits of therapy and to live as well as possible with the effects of the disease and its treatment.

Supportive care is not a distinct specialty and may be delivered in part by the patient's family and other carers, rather than by professionals. It includes:

- Self-help and support
- Information
- Psychological support
- Social support
- Spiritual support
- Rehabilitation
- Symptom control
- Terminal care
- Bereavement support and care

Palliative care embraces many elements of supportive care, although there are well-defined areas of expertise within specialist palliative care to which patients and carers may need access. National Institute for Clinical Excellence (NICE) (2004) define palliative care as 'the active holistic care of patients with advanced progressive illness. Management of pain and other symptoms and provision of psychological, social and spiritual support is paramount. The goal of palliative care is achievement of the best quality of life for patients and their families. Many aspects of palliative care are also applicable earlier in the course of the illness in conjunction with other treatments.'

Palliative care is provided by two distinct groups of health and social care professionals:

1. Non-specialist palliative care services – These are delivered by the professionals providing the day-to-day care for cancer patients either in the community or in hospital. Those providing such care should be able to assess the care needs and information needs of patients and their families or carers and know when and how to seek advice from or refer to specialist palliative care services.
2. Specialist palliative care services – These are provided by multi-professional care teams who should be able to provide
   - assessment, advice and care for patients and families in all care settings, including home, hospital and care home;
   - specialist inpatient care (hospital or hospice);
   - intensive coordinated home care for patients with complex needs who wish to remain in their own home;
   - day-care facilities;
   - advice and support to all people involved in a patients care;
   - bereavement support;
   - education, training and research.

The specialist palliative care team includes palliative medicine consultants and nurse specialists, together with physiotherapists, occupational therapists, dietitians, pharmacists, social workers and others able to provide physical, spiritual and psychological support. The expanding field of paediatric palliative care has shown the need for such services directed towards children with serious illness.

The prevalence of symptoms in advanced cancer varies according to tumour type and site, but common symptoms would include:

- Pain
- Weight loss
- Fatigue and general weakness
- Anorexia
- Insomnia
- Constipation
- Depression and anxiety
- Nausea and/or vomiting
- Breathlessness

Pain is a common symptom and deserves special mention. It is estimated to be suffered by 50–70% of cancer patients and is the most feared symptom. Inadequate pain assessment has been shown to be the greatest barrier to effective control. Many patients have more than one pain type or site. Careful assessment of each pain at each site, paying particular attention to nature and severity, frequency and precipitating or relieving factors, will ensure that the pain is treated appropriately. This would normally involve the use of analgesics, which not only necessitates regular review of the patient to assess response and allow titration of dose but also necessitates anticipation and control of the side effects of such treatment. Some patients may benefit from other forms of relief including co-analgesics (such as non-steroidal anti-inflammatory drugs, steroids or drugs which affect nerve conduction), surgery or radiotherapy, bisphosphonate therapy, transcutaneous electrical nerve stimulation (TENS), epidural infusion, nerve/ganglion block, cordotomy, acupuncture or relaxation therapy.

Moderate-to-severe pain in cancer usually responds at least partially to treatment with opioids (morphine and related drugs). Constipation, nausea, sedation and dry mouth are classic side effects but may reduce in severity after the initial introductory period, although prophylactic laxatives are usually prescribed. Toxicity can occur, most commonly manifest, as confusion/agitation, vivid dreams and hallucinations to profound sedation and respiratory depression. This may be seen when the dose has been increased too far or too rapidly, or not reduced following other successful treatment, e.g. radiotherapy, or by accumulation of the drug caused by the introduction of other medication or by the changes in the ability to clear the drug due to changes in renal function, including dehydration. A few patients are genuinely intolerant of individual opioids and demonstrate toxicity even at low doses. Using an alternative opioid may help this.

Occasionally, patients or health professionals are deterred from using opioids for fears about addiction and tolerance, i.e. loss of clinical effectiveness over time. Physical dependence may be a feature of opioid use for chronic pain, but psychological dependence is unlikely. The concerns regarding tolerance are unfounded and increases in dose are usually in response to a change in the clinical condition of the patient. These concerns must not be an obstacle to effective pain relief.

Patients move frequently between locations (home, hospital and hospice), between care teams (primary care, cancer care and palliative care) and between providers (NHS, local authority and the private and voluntary sectors). Coordination amongst these care teams and services is necessary to provide continuity of care. This largely relies on timely communication, including palliative care representation at site-specific multidisciplinary meetings and case conferences. The plans for single integrated electronic patient records should prove to be helpful.

Summary

Cancer and its increasingly intensive treatment have a major impact on patients, family and carers and their ability to continue with their usual daily activities. NICE (2004) defines cancer rehabilitation as attempting to maximise patients' ability to function, to promote their independence and to help them adapt to their condition. It offers a major route to improving their quality of life, no matter how long or short the timescale. It aims to maximise dignity and reduce the extent to which the cancer interferes with an individual's physical, psychosocial and economic functioning. The importance of rehabilitation services in improving patients' lives is gaining more recognition and they are increasingly being seen as integral to patient care.

References

Cancer Research UK (2005). *Lifestyle and cancer risk in the UK population.* Retrieved 31 October 2007 from http://info.cancerresearchuk.org/cancerstats/causes/lifestyle/

Greene, F. L., Page, D. L., Fleming, I. D., Fritz, A. G., Balch, C. M., Haller, D. G. & Morrow, M. (Eds.) (2002). *AJCC cancer staging manual* (6th ed.). New York: Springer-Verlag.

National Council for Hospice and Specialist Palliative Care Services (2002). *Definitions of supportive and palliative care.* Briefing paper 11. London: National Council for Hospice and Specialist Palliative Care Services.

National Institute for Clinical Excellence [NICE] (2004). *Guidance on cancer services: improving supportive and palliative care for adults with cancer – the manual.* London: National Institute for Clinical Excellence.

Office for National Statistics (2006). *Cancer statistics – registrations of cancer diagnosed in 2004, England.* Series MB1, No. 35. London: Office for National Statistics.

Steel, G. G. (Ed.) (2002). *Basic clinical radiobiology* (3rd ed.). London. Hodder Arnold.

World Health Organization (2006a) *Fact sheet No 297: cancer* [online]. Retrieved 31 October 2007 from http://www.who.int/mediacentre/factsheets/fs297/en/

World Health Organization (2006b) *Cancer control: knowledge into action: WHO guide for effective programmes.* Geneva: World Health Organization.

Chapter 2
REHABILITATION IN ONCOLOGY AND PALLIATIVE CARE

Jane Rankin and Dr Jacqueline Gracey

Learning outcomes

Having read this chapter the reader will be able to:

- Describe what is meant by cancer rehabilitation and be able to discuss the allied health professions' role in rehabilitation and symptom management
- Discuss the political background to the development of cancer services and understand the role that cancer networks can play in developing cancer services
- Discuss the many issues that impact on quality service provision in both generalist and cancer specialist fields including the need for oncology and palliative care in undergraduate and postgraduate education

Introduction

This book is designed to review the common cancers and their associated problems in order to highlight the potential roles and joint working of the allied health professions (AHPs) in this speciality. Each chapter is evidence based and provides case studies to demonstrate the integration of AHP services within and between the various care settings, such as cancer centres, local hospitals, the community and voluntary sectors. Whilst being of benefit to clinicians, this chapter will also inform managers, commissioners, academics, researchers and students of the huge impact that AHP staff can have in this field, highlighting areas of unmet need and underprovision which would benefit from additional education and resources.

Rehabilitation brings added value to supportive and palliative care. It is a myth that it is somehow an optional extra (Crompton, 2000). Common misconceptions are challenged, including the belief that rehabilitation for people with life-threatening diseases is wasteful of resources and that it can be acceptable only if measurable improvement or restoration of function occurs. The ethos should be to facilitate patients to live as independently as possible whilst, at times, preparing to die. The rationale for this report was supported by the National Cancer Director, Professor Mike Richards, as it highlighted the need for development of a support service strategy as one of the priorities of the National Cancer Modernisation Programme. Importantly, it identified rehabilitation as an essential component.

Cancer rehabilitation

Cancer rehabilitation, although a relatively new concept, is now recognised as an essential component of the cancer journey. In curative treatment planning it is no longer acceptable to kill cancer cells alone; care must also be delivered to the patient and carers to help them to cope with the effects of the disease and the medical interventions. Quality of life is now an integral component of all medical trials supporting the need for effective treatment and minimisation of the associated side effects. As medical management continues to progress, radiotherapy and chemotherapy may be increasingly delivered concurrently, thereby increasing the levels of potential toxicity and related side effects. Some of these effects are short lived, e.g. reduced white cell count and associated infections, whilst others may be long-term problems, such as cancer-related fatigue (CRF). Patients may therefore need more support and rehabilitation to regain pre-disease status. Survivorship, both physical and psychological, is gradually becoming recognised alongside extended life gains.

Palliative care is based on the holistic management of symptoms and is now accepted to be more than the administration of analgesia. Recent developments in medical care not only demonstrate increasing success in curing cancers but also offer life-lengthening opportunities where the disease is controlled rather than cured and patients with active cancer live longer (Rosen *et al.*, 2006). As a result, cancer is now recognised as a chronic illness, and the necessity for development of supportive care has become paramount in all care settings.

Cancer rehabilitation can be defined as:

A dynamic, ongoing health-orientated process designed to promote maximum levels of functioning in individuals with cancer related health problems' and is an ethical commitment by cancer care providers (Watson, 1992).

It aims to improve quality of survival so that patients will be as comfortable and productive as possible and can function at a minimum level of dependency regardless of life expectancy (Dietz, 1981). As such, prognosis ceases to be a contradiction for rehabilitation and becomes purely a consideration for intervention planning.

Dietz (1980) describes four recognised cancer rehabilitation stages:

- Preventative: reducing the impact of expected disabilities and assistance in learning to cope with any disabilities
- Restorative: returning the patient to pre-illness level without disability
- Supportive: in the presence of persistent disease and the continual need for treatment, the goal is to limit functional loss and provide support
- Palliative: further loss of function, put in place measures which eliminate or reduce complications and to provide support (symptom management)

The placement of AHPs in cancer services, in both the curative and palliative care settings, is an essential prerequisite for the further development of rehabilitation. AHPs have an underutilised arsenal of skills and knowledge that can provide timely, holistic, patient-centred care for these patient groups. AHPs interact with patients in many settings and are currently part of specialist teams working in cancer centres, cancer units or general medical units, in nursing and residential homes and in the community. Similarly, AHPs may work in palliative care in the aforementioned areas or in specialised settings including hospices and day care. This provides support at all stages of the cancer pathway and in all care settings, from prevention, diagnosis and treatment to palliative and terminal care.

AHPs aim to improve quality of life, so that lives are as comfortable, productive and independent as possible. This applies even if life expectancy is short. As change or deterioration can happen frequently, rapidly or unexpectedly, there is a need to have sufficient resources to react in a timely manner and to reassess continuously to ensure that priorities and goals are realistic and achievable. The field of oncology requires all health professionals to be particularly responsive and able to plan ahead to assess changing needs in line with medical and functional status. The principles of cancer rehabilitation, as defined by Habeck *et al.* (1984, cited in Fulton, 1994), are integral to the work of all the professions:

- Comprehensive care is provided to address the needs (economic, physical, psychological and social vocational factors) of the whole person.
- A team approach is used to achieve coordinated interprofessional care.
- The unit of care includes both the patient and the family/main carers.
- Goals are derived from the effects of the medical problem in accordance with prognostic expectations.
- Intervention occurs as soon as the likelihood of disability is anticipated.
- Rehabilitation needs must be assessed on a continuing basis and met throughout all stages of care.
- Education is a major component of the process.

In order to understand the developing need for further specialist and generalist AHP service provision, it is necessary to review the government's objectives and other associated factors.

The development of cancer services (political context)

The *Policy Framework for Commissioning Cancer Services Review* (Calman & Hine, 1995) highlighted the initial direction of cancer services development in England and Wales including the integration of rehabilitation from diagnosis onwards. Other principle goals of this report included:

- Access to uniformly high quality of care from primary to tertiary settings via cancer networks

- Dedicated specialist staff
- Public and professional education to aid early recognition of symptoms and screening programmes
- Improved patient information and communication
- Patient-centred care
- Primary care teams recognised as a central element in care
- Outcomes monitoring
- Recognition of the need for psychological support

This was supported by other regional specific documents for Scotland and Northern Ireland which further developed these themes, including that of increased specialisation in cancer management for all professions, a more definite multi-professional approach and research-based services (Campbell, 1996). However, despite the rapid and dynamic changes that occurred post-Calman–Hine, it was recognised that inequalities still existed accessing high-quality services. In response, the government produced the *NHS Cancer Plan* (Department of Health [DH], 2000), which aimed to ensure that every person with cancer could access the best available treatments, including multi-professional team support and care. It also identified the need to develop services beyond the cancer centres and units to ensure a continuum of care.

This was facilitated by the development of regional cancer networks to create a patient-centred service promoting health and well-being, delivering effective treatment, care and support, securing user involvement, fostering cultural change and practice and developing leadership and productive teamwork. Cancer networks can engage with all stakeholders to support and develop expert tumour management in pathology-related teams (e.g. lung cancer) and also professional and intervention-specific groups such as pharmacy or AHPs and supportive and palliative care. Specific groups or teams interact to share expertise and problem solve in order to promote multidisciplinary working and equitable provision of high-quality services (Northern Ireland Cancer Network, 2006). It is hoped that the continued roll out of electronic patient records will promote network-wide seamless communication and care, particularly for palliative 'out-of-hour' domiciliary care.

In order to recruit and retain this skilled workforce, the Cancer Care Workforce Team (DH, 2003), in conjunction with the National Workforce Development Board, produced a national strategy prioritising the plan for additional staffing (including AHPs), new ways of working and meeting the continual professional development needs of existing staff. Progress has been made in recruiting medical, nursing and radiography staff, specifically in diagnostics and staging. However, the numbers of specialist AHPs have not, as yet, increased in line with other professions. Whilst new service developments have been announced, in *Investment in Cancer 2001/02 and 2003/04* (DH, 2005), including improvements in lymphoedema services, it does not specify AHP gains and yet quotes the NHS Workforce Census Plan to have a target of 6500 new AHPs by 2004.

In 2006, *Future Trends and Challenges for Cancer Services in England* commended the changes resulting from the cancer plan especially the increasing survival rates, falling death rates, streamlined and timely clinical pathways and increasing access to specialist teams. However, it challenged current service provision with new factors that must be considered as development continues (Rosen *et al.*, 2006). These include:

- Cancer is more common in the elderly population. The proportion of over 65s will increase from 16% (in 2004) to 23% by 2031. Demographic and epidemiological trends predict a continued increase in the population with cancer diagnoses (Office for National Statistics, 2006, cited in Rosen *et al.*, 2006).
- New cancer treatments are encouraging new routes of care delivery in the community with significant impact on primary care resources.
- Other papers, including *Our Health, Our Care, Our Say: A New Direction for Community Services* (DH, 2006a), also impact on how and where the population want services to be delivered and the gradual shift towards community care settings and the choice to die at home (DH, 2004a).

The 2006 paper also cites the National Audit Office (National Audit Office [NAO], 2005a) report *Tackling Cancer: Improving the Patient Journey*, which highlights the continued lack of supportive and palliative care services and specifically recommends an improvement in end-of-life care. Currently, over 50% of all patients wish to die at home; however, less than 20% are actually facilitated to do so (DH, 2004a). This has been addressed to some degree by the *Building on the Best: End of Life Care Initiative* (DH, 2004a), which aims to improve care at this emotional time through the use of specialist assessment tools, including the Gold Standards Framework and The Liverpool Care Pathway for the Dying. The tools address best hospice-type care and allow the transfer of these skills to other settings, including hospitals, the community and care homes. Nationally, this change may be a slow development process as it challenges the traditional care management culture. The preferred place of care's patient-held record also encourages health care staff to monitor and facilitate patient choice over where to be cared for and to die (National Health Service [NHS], 2006).

This planned move from acute to community for end-of-life care does, however, have significant financial, ethical and potentially legal consequences. Questions must be asked regarding the potential situation where current services discuss and agree a home care plan with a patient and family, but ultimately are not be able to deliver the agreed service. This has the potential to turn a failed well-meaning intervention into an emotional and traumatic episode of care. The debate over location choice versus medical appropriateness must also be considered. It is also essential that supportive and palliative care do not get lost in the whole current end-of-life care debate.

Further management issues are also raised, such as the acknowledgement of urgent referrals from general practitioners for patients with suspected cancer. Statistics from the DH (2006b) suggest that general practitioners do not necessarily recognise cancer symptoms and initiate the secondary referrals and diagnostic tests. *The NHS Cancer Plan: A Progress Report* (NAO, 2005b) reports that almost 90% of patients are waiting for a maximum of 1 month and 78% are waiting less than 2 months from diagnosis to treatment. This group of patients with cancer-suggestive symptoms, e.g. rapid weight loss, fatigue and shortness of breath, may not be receiving symptom-specific care, whilst the initial referrals to secondary resources, and later diagnostic tests, occur. Many such symptoms can be managed by AHPs and have the potential to make the waiting period more manageable, improve quality of life, prepare the patient for potential cancer treatment and, at times, prevent early hospital admission.

In an attempt to highlight the need for continued supportive service development, the National Institute for Health and Clinical Excellence (National Institute for Clinical Excellence [NICE], 2004) produced *Guidance on Cancer Services: Improving Supportive and Palliative Care for Adults with Cancer*. This is intended to complement the series of guidance manuals on specific cancers and provides evidence-based recommendations on service models most likely to lead to high-quality services and care (DH, 2004b). A key recommendation states:

> *Commissioners and providers, working through Cancer Networks, should institute mechanisms to ensure that patient's needs for rehabilitation are recognised and that comprehensive rehabilitation services and suitable equipment are available to all patients in all care locations. A four-level model for rehabilitation services is the suggested model for achieving this.*

A similar recommendation is made for complementary therapies.

The National Cancer Network AHP Lead Forum (2007) has built on the initial NICE four-level version by producing a new model of cancer rehabilitation assessment and support. They have defined the levels of experience, knowledge and role requirements relating to the posts in specific oncology settings, thus providing a more effective means of establishing baseline service reviews (Table 2.1).

The drive to strengthen supportive patient care following the NICE (2004) document has been continued with the development of the Holistic Common Assessment of Supportive and Palliative Care Needs for Adults with Cancer (Cancer Action Team, 2007). This assessment aims to identify specific needs and be the catalyst for further specialist assessment and treatment and focuses on items of particular concern to the patient. It is divided into five domains:

- Background information and assessment preferences
- Physical needs
- Social and occupational needs
- Psychological well-being
- Spiritual well-being

As such, it provides the potential to ensure appropriate and timely referrals to all supportive services and aspires to encourage the adoption of a unified approach to assessment and record keeping.

The cancer pathway

AHPs have a vital role in the cancer pathway from pre-diagnosis to cure or end-of-life care. Each stage requires a variation in approach, goal setting, treatment modification

Table 2.1 Model of rehabilitation assessment and support: definitions of the levels.

Those involved at each level and their functions are as follows:

Level 4

- It involves advanced practice and expert AHPs who work mostly or exclusively with patients who have cancer (more than 75% of their clinical caseload)
- They will provide clinical leadership and expert advice
- Practitioners with the skills to provide level 4 care will have received higher level training (possibly accredited) and as part of their role may provide postgraduate training within the specialty
- They will be highly experienced, advanced or consultant practitioners with a defined amount of experience

Level 3

- It involves experienced AHPs with specialist levels of training in rehabilitation techniques and approaches to managing patients with cancer
  or
  are specialist AHPs in other clinical fields but who can apply their advanced knowledge of rehabilitation to patients with cancer
- They will deliver interventions which require knowledge of the impact of the disease and its treatment. They may have a varied caseload of which 25–75% of their clinical caseload is focused on cancer and palliative care

Level 2

- AHPs at level 2 deliver routine assessments of rehabilitation needs and interventions. They will be a registered allied health professional. Patients with cancer form a small percentage of what is often a mixed caseload. Patients will be referred to a more experienced colleague according to need
- AHPs working at this level will have a basic understanding of cancer and the impact of the disease and its treatment

Level 1

- This involves anyone who identifies a rehabilitation need, makes referrals and provides day-to-day care. It may include health and social care professionals, the patient and the carer. Patient's needs are assessed using an agreed assessment tool with basic interventions initiated by a health care professional. Health care assistants and assistant practitioners working under the guidance of a health care professional can also provide care at this level
- Referrals may be made to the next appropriate level of care. Because rehabilitation is about the ability to function and perform everyday activities, it is hard to quantify the providers of rehabilitation input at this level

National Cancer Network AHP Forum (2007).

and accepted outcomes. It is therefore important to understand the differences in the ethos of each potential intervention.

Curative/radical care

This describes the dynamic approach required to treat the patient whose cancer treatment is aiming to kill all cancer cells in order to produce a cure. The potential side effects are severe as healthy cells are also damaged or killed. Rehabilitation goals will be to return the patient to pre-cancer status, but will need to be cognisant of the daily variation in the patient's condition caused by the aggressive medical intervention.

Supportive care

'…helps the patient and their family to cope with cancer and treatment of it from pre-diagnosis, through the process of diagnosis and treatment, to cure, continuing illness or death and into bereavement. It helps the patient to maximize the benefits of treatment and to live as well as possible with the effects of the disease. It is given equal priority alongside diagnosis and treatment' (National Council for Hospice and Specialist Palliative Care Services [NCHSPCS], 2002).

Palliative care

'…the active holistic care of patients with advanced progressive illness. Management of pain and other symptoms and provision of psychological, social and spiritual support is paramount. The goal of palliative care is achievement of the best quality of life for patients and their families. Many aspects of palliative care are also applicable in the course of the illness in conjunction with other treatments' (NCHSPCS, 2002).

End-of-life care

'…requires an active compassionate approach that treats, comforts and supports individuals who are living with or dying from progressive or chronic life threatening conditions.

Such care is sensitive to personal, cultural and spiritual values, beliefs and practices and encompasses support for families and friends up to and including the period of bereavement' (Ross *et al.*, 2000, cited in DH, 2006c).

Despite these specific definitions, there is potential movement from one stage to another, which should be boundary free. Processes should be in place to facilitate all levels of communication and coordination between the various care settings and professions (DH, 2004c). For example, a patient diagnosed as having a potentially curative cancer may progress to disease recurrence and need supportive and palliative care. The dramatic developments in medical management have also allowed the period from diagnosis of an incurable cancer (palliative treatment) to death to be dramatically extended. This life-lengthening process, whilst providing an extended period of reasonable health, can result in the patient experiencing more episodes related to progressive disease. For example, a patient with recurrent breast cancer may experience bone, lung and brain secondaries alongside treatment-related conditions such as lymphoedema and cancer-related fatigue. The management of such a patient can be very complex, requiring expertise in the various fields of orthopaedics, respiratory care, neurology and lymphoedema management. Specialist knowledge of the disease, its staging, pathology and diagnostic tools and potential recurrence patterns allow the specialist health care professional to anticipate problems and to monitor and prepare for them. In other words, people are now living, rather than dying, with cancer. This has important implications for service provision.

The role of 'the AHP' in oncology and palliative care

The oncology AHP must have knowledge of the disease, its progression and the impact of available cancer treatments. Adopting a rehabilitation approach redirects the emphasis away from the actual disease to the rehabilitative potential of each individual cancer patient and his/her family or carers' needs (Fulton, 1994). The focus of the therapy intervention is the physical and functional consequence of the disease and its treatment rather than the pathological condition (Fulton & Else, 1997).

The psychological aspects of cancer care must also be considered. This has importance for all professions as many cancer patients experience anxiety/depression around the time of diagnosis and initial cancer treatment. AHPs can provide general psychological support and, as such, require advanced skills to communicate effectively and compassionately. This is of particular importance when dealing with patients and carers during end-of-life care. AHPs that have regularly cared for patients through supportive and palliative care may also develop an emotional bond to the patient and carers.

AHPs have a unique role to play in this specialist field. Each will now be described briefly:

Occupational therapy

'Occupational therapy (OT) focuses on the nature, balance, pattern and context of occupations and activities in the lives of individuals, family groups and communities. It is concerned with the meaning and purpose that people place on occupations and activities and with the impact of illness, disability or social or economic deprivation on their ability to carry them out. The main aim of occupational therapy is to maintain, restore or create a match, beneficial to the individual, between the abilities of the person, the demands of their occupation and the demands of the environment, in order to maintain or improve the client's functional status and access to opportunities for participation' (Health Professions Council, 2006).

As well as assessing an individual's physical disabilities, occupational therapists address lifestyle management and work with people with cancer and their family/carers to achieve balance in life and enabling individuals to assess their priorities. This includes social and spiritual issues, helping them find a meaningful occupation, considering cultural influences and linking hospital or hospice care and living at home. Equipment provision may also be necessary to aid independence.

Physiotherapy

'Physiotherapy is a health care profession concerned with human function and movement, and maximising potential. It uses physical approaches to promote, maintain and restore physical, psychological and social well-being, taking account of variations in health status. It is a science-based profession committed to extending, applying, evaluating and reviewing the evidence that underpins and informs its practice and delivery. The exercise of clinical judgment and informed consent is at its core' (Chartered Society of Physiotherapy [CSP], 2002).

The Association of Chartered Physiotherapists in Oncology and Palliative Care (ACPOPC, 1993) considers the main aim of physiotherapists working with patients with cancer to be:

'...assisting these individuals to minimise some of the effects which the disease or its treatment has on them. It is often possible to improve their quality of life, regardless of their prognosis by helping them to achieve their maximum potential or gain relief from distressing symptoms.'

The oncology physiotherapist aims to improve overall quality of life through restoring function, reducing disability and pain and increasing conditioning and mobility (McDonnell & Shea, 1993, cited in CSP, 2003). Knowledge of functional anatomy and ergonomics facilitates the management of these complex multi-pathology cases.

Nutrition and dietetics

Dietitians are uniquely qualified to translate scientific information about food into practical dietary advice. As well as providing impartial advice about nutrition and health, dietitians also advise about food-related problems and treat disease and ill health (British Dietetic Association [BDA], 2006).

The aim of the oncology dietitian is 'to optimise the nutritional status and quality of life of those patients who are malnourished or at risk of malnutrition as a result of their illness or treatment they are receiving' (BDA Oncology Group, 2002). Optimising nutritional status is an important goal for any anti-cancer treatment. Adequate nutrition can improve tolerance and response rate to radiotherapy and combination of chemotherapy and radiation, improve immune status, increase wound healing and reduce complications. The role of nutritional support is therefore a crucial component of cancer care (BDA Oncology Group, 2002).

Speech and language therapy

Speech and language therapists (SLTs) specialise in the assessment, diagnosis and treatment of patients who have communication and/or swallowing disorders. These can occur as a direct result of disease or cancer treatment. SLTs aim to provide the support and intervention necessary to improve these aspects of the patient's quality of life. Although SLTs often work as key members of a head and neck cancer team, they also provide a service to many other teams in oncology where communication and swallowing disorders occur.

Communication disorders include low speech volume, hoarseness and restricted oral movement. This loss of spontaneous, effortless speech can add to the patient's feelings of isolation and frustration. Care includes teaching compensatory techniques and modification to the environment to provide the best outcome for the patient. Additionally, swallowing disorders are associated with a number of potential risks to patients including poor nutrition and aspiration. To improve assessment and management SLTs may utilise instrumental assessment, including video fluoroscopy or fibreoptic endoscopic evaluation of swallowing.

Podiatry

The role of the podiatrist is developing in cancer rehabilitation: assessing, diagnosing and treating lower leg and foot problems in order to promote and maintain mobility. This may involve a biomechanical assessment of the lower limbs to evaluate foot function. Off-loading the foot, via specialist footwear or orthotics, may be required to maximise function and reduce pain for specific tumours of the lower limb.

Problems may arise as a result of cancer treatment; e.g. common foot problems may be exacerbated due to immunosuppression, a foot wound progressing to an infected wound and peripheral neuropathy causing numbness, tingling and pain in the extremities. There are many side effects of chemotherapy that manifest in the feet, including peripheral neuropathy, palmar–plantar erythrodysesthesia and nail conditions such as onycholysis (separation or loosening of a fingernail or toenail from its nail bed) and onychodystrophy (malformation of the nail). After radiotherapy, skin can behave as though it has been sunburned: hypersensitive, weeping, breakdown or ulcerating. This is an important consideration especially if there is a history of diabetes or peripheral vascular disease. Lymphoedema also provides a challenge and may require podiatric input when it affects the feet and lower legs.

The podiatrist can also play a key role in the recognition of neoplastic changes to the foot, including melanoma, Kaposi's sarcoma, basal and squamous cell carcinoma.

Evaluating therapy interventions: outcome measures

An outcome measure provides information regarding any change in health status from one point in time to another. This requires multiple measurement points set against a baseline which should be pre-intervention. As the use of outcome measures becomes routine in all aspects of patient care, the field of oncology and palliative care must also demonstrate clinical effectiveness in order to shape modern, safe, effective and timely practice and produce evidence to support the requirement for new resources in areas of unmet need. This is of particular relevance with the current changes in cancer management and the resulting life-lengthening medical outcomes. The challenge, therefore, is to assess AHP management, incorporating holistic care, a variety of potential disease presentations, potential disease spread and 'managed deterioration'.

The World Health Organization (World Health Organization [WHO], 1980) developed the concept that illness can be considered at four levels:

- Pathology.
- Impairment – the immediate consequence of the pathology as perceived by the patient. Suitable assessment tools include tape measures, scales and gonimeters.

Table 2.2   Cancer-related outcome measures.

Cancer rehabilitation evaluation system – short form (CARES-SF)
Multi-dimensional questionnaire
   Assesses the day-to-day problems and rehabilitation needs of the person with cancer:

Physical	Psychological
Medical interaction	Marital
Sexual problems	

Self-report (rated on a scale 0–4)
Fifty-nine items (original format has 139 items)
High level of reliability and validity (Schag *et al.*, 1991)

Functional assessment of cancer therapy scale – general (FACT-G)
Measures health-related Q of L in cancer patients who are receiving therapy
Twenty-eight-item self-report tool (scale 0–4)
Multi-dimensional:

Physical	Functional
Social	Emotional well-being
Patient–physician relationship	

High level of reliability and validity (Cella *et al.*, 1993)

Edinburgh rehabilitation status scale (ERSS)
Measures four dimensions in which change may occur in the course of a disability illness or during rehabilitation:

Independence	Activity
Social integration	Effects of symptoms on lifestyle

Useful as profession-specific or group tool
Completed by a clinician

Not specifically designed for cancer patients but found to be appropriate (Affleck *et al.*, 1988).

- Disability – the external behavioural consequence of the disease. Assessment tools such as a timed walk test and various activities of daily living assessments are appropriate.
- Handicap – 'represents socialisation of an impairment or disability, and as such, it reflects the consequences for the individual, whether cultural, social, economic and environmental, that stem from the presence of impairment and disability' (WHO, 1980). It must therefore be measured using a multi-dimensional tool which will address all areas.

Specific outcome measures are available for individual professions; however, Tables 2.2 and 2.3 show a selection of generic multi-dimensional, holistic tools for cancer-related issues and palliative care.

Education and research

As rehabilitation in cancer care evolves, the implications are far reaching for educational research and development. AHPs need to be more aware of the statistics related to cancer survivorship and the role they can play in the long-term management of patients. This must be delivered at an early stage in professional careers. An education at both undergraduate and postgraduate level is the key to the development of

Table 2.3 Palliative-care-related outcome measures.

The Spitzer QL index

Designed to enhance Q of L for patients with terminal cancer

Interview format

Topics – activities, living, health, support and outlook on life (Spitzer *et al.*, 1981)

Hospice Q of L index (HQLI)

Designed to assess the overall Q of L of hospice patients

Twenty-five-item self-report questionnaire

Four major categories:

    Physical/functional

    Psychological

    Social/spiritual (relationships)

    Financial

Has only been validated for inpatient hospice setting (McMillan, 1996)

Edmonton functional assessment tool

Further development and validation for use in palliative care (EFAT-2)

    Designed to assess physical impairment and functional performance of patients in palliative care

    Assesses ten functional activities important to patients even in the terminal stages of their illness (Kaasa & Wessel, 2001)

---

high-quality cancer care for patients and their families and furthermore will enhance the continued professional development of AHPs. As such, cancer networks need to agree an education and training programme to meet the levels of rehabilitation interventions required. In order to provide the skilled workforce, recommended by the DH guidance (DH, 2004b), there is an emphasis on determining and ensuring that education and training are available at appropriate levels for all grades of staff. Education is graded in four levels (basic intervention to highly specialist care), which relate to Table 2.1 (National Cancer Network AHP Leads Forum, 2007). The training prerequisite supports the initial recommendations from Calman–Hine and other regional documents regarding specialist advanced skills for those working specifically in oncology. This currently is difficult to source as the majority of AHP undergraduate programmes do not contain oncology and palliative care modules.

Professional and regulatory bodies for health care professionals must adopt cancer within their core curriculum and incorporate it into a spiral curriculum building knowledge and skills at an undergraduate level so that AHP management of patients throughout their cancer journey is embedded in practice. A study by Wood and Ward (2000), using a qualitative methodology, reported the cancer education needs for non-specialised staff. Key areas of need included:

- An overview of cancer, what it is and how it affects patients
- Cancer treatments and side effects
- Communication skills
- Physical and practical issues
- Care organisation, referral routes and roles of staff
- Death and dying issues

It was reported that such training needs are not simply an issue for nursing and AHPs but for other staff groups, such as health care assistants, who often have most contact with cancer patients as they are frequently involved in personal care.

The engagement of undergraduate students is vital not only through university education in areas described by Wood and Ward (2000), but also as part of practice-based learning in the form of oncology and palliative care student placements. Interprofessional practice placements, if facilitated appropriately, should help to develop the multidisciplinary teams that are essential for integrated patient pathways to provide seamless care to patients.

Unfortunately, there are currently no clearly defined career pathways linked to post-registration education and training programmes for AHPs wishing to develop their clinical expertise in cancer care. Some multi-professional postgraduate education is available from Macmillan, Marie Curie and a few universities on a limited basis. This limits the options for those clinicians working at level 4 who should have access to post-entry education (postgraduate diplomas, masters and doctorates) in order to support their development and research. The further establishment of such programmes would enhance the knowledge and skills of practitioners at all levels and encourage movement into extended scope and highly specialist consultant roles. There are significant resource implications regarding the education and training requirements of health care professionals working in cancer care. NICE (2004) estimated significant costs for implementing the four-level model of rehabilitation assessment and support. However, it is only via the cancer networks that true costs can be established and business cases made to support the recommendations of this guidance.

AHP research is still a developing area. As the evidence base develops within these professions, so too will research in the field of cancer rehabilitation. Research is needed to explore the role, components and outcomes of rehabilitation, including the contribution of AHPs. Additionally, research is needed to determine what models of rehabilitation are most effective for different patient groups and how these are best integrated with other services (NICE, 2004).

Cancer is a top government priority and research into all aspects of cancer is essential to decrease the burden of the disease. The DH has taken important strategic action to ensure that research efforts are focused on achieving the maximum benefits for patients. The NHS Cancer Plans and related documents are the main framework for all cancer research activities (DH, 2000). These advocate that all involved in the funding and delivery of cancer research produce definitive proposals for a National Cancer Research Institute (NCRI) and supporting networks. The NCRI is a partnership between government and the voluntary and private sectors. The formation of the NCRI has led to the development of a coordinated view of research and global networks, with partners such as the National Cancer Institute (NCI) in the USA. This government support is not specifically aimed at science projects, but for other areas and specific programmes of cancer research in areas of high priority, including epidemiology, prevention, screening, genetics, primary care and supportive and palliative care. Additionally, the NCI portfolio, known as ensuring the best outcomes for all, addresses key issues including quality of cancer care, survivorship and health disparities (National Cancer Institute [NCI], 2006). The infrastructure and networks for cancer research must therefore be established to facilitate AHPs to engage in research in areas such as prevention, primary care and supportive and palliative care.

There are opportunities for AHPs to undertake both quantitative and qualitative research in this area of practice; however, engagement in such research can be problematic due to pressures of clinical workload and a lack of expertise in sourcing adequate funding. Opportunities for funding favour both researchers and institutions which hold established track records of research excellence. There have been significant developments such as the formation of the Research Forum for Allied Health Professionals (RFAHP). This is a multi-professional body that has been in existence for 5 years and has developed strategic aims which include:

- To be the primary point of contact for matters relating to AHP research information and communication
- To enhance the research capacity and productivity of the AHPs; to contribute to national, regional and local research and development initiatives to reflect the full spectrum of health and social care
- To influence the funding of AHPs research through lobbying fenders and policy setting bodies; to promote opportunities for multidisciplinary collaboration
- To facilitate evidence-based practice through the promotion of research sensitivity

The formation of such groups is a positive step in developing research for AHPs. The group's very long-term vision aims to have all AHP practice knowledge and evidence based by the year 2100, within a respected culture of high-quality research. AHPs are therefore emerging professions developing research in a relatively emerging area of practice. There are of course other research forums including the Palliative Care Research Society (www.pcrs.org.uk) which aims to promote research amongst all health care professionals. The engagement of AHPs in such research provides both challenge and opportunity. Research priorities have been set regarding the need to improve the patient experience and, in particular, to ensure the maximum effectiveness of such work carried out by the NHS (Strategic Priorities in Cancer Research and Development, 1999). AHPs should feel compelled to accept this challenge.

Health professionals must also utilise existing research to plan for the future. The DH is a supporter and major founder of the Cochrane Collaboration. This database now contains over 50 systematic reviews related to cancer from around the world. It is hoped that reviews on rehabilitation in the cancer population will soon become available as protocols are currently being established in this area. Additionally, it is hoped that the DH will commission further reviews to ensure that future cancer guidance from NICE is informed by current evidence. To ensure that this progress continues, AHPs must engage in research and reflect its outcomes in practice.

In conclusion, the development of education at both undergraduate and postgraduate levels is vital to the future practice of AHPs in oncology and palliative care. Managers, commissioners, professional bodies and AHP clinicians must together ensure that resources to facilitate education and research are prioritised and made available to allow the document *Fulfilling Lives – Rehabilitation in Palliative Care* (Crompton, 2000) to become a reality.

Future service provision

The *NHS Cancer Plan and New NHS: Providing a Patient-Centred Service* (DH, 2004b) continues to target inequalities and promotes prevention as well as cure. It states that more than half of all cancers may be prevented through measures to reduce smoking, improve diet and increase physical activity. Its findings include:

- Smoking is the most important cause of cancer and accounts for one-third of cancer deaths.
- Obesity is now recognised as a major risk factor for some cancers, particularly breast, bowel and renal cancers.
- Increasing levels of physical activity will help to reduce obesity and can directly reduce the risk of some cancers (DH, 2004b).

AHPs have core skills in areas such as exercise, respiratory care and nutrition which should be utilised to address prevention and promotion of healthy self-management. This is a relatively new challenge for therapy professions where intervention has traditionally been reactive rather than proactive. Health promotion, informal screening and common cancer symptom recognition are all within the AHP remit.

Traditionally, the government has primarily addressed cancer treatment issues; however, this new approach concentrates on reducing future numbers of potential cancer patients. The increasing levels of risk factors identified in the population make this target for early detection and prevention vital for future service provision. If the estimated increase in population continues and the current rates of diagnosis are maintained, current health economics may fail as demand outstrips resources.

Modern cancer service provision is based on regional networks, ideally providing an equitable, quality, seamless service to all cancer-tumour-specific groups (breast, gynaecological, lung etc.) in all care settings. The combination of the predicted changes in demography, the increase in numbers of cancer survivors and the life-extending medical outcomes will have significant impact on the need for projected future rehabilitation services. The actual demand for cancer rehabilitation in all care settings can therefore only rise (Rosen *et al.*, 2006). This will be particularly significant in areas where cancer care has not traditionally been provided, such as the community. Balance will need to be maintained between concentrating expertise in centres of excellence for complex activity and planning to skill up generic clinicians working with patients undergoing advancing cancer treatments in other locations. This will impact on all service providers and education establishments.

Progressively, multi-professional cancer management teams are becoming tumour site specific in their format in order to increase expertise and overall outcomes. Whilst this move was initiated by the medial practitioners, the nursing profession has reproduced the model and it is now common to have clinical nurse specialists dedicated to specific tumour teams. AHPs also have specialist knowledge in this field within their own professional groups and should be encouraged to specialise and integrate further as dedicated team members to provide a more holistic package of expert care working at level 4 in the NICE model (Table 2.1). For example, the head and neck cancer specialist team should now have dedicated specialist speech and language therapists, dietitians, physiotherapists, occupational therapists and radiographers working alongside doctors and nurses. This model is reproducible for other tumour groups and palliative care.

There are, currently, no guidance figures for staffing cancer services; AHPs are however recognised as integral players in the cancer management teams in the various NICE tumour-specific guidance documents. This is particularly noted in *Improving Supportive and Palliative Care for Adults with Cancer* (NICE, 2004), which also highlights the lack of review or development of the role of the AHP oncology clinical specialist or consultant.

The Department of Health and Children for Ireland (2001) has produced palliative care resource guidance. This recommends at least one whole time equivalent (WTE) physiotherapist and occupational therapist per ten beds in a specialist palliative care inpatient unit, and one WTE physiotherapist and occupational therapist per 125 000 per head of population for community services specialising in palliative care. It also recommends specific SLT and dietetics sessions for all inpatient palliative care units. As the modern role of the hospice continues to evolve, it is likely that day hospital and outpatient services will face higher levels of demand. Palliative care in England and Wales, particularly in the community and voluntary sectors, received a budget of 50 million pounds per annum from 2003 to address inequalities, including shortages of experienced professionals, and to raise confidence regarding joint service arrangements with the voluntary sector (DH, 2000).

As bed-usage pressures continue to increase, cancer centres and units will have their bed usage limited to curative cancer treatments or emergency admissions alone. Progressively, the current flexibility of having delayed discharges to permit extended rehabilitation or due to lack of discharge location will not be acceptable. This lack of acute cancer/palliative care drop-down rehabilitation beds will continue to impact on both the community and voluntary sectors. The projected change to the delivery of cancer care will affect all AHPs who may come into contact with people with cancer in both dedicated facilities and other environments. Managers and commissioners will be challenged to ensure adequate skilled service provision to this vulnerable and growing patient group.

Published late in 2007, the Cancer Reform Strategy (DH) delivers proposals for the further development of modern cancer services. Key elements include increased focus on prevention, extended screening, faster treatment and extended services for the increasing numbers of people surviving with cancer. This document acknowledges the potential physical or psychological side effects resulting from the diagnosis or cancer treatment in those cured from or living with cancer and the ensuing holistic needs. Lymphoedema and brachial plexopathy are mentioned as common examples of long-lasting and potentially debilitating problems. This has prompted the National Cancer Director to plan for and lead a new Cancer Survivorship Initiative, in collaboration with some of the cancer charities, to investigate how these needs will be met on an individual basis. This will include provision of rehabilitation programmes, nutritional advice and back-to-work support.

A further recommendation states that commissioners should ensure that the NICE (2004) guidance on supportive and palliative care is implemented by December 2008 supported by the work of the Cancer Action Teams. Supporting projects include the cancer rehabilitation measures designed to facilitate local developments regarding cancer network structure (rehabilitation lead and group) and function including baseline service mapping and the agreement of rehabilitation guidelines for tumour-specific groups.

The reform strategy will also establish a new annual NHS Cancer Patient Experience Survey Programme designed to produce local information and drive future service improvements.

Key learning points

- Cancer is now considered to be a chronic disease, with patients 'living with' rather than just dying of cancer.
- Cancer treatments are improving rapidly, thus necessitating the need for rehabilitation and symptom management.
- More cancer treatments will be delivered in the community setting, thereby requiring development of generalist and specialist domiciliary cancer AHP resources.
- Currently, there is limited provision of cancer care education both at an undergraduate and postgraduate level. Universities and other institutions must develop specialist training for those staff working in oncology and palliative care as clinical specialists, AHP consultants and researchers.
- Increasing prevalence rates signify the need for reassessment of current AHP resources and an urgent review to guarantee future-efficient and effective service provision in both the generalist and specialist fields.

References

Affleck, J. W., Aitken, R. C., Hunter, J. A., McGuire, R. J. & Roy, C. W. (30 January 1988). Rehabilitation status: a measure of medicosocial dysfunction. *The Lancet*, 1, 230–233.

British Dietetic Association [BDA] (2006). Retrieved 30 November 2006 from www.bda.uk.com

British Dietetic Association [BDA] Oncology Group (2002). *The state registered dietitian's role in oncology: working with patients with cancer.* Birmingham: British Dietetic Association.

Calman, K. & Hine, D. (1995). *A policy framework for commissioning cancer services.* London: Department of Health.

Campbell, H. (1996). *Cancer services – investing for the future.* Belfast: Department of health and Social Services.

Cancer Action Team (2007). *Holistic assessment of supportive and palliative care needs for adults with cancer: assessment guidance.* London: St Thomas' Hospital.

Cella, D. F., Tulsky, D. S., Gray, G., Sarafian, B., Linn, E., Bonomi, A., Silberman, M., Yellen, S. B., Winicour, P., Brannon, J., Eckberg, K., Lloyd, S., Purl, S., Blenowski, C., Goodman,

M., Barnicle, M., Stewart, I., McHale, M., Bonomi, P., Kaplan, E., Taylor, S., IV, Thomas, C. R., Jr & Harris, J. (1993). The functional assessment of cancer therapy scale: development and validation of the general measure. *Journal of Clinical Oncology, 11*, 570–579.

Chartered Society of Physiotherapy [CSP] (2002). *Curriculum framework for qualifying programmes in physiotherapy.* London: Chartered Society of Physiotherapy.

Chartered Society of Physiotherapy [CSP] (2003). *The role of physiotherapy for people with cancer-CSP position statement CSP 99.* London: Chartered Society of Physiotherapy.

Crompton, S. (2000). *Fulfilling lives-rehabilitation in palliative care.* London: National Council for Hospice and Specialist Palliative Care Services.

Department of Health [DH] (2000). *The National cancer plan: a plan for investment, a plan for reform.* London: Department of Health.

Department of Health [DH] (2003). *Cancer CGWT.* Retrieved 3 July 2006 from www.dh.gov.uk/PolicyAndGuidance/HealthAnd SocailCareTopics/Cancer

Department of Health [DH] (2004a). *Building on the best: end of life care initiative.* Retrieved 3 July 2006 from www.dh.gov.uk/PublicationsAndStatistics/

Department of Health [DH] (2004b). *The NHS cancer plan and the new NHS: providing a patient-centred service.* Retrieved 3 July 2006 from www.dh.gov.uk/publications

Department of Health [DH] (2004c). *Cancer in primary care: a guide to good practice.* Retrieved from www.modern.nhs.uk/cancer/primarycare

Department of Health [DH] (2005). *Investment in cancer 2001/02 and 2003/04.* Retrieved 3 July 2006 from www.dh.gov.uk/Publications

Department of Health [DH] (2006a). *Our health, our care, our say: a new direction for community services.* London: Department of Health.

Department of Health [DH] (2006b). *England summary – cancer waiting times: monitoring the one month wait target from diagnosis to treatment for all cancers.* Retrieved 27 June 2006 from www.performanve.doh.gov.uk/cancerwaits/2005/q3/part6.html

Department of Health [DH] (2006c). *Introductory guide to end of life care in care homes.* Retrieved 24 October 2006 from www.endoflifecare.nhs.uk

Department of Health [DH] (2007). *Cancer reform strategy.* Retrieved 5 December 2007 from www.dh.gov.uk

Department of Health and Children (2001). *Report of the National advisory committee on palliative care.* Dublin: Department of Health and Children.

Dietz, J. H. (1980). Adaptive rehabilitation in Cancer. *Postgraduate Medicine, 68* (1), 145–153.

Dietz, J. H. (1981). *Rehabilitation in oncology.* New York: John Wiley.

Fulton, C. L. (1994). Physiotherapists in cancer care: a framework for rehabilitation of patients. *Physiotherapy, 80* (12), 830–834.

Fulton, C. L. & Else, R. (1997). Rehabilitation in palliative care: physiotherapy. In: D. Doyle, G.W.C. Hanks & N. McDonald (Eds.), *Oxford textbook of palliative medicine.* Oxford: Oxford University Press.

Habeck, R. V., Romsaas, E. P. & Olsen, S. J. (1984). Cancer rehabilitation and continuing care: a case study. *Cancer Nursing, 7*, 315–319.

Health Professions Council (2006). Retrieved 30 October 2006 from www.hpc-uk.org/aboutregistration/professions

Kaasa, T. & Wessel, J. (2001). The edmonton functional assessment tool: further development & validation for use in palliative care. *Journal of Palliative Care, 17* (1), 5–11.

McDonnell, M. E. & Shea, B. D. (1993). The role of physical therapy in patients with metastatic disease to bone. *Back and Musculoskeletal Rehabilitation, 3* (2), 78–84.

McMillan, S. C. (1996). *Quality of life assessment in palliative care.* Retrieved 11 March 2005 from www.moffitt.usf.edu/pubs/ccj/v3n3/article4.html

National Audit Office [NAO] (2005a). *Tackling cancer: improving the patient journey.* London: The Stationery Office.

National Audit Office [NAO] (2005b). *The NHS cancer plan: a progress report*. London: The Stationery Office.

National Cancer Institute [NCI] (2006). Retrieved 5 December 2007 from http://researchportfolio.cancer.gov/

National Cancer Network AHP Forum (2007). *Chair network leads: Jackie turnpenney*. Retrieved 28 August 2007 from jackie.turnpenney@manchester.nhs.uk

National Council for Hospice and Specialist Palliative Care Services [NCHSPCS] (2002). *Definitions of supportive and palliative care*. Briefing paper 11. London: National Council for Hospice and Specialist Palliative Care Services.

National Health Service [NHS] (October 2006). *End of life care programme*, Issue 5. Leicester: National Health Service. Retrieved 15 January 2007 from www.endoflifecare.nhs.uk

National Institute for Clinical Excellence [NICE] (2004). *Guidance on cancer services: improving supportive and palliative care for adults with cancer*. London: National Institute for Clinical Excellence.

Northern Ireland Cancer Network (2006). *Cancer network values*. Belfast: Department of Health, Social Services and Public Health.

Office for National Statistics (2006). National projections. Retrieved 10 March 2008 from www.statistics.gov.uk/cci/nugget.asp?id=1352

Rosen, R., Smith, A. & Harrison, A. (2006). *Future trends and challenges for cancer services in England-a review of literature and policy*. London: King's Fund/Cancer Research UK.

Schag, C. A., Ganz, P. A. & Heinrich, R. L. (1991). Cancer rehabilitation evaluation system – short form (CARES-SF). *Cancer*, 68, 1406–1413.

Spitzer, W. O., Dobson, A. J., Hall, J., Spitzer, W. O., Dobson, A. J., Hall, J., Chesterman, E., Levi, J., Shepherd, R., Battista, R. N. & Catchlove, B. R. (1981). Measuring the quality of life of cancer patients. *Journal of Chronic Diseases*, 34, 585–597.

Strategic Priorities in Cancer Research and Development (1999). Retrieved 2 December 2007 from http://science.cancerresearchuk.org/

The Association of Chartered Physiotherapist in Oncology and Palliatives Care (1993). *Guidelines for good practice*, London: Chartered Society of Physiotherapy.

Watson, P. G. (1992). The optimal functioning plan: a key element in cancer rehabilitation. *Cancer Nursing*, 15, 254–263.

Wood, C. & Ward, J. (2000). A general overview of the cancer education needs of non specialist staff. *European Journal of Cancer Care*, 9, 191–196.

World Health Organization [WHO] (1980). *The International classification of impairments, disabilities and handicaps*. Geneva: World Health Organization.

SECTION 2
THE MULTI-PROFESSIONAL MANAGEMENT OF SPECIFIC TUMOUR TYPES

Chapter 3

MULTI-PROFESSIONAL MANAGEMENT OF PATIENTS WITH BREAST CANCER

Melanie Lewis, Iona Davies and Jill Cooper

Learning outcomes

After reading this chapter the reader should be able to:

- Describe the clinical presentation, diagnosis, investigations and treatment options for breast cancer
- Discuss the possible symptoms and problems that can occur with patients undergoing treatment
- Critically discuss the multi-professional approaches of allied health professionals in the treatment of patients with breast cancer
- Discuss the physical and psychological difficulties which may face patients with breast cancer throughout the cancer journey

---

Introduction

Breast cancer is the most common cancer in women in the UK, accounting for one in four of all female cancers and 16% of all cancers (Cancer Research UK [CRUK], 2006). It is the second most common cancer in the UK after non-melanoma skin cancer and over 44 000 new cases are diagnosed every year (CRUK, 2006).

It claims the lives of 12 400 women each year in the UK, but is rare in men, with approximately 300 new cases being diagnosed annually (CRUK, 2006). Earlier detection and improved treatment have resulted in death rates in the UK falling by 20% in the last 10 years, and of those women diagnosed with breast cancer today, 60% are likely to survive for at least 20 years (CRUK, 2006).

Cancer survival rates commonly refer to a 5-year period, because 1-year survival gives only a very short term view of prognosis and progress, and for 10-year survival and beyond, one has to look at people diagnosed a long time ago (Coleman *et al.*, 2004). Recurrence is most likely to occur in the lymph nodes (axilla or supra clavicular), skin surrounding wound sites, bone, lung, liver and brain (Tobias & Eaton, 2001). Patients could also have another primary tumour in the remaining breast.

Table 3.1 Risk factors for developing breast cancer.

Gender	Predominantly a female disease: 135 women to 1 male
Age	Risk increases with age
Hormonal factors	Uninterrupted menstrual cycles – early menarche and late menopause with no breaks for pregnancy
Reproductive history	The younger the woman when she begins childbearing, the lower her risk of breast cancer. More full-term pregnancies and breast feeding can also lower the possibility of developing breast cancer
Exogenous hormones	The contraceptive pill and hormone replacement therapy slightly increase risk
Family history	Previous primary diagnosis of breast cancer and a first-degree relative (mother or sister) diagnosed with breast cancer
Obesity	Body mass over 30 and a diet high in fat, especially animal fat
Other factors	Lack of physical activity, excess alcohol consumption and a higher socioeconomic status

Treatment for recurrence is usually oncology led and depends on the individual patient case. Allied health professional (AHP) interventions for the management of metastatic disease will be discussed in later chapters, focusing on musculoskeletal and neurological issues and specific symptoms.

AHPs have an important role in the management of patients with breast cancer, addressing patients' physical, functional and psychosocial needs (Vockins, 2004). Multi-professional working in oncology should provide a seamless service from diagnosis to recovery and support patients in maintaining their independence and autonomy (National Institute for Clinical Excellence [NICE], 2002). As survival rates continue to improve (Office for National Statistics, 2004), AHP service provision needs to be proactive to avoid potentially debilitating costly side effects of cancer and its treatment (National Council for Hospice and Specialist Palliative Care Services [NCHSPCS], 2000).

Aetiology

Table 3.1 demonstrates the risk factors for developing breast cancer.

Incidence and prevalence

Breast cancer is strongly related to age. Incidence increases with age, with the greatest rate of increase prior to menopause (CRUK, 2006). More than 80% of cases occur in women aged 50 years and over (CRUK, 2006), the highest numbers of cases being in the 50–64 age group and it is these women who are targeted for the national screening programme in the UK. In 2004, routine screening was extended to include women up to the age of 70 from 2004 (CRUK, 2006).

Although it is rare for teenagers and women in their early 20s to be diagnosed with breast cancer, this form of cancer is the most commonly diagnosed cancer in women under 35 in the UK (CRUK, 2006). Statistics are available on the regularly updated Cancer Research Campaign website (CRUK, 2006).

Geographic variations show that, worldwide, more than a million women are diagnosed with breast cancer every year, accounting for 10% of all new cancers and 23% of female cancers (Ferlay *et al.*, 2002). The incidence rates vary considerably, the highest rates being in the developed world and the lowest rates in Africa and Asia. This may be due to difficulties in obtaining accurate statistics in these areas, or other theories relating to dietary and environmental factors have been proposed (Ziegler *et al.*, 1993). Migrants from low- to high-risk countries acquire the risk of the host country within two generations (Ziegler *et al.*, 1993).

Cancer genetics

Variations of the *ATM*, *BRCA1*, *BRCA2*, *CHEK2* and *RAD51* genes all increase the risk of developing breast cancer. The *AR*, *DIRAS3*, *ERBB2* and *TP53* genes are also associated with breast cancer (Genetics Home Reference, 2007).

These genes provide instructions for making proteins that help to regulate the growth and division of cells. Some of these proteins are involved in detecting and repairing damaged DNA. Others help the cell respond to external signals, such as hormones and growth factors. When a gene mutation alters the structure or function of these proteins, cells in the breast can grow and divide uncontrollably and form a tumour. *BRCA1* and *BRCA2* are major genes related to hereditary breast cancer. People who have inherited certain mutations in these genes have a higher risk of developing breast cancer, ovarian cancer and several other types of cancer over their lifetime (Genetics Home Reference, 2007).

The way that breast cancer risk is inherited depends on the gene involved. For example, mutations in the *BRCA1* and *BRCA2* genes are inherited in an autosomal-dominant pattern, which means one copy of the altered gene is sufficient to increase the chance of developing cancer. In other cases, the inheritance of breast cancer risk is unclear. It is important to note that people inherit an increased *risk* of cancer. Not all people who inherit mutations in these genes will develop cancer.

Somatic mutations (genetic changes that occur only in breast cancer cells) occur during a person's lifetime and are not inherited (Genetics Home Reference, 2007). In the UK, if individuals are aware of a strong family history of breast cancer, they may be screened at a genetic or breast family history clinic from an early age, i.e., in their 20s rather than wait for the screening programme in their 50s (Tobias & Eaton, 2001).

Diagnosis

Tobias and Eaton (2001) describe the most common symptoms of breast cancer as:

- Lump 90%
- Painful lump 20%

Table 3.2 Clinical staging of breast cancer.

Stage I	Tumour up to 2 cm No lymph nodes affected No evidence of spread beyond the breast
Stage II	Tumour between 2 and 5 cm and/or Lymph nodes in axilla affected No evidence of spread beyond the axilla
Stage III	Tumour more than 5 cm Lymph nodes in axilla affected No evidence of spread beyond the axilla
Stage IV	Tumour of any size Lymph nodes in axilla often affected Cancer has spread to other parts of the body

- Nipple change 10%
- Nipple discharge 3%
- Skin contour change 5%

The majority of women diagnosed with breast cancer have presented to their general practitioner (GP) with a breast lump (Tobias & Eaton, 2001). Referral is then made to a breast clinic where the diagnosis is confirmed, or excluded, by fine-needle aspiration. The fine needle and syringe extract a tiny volume of material for examination. If the aspiration test confirms cancer, the treatment options are discussed with the patient.

Many breast cancers are also detected by mammography before any symptoms are noticed and women in the UK aged 50 and over are encouraged to attend for breast screening (NICE, 2002). Whilst the screening does not diagnose the disease, it enables those who are tested positive to be called back for further diagnostic tests to determine whether they do have the disease (CRUK, 2006).

Table 3.2 describes the clinical staging of breast cancer.

Treatment options

Table 3.3 demonstrates the pathology of breast cancer and treatment options.

Chemotherapy
- Neoadjuvant chemotherapy refers to first-line chemotherapy which is given for a large breast tumour to shrink it prior to surgery, thus avoiding the need for mastectomy.
- Adjuvant chemotherapy refers to chemotherapy which is given after local treatment for the tumour (surgery or radiotherapy) to reduce the risk of metastatic disease and improve disease-free survival.
- Palliative chemotherapy is given to improve quality of life, so the benefits must outweigh the side effects (Harmer, 2003).

Table 3.3 Breast cancer pathology.

Breast cancer	Possible treatment
Ductal carcinoma in situ (DCIS) Known as pre-invasive or non-invasive carcinoma. Cancerous cells found within the mammary ducts that are usually contained. Does not cause metastatic spread. Cure is almost always likely with treatment	Surgery – most common to have wide local excision (WLE) or mastectomy if the DCIS is large. Axillary surgery unlikely unless large DCIS seen. Radiotherapy – if high grade Hormonal therapy – if DCIS has OR cells present
Lobular carcinoma in situ (LCIS) LCIS does not develop into full breast cancer. Cell changes occur in the linings of the lobules in the breast. Usually seen in both breasts and like DCIS does not usually spread	Surgery – not usually needed Hormonal therapy – currently clinical trials are investigating the effects of tamoxifen and Arrimidex on the reduction of LCIS developing into breast cancer
Infiltrating ductal carcinoma (invasive) Most common invasive breast cancer diagnosed. Cancer cells commonly invade other breast tissue. Can spread typically to bone, lung and liver Tubular carcinoma (invasive) Infiltrating lobular carcinoma (invasive) Medullary carcinoma (invasive) Plus many others	The breast cancer multidisciplinary team including surgeons, pathologists, radiologists and oncologists will decide all treatments Surgery – mastectomy or WLE Chemotherapy – neo or adjuvant Radiotherapy – to surrounding area. Hormonal therapy – including Herceptin if HER+
Inflammatory breast cancer Rare and most aggressive cancer. High probability of axillary spread	
Paget disease Adenocarcinoma of the nipple with eczema skin changes. Usually associated with DCIS	

Silva & Zurrida (2005).

Radiotherapy

Breast irradiation is a major part of the radiotherapy workload in the UK, accounting for approximately 30% of all radiotherapy resources (CRUK, 2006). It is used:

- As an early treatment following wide local excision to complete the treatment by killing off remaining cancer cells
- As a treatment for locally advanced breast cancer to shrink a large, inoperable tumour
- As a treatment for metastatic breast cancer to enhance quality of life by reducing the tumour bulk, reducing the amount of dying tissue and reducing the possibility for infection and odour (Burnet, 2003)

Surgery

Clinical and pathological features of breast cancer influence the type of surgery used. These include position and size of the cancer, the size of the host breast, the completeness of any initial excision, the histological grade, age, the presence of an extensive in situ component and lymphovascular invasion (Harmer, 2003).

- Excision biopsy – It may be required if clinical examination, imaging, cytology and/or core biopsy are inconclusive, to remove the lump.
- Lumpectomy – The tumour is removed with clear margins of normal tissue. Sizes of margins depend on local guidelines.
- Quadrectomy – It is similar to lumpectomy but a larger margin of normal tissue is removed.
- Central excision – Nipple is removed.
- Simple mastectomy – Only the breast is removed.
- Modified radical mastectomy – The breast and lymph nodes are removed but not chest wall muscles.
- Total radical mastectomy – It is less frequently used, and involves excision of the breast, pectoralis major and minor plus complete axillary lymph node clearance (Harmer, 2003).

Breast reconstruction aims to recreate a breast mound, and is performed either as a primary procedure at the same time as a mastectomy or as a delayed secondary procedure (Futter *et al.*, 2002). For this either prosthesis or autogenous tissue is used, as described in Table 3.4. The aim is to provide symmetry and so it may be necessary to operate on the unaffected breast to achieve comparable shape and size.

Axillary lymph node surgery. There are approximately 20–30 lymph nodes in the axilla. Axillary node sampling and sentinel node biopsy (SNB) are used when lymph nodes are suspected as negative and the tumour is contained within the breast. SNB involves lymphatic mapping to identify the first lymph node (sentinel node) that receives lymphatic drainage from the affected breast. If the SNB is positive for tumour cells, then further axillary management is carried out (Ronka *et al.*, 2004). When lymph nodes are removed, there is the risk of lymphoedema (Chapter 11).

Hormone therapy

Hormones are substances that occur naturally in the body where they control the growth and activity of normal cells. Although they do not usually affect cancer cells, in breast cancer the situation is different.

The female hormones oestrogen and progesterone are naturally produced by the ovaries before menopause. After the menopause, oestrogen is made in much smaller amounts by the adrenal glands. These hormones affect the growth of some breast cancer cells. This means that drugs or treatments that block the effects of hormones, or lower the levels of oestrogen and progesterone, can be used as a treatment for some types of breast cancer (CRUK, 2006).

If breast cancer cells are oestrogen receptor (OR or ER) positive, hormone therapy such as tamoxifen followed by aromatase inhibitors such as Arimidex may be indicated. Tamoxifen is commonly given for 5 years after all chemotherapy has finished.

Table 3.4 Types of breast reconstruction.

Prosthetic reconstruction	Breast mound is achieved by a tissue expander, which is gradually inflated until the desired shape and volume is achieved, or by a preformed prosthesis. It is inserted into a pocket created between the rib cage and pectoral muscles
Autogenous reconstruction	Flap of tissue with its blood supply can be taken from the back, buttock or abdomen to create a breast mound and can be pedicled or free flap
Latissimus dorsi flap	Section of muscle with overlying skin is dissected and rotated around its blood vessel to its new position. For larger breasted women, a latissimus dorsi flap can be used in conjunction with a prosthesis
Transverse rectus abdominis myocutaneous flap (TRAM)	Stomach fat, skin, underlying muscle and blood supply are dissected and mobilised to form a breast mound
Deep/superficial inferior epigastric perforator (DIEP/SIEP)	These have evolved from the TRAM flap. Utilises the stomach, skin and fat but leaves the underlying muscle untouched
Superior/inferior gluteal artery perforator flap	Fat and overlying skin from either the upper or lower part of the buttock region can be utilised to reconstruct the breast mound
Nipple reconstruction	Performed as a secondary procedure once the reconstructed breast has settled to ensure correct alignment of the nipple. Possible donor sites include the skin from the inner thigh, behind the ear, axillary dog ears and the remaining nipple
Tattooing	Intradermal pigmentation can be used to achieve nipple/areola colouration
Mammoplasty	Commonly referred to as breast reduction and involves a reduction in the volume of the breast and uplift
Mastoplexy	Breast is uplifted but the volume remains unchanged

Arimidex is given to post-menopausal women. Both are given in early stage breast cancers to prevent recurrence (Tobias & Eaton, 2001).

Hormonal medication can cause hot flushes, night sweats, weight gain, loss of libido and vaginal dryness, all of which affect quality-of-life issues, including physical, body image, sexuality, psychological and emotional, and AHPs need to be aware of these effects in their treatment programmes (Shearsmith-Farthing, 2001).

Pre-treatment interventions of AHPS

In most hospital settings, AHPs do not routinely see breast cancer patients prior to treatment; however, a pre-assessment is beneficial to provide baseline information by which treatment outcomes can be evaluated. This is particularly pertinent for pre-operative measurements for lymphoedema (using tape measure or bioimpedance), associated quadrant dysfunction and postural adaptations. Verbal advice and post-operative information should be reinforced with written literature. Skalla *et al.* (2004) stated that accurate and relevant information leaflets could decrease emotional distress plus improve self-coping strategies.

The potential side effects experienced by patients during chemotherapy differ greatly from patient to patient, depending on their tolerance to drug regimes and the drugs utilised in their disease management.

Physiotherapists and occupational therapists (OTs) have extensive anatomical knowledge and use a problem-solving approach, which makes them ideally suited to assess patients pre-operatively.

The physiotherapy assessment should include:

- Full examination of any existing neurological and musculoskeletal as well as medical and psychosocial problems that may affect post-operative outcomes
- Identification of potential risk factors for post-operative complications including respiratory disorders
- Specific and relevant information and advice for patients with breast cancer plus leaflets on post-operative exercise routines.

OTs should assess functional independence, including the ability to wash, dress and carry out basic self-care activities. The basic ability to care for one's self is vital to patients' self-esteem and well-being. The OT enables an individual to maximise her quality of life by addressing difficulties in occupational performance (Vockins, 2004). Early intervention ensures that the individual's optimum independence is achieved by assessing and analysing:

- Pre-morbid factors, e.g. age, other medical conditions and disabilities
- How these will influence and potentially affect recovery from surgery
- The need for equipment and adaptations to assist in functional independence
- Psychosocial factors requiring intervention relating to anxiety and body image which may alter the individual's ability to be independent

Post-treatment interventions of AHPs

Current practice in the UK is that patients will be kept in hospital for a minimum of 2–5 days and discharge is usually dependent on surgeons' protocols and patients' post-operative recovery (NICE, 2002).

AHP intervention for physical sequelae of treatment

Shoulder range of movement

There are many studies reporting decreased shoulder mobility and strength after breast cancer treatment. Johansson *et al.* (2001) stated that at 6-month post-surgery,

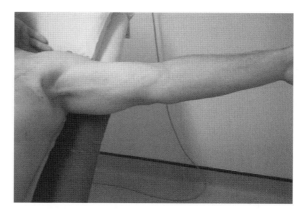

Figure 3.1 Cording.

61% of patients had reduced internal rotation, 41% decreased abduction, 34% limited external rotation and 33% restricted flexion. Contributory factors included cording (described below in axillary web syndrome), stiffness in the tissues and pain. Macleod and Koelliing (2003) suggest that shoulder mobility problems are probably due to damage to the rotator cuff muscles rather than the glenohumeral joint.

Axillary web syndrome or 'cording' refers to palpable taut cords that can occur in the axilla and can extend down to the cubital fossa or even to the base of the thumb (Figure 3.1). There are typically two or three cords present which result in pain and limited shoulder mobility, particularly abduction (Moskovitz *et al.*, 2001). According to Leidenius *et al.* (2003) 72% of patients undergoing axillary clearance and 20% of patients having SNB were found to have cording and it is hypothesised that these cords are actually caused by a disruption of the superficial lymphatics and vessels by stasis or hypercoagulation.

There is very little evidence to guide the management of cording and much research needs to be done in this area. The two papers mentioned above suggest that cording will resolve spontaneously within 3 months, but clinical experience suggests that cording can be expedited with a range of physiotherapy techniques (Fourie & Robb, 2008). Modalities which have been used are soft tissue massage and stretches combined with passive and active physiological movements. Occasionally, during activities of daily living or physiotherapy, the cords can 'snap' and do not reform. This is often associated with an increase in range of movement.

Patients should routinely receive verbal and written instructions on mobility exercises, scar mobilisation and postural guidance from the physiotherapist. General upper-limb mobility and specific exercises can improve shoulder function. Seromas are tumour-like collections of clear body fluid in the tissues. Some centres restrict shoulder movement to 90° and stop exercises until the drains are removed to decrease the risk of seroma formation and promote tissue healing (Clodius, 2001; Schultz *et al.*, 1997). It is claimed that SNB as an alternative to axillary clearance will reduce shoulder mobility problems (Leidenius *et al.*, 2003).

The OT assesses the functional consequences and provides a treatment programme, adaptive equipment and compensatory techniques to overcome any disability (Cooper, 2006).

Pain

Patients will experience varying levels of post-operative pain, which can usually be controlled with analgesics and adjuvant drugs. However, some patients may develop complex chronic pain syndromes secondary to biomechanical, behavioural, emotional and sociocultural influences. Post-mastectomy neuritis results from severance of branches of the intercostal brachial nerves during surgery. Ververs *et al.* (2001) cited that 20% of patients reported pain and numbness at 6-month post-surgery. Karki *et al.* (2005) found that 25% of patients experienced pain at 6 months and 29% at 1-year post-operatively and that patients undergoing a lumpectomy experienced more pain in the axilla and chest wall/breast area than mastectomy patients.

It is essential that physiotherapists and OTs are aware that patients with high levels of acute pain may be more likely to develop chronic pain and other problems (Jung *et al.*, 2003).

Although the evidence base is limited, physiotherapy modalities such as transcutaneous electric nerve stimulation (TENS) (Robb *et al.*, 2006), muscle balance techniques and soft-tissue and joint mobilisations may help alleviate pain. OT and physiotherapy approaches including relaxation techniques and alternative and cognitive therapies may also be effective in pain relief and are discussed more fully later in this chapter and in Chapter 15. Robb *et al.* (2006) reported on a cognitive–behavioural therapy (CBT) pain management programme for cancer patients with chronic treatment plan in which treatments included education, relaxation, exercise training and goal setting. Although this was a small preliminary study, there was a significant trend towards improvement in anxiety and depression, fitness and coping with pain.

Syrjala *et al.* carried out a controlled clinical trial to compare imagery relaxation and cognitive–behavioural training and concluded that the relaxation arm of the study coped better with disease- and treatment-related pain.

In summary, pain can affect physical function and reduce activities of daily living, thereby influencing quality of life and overall survivorship. Patients may also have to learn to live with chronic discomfort.

Peripheral neuropathy

This is the general term denoting functional deterioration in the body's outlying nervous system and may be a side effect of chemotherapy, or the direct effect of tumour, surgery spinal cord compression or lymphoedema. Consequently, it may be temporary or permanent. The symptoms usually resolve once the drugs are metabolised and the treatment finished (Cooper, 2006). It may impact on mobility, dexterity, pain and hand function, and needs OT and physiotherapy management in order to maintain range of movement, strength and functional independence and avoid atrophy and injury due to sensory loss.

Cook and Burkhardt (1994) describe how chemotherapy can cause demyelinisation of the nerve fibres and how large-fibre sensory nerves are affected. The resulting symptoms are muscle cramps and/or electric shocks, suggesting damage to the posterior column or spinal dorsal nerve column. Partial denervation may result in paraesthesias, hyperaesthesias and complaints of clumsiness when attempting to sustain a grip and impairment or loss of proprioception (Holden & Felde, 1987). Difficulties with functional tasks are often reported, as well as weakness and atrophy of intrinsic and extrinsic muscle groups, a loss of integrity of the palmar arches and a decreased range of motion of the joints (Cooper, 2006). There is also an increased risk of injury due to sensory changes.

Patients with breast cancer experiencing peripheral neuropathy seldom have a typical pattern and, as with all patients regardless of their disability, their functional problems will be unique (Cooper, 2006). This must be considered when selecting the treatment modality, which may include:

- Assessment and analysis of the anatomical and physiological effect of the neuropathy plus its emotional and psychological impact
- Assessment of how it impacts on the whole body as well as the isolated hand or arm
- Treatment programme for hand function as well as full assessment for self-care, domestic and/or work activities and hobbies
- Provision of assistive devices and compensatory techniques
- Provision of static or dynamic splinting to optimise function or provide correct positioning if there is no active movement
- Provision of sling for comfort or protection
- Patient education on safety and protection of the desensitised hand
- Oedema control techniques (Cook & Burkhardt, 1994)

Radiation-induced brachial plexopathy

Radiation-induced brachial plexopathy (RIBP) is a rare side effect of radiotherapy and describes irreversible damage to the brachial plexus due to ionising radiation for treatment of breast cancer (Royal College of Radiologists [RCR], 1995). It is estimated to have affected 1% of patients treated with radiotherapy at that time (RCR, 1995). Supraclavicular and/or axillary irradiation may cause oedema and fibrous tissue to constrict the brachial plexus, the neurolemmal sheath undergoes varying degrees of fibrous thickening, and hyalinisation and obliteration of blood vessels cause further ischaemia of nerve fibres (RCR, 1995). The symptoms may present 6 months to 20 years after treatment, most commonly 2- to 5-year post-radiotherapy with symptoms including:

- Numbness of fingers
- Wasting of lumbricals
- Neuropathic pain in hand, arm and/or shoulder
- Lymphoedema and/or atrophy
- Loss of motor power and normal movement (Cooper, 1998)

The management of patients with RIBP needs a multidisciplinary, patient-centred approach (Davis, 1995). Due to its degenerative and progressive nature, constant

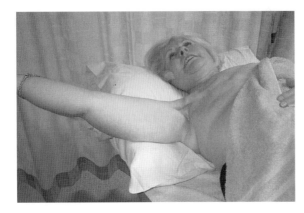

Figure 3.2 Scarring.

re-evaluation is essential. Treatment should address the physical, psychological, functional, emotional and social aspects, particularly the issues addressed in previous section.

Scar management

Scar formation is the normal response to injury, including surgery (Karki *et al.*, 2005), and the aim of scar management is to produce a strong mobile scar. The use of corrective scar tissue mobilisation has been advocated but there is currently little evidence available. Fourie (2006) suggests that early active movement coupled with tissue massage/mobilisation will encourage the alignment of collagen fibres along the lines of stress. This reduces the formation of excessive cross-link fibres and adhesions responsible for the restriction of gliding planes. Figure 3.2 shows restriction of movement from scar adhesions and Figure 3.3 potential reconstruction scarring. Massage is also thought to reduce scar hypersensitivity and helps patients to overcome their fear of the operated area (Fourie, 2006).

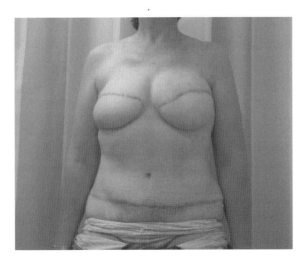

Figure 3.3 Reconstruction scarring.

Silicone gel and elastomers to hydrate and soften the surgical scar can also be utilised as a treatment tool (Mustoe *et al.*, 2002). Hypertrophic or kelloid scars may require pressure therapy, steroid injections or laser therapy.

Lymphoedema

Lymphoedema is the accumulation of lymph fluid in the tissues, resulting in swelling, and is caused by obstruction of the lymphatic vessels. This is discussed in detail in Chapter 11. Figure 3.3 shows lymphoedema of the breast.

Skin changes

Up to 90% of patients receiving radiotherapy experience skin changes, which include burns or erythema, dryness, flaky and peeling skin, pigmentation alterations and sensory changes, such as numbness and burning sensations (Burnet, 2003). There is limited evidence on optimum skin-care regimes, but washing the area gently with neutral pH soap, moisturising and hydrating the area does have a positive effect on healing time (Naylor *et al.*, 2001). Simple and non-perfumed creams or aloe-vera gel are often recommended.

Posture

Patients can experience significant postural problems post-operatively due to prolonged protraction of the shoulder joint, secondary to tightness of the pectoral major muscles (Karki *et al.*, 2005). If the patient wears an external breast prosthesis, the correct type, weight and size of prosthesis must be fitted to ensure that it does not strain the trapezius muscle and cause posture-related musculoskeletal damage (Roberts *et al.*, 2003). It is essential that patients wear the correct-size bra and be re-measured regularly, as normal lymphatic drainage can be compromised by incorrectly fitting underwear (Roberts *et al.*, 2003).

Cancer-related fatigue

Cancer-related fatigue (CRF) is widely recorded to affect patients with all cancer diagnoses irrelevant of treatment type or staging (Richardson, 2004) and is discussed in detail in Chapter 12.

Nausea

Nausea is mainly management by medication (anti-emetic drugs) but patients experiencing anticipatory nausea may benefit from relaxation techniques/hypnosis. Acupuncture or TENS may also be beneficial. Molassiotis (2000) reported on a pilot study using progressive muscular relaxation in which this training was an effective adjuvant method in decreasing nausea and vomiting in chemotherapy patients, which had the effect of reducing anxiety. Mucositis or oral dryness and ulcers are common side effects of chemotherapy and affect taste, speech and swallowing. Sucking ice chips and prophylactic use of antifungal preparations may be useful in alleviating symptoms (Worthington & Clarkson, 2002).

Weight gain/loss

This affects a high percentage of patients receiving chemotherapy. Many report weight gain, although some of this may be attributable to increased calorie intake and reduced activity in addition to the direct effect of the medication. A significant percentage, however, experience weight loss secondary to nausea and altered appetite. All require information on healthy diets to help them maintain a stable weight, control flushes and protect against osteoporosis.

Hair loss/nail damage

This can have a major impact on a patient's body image and self-esteem at a time when they are already vulnerable and is an important issue about which AHPs need to be aware in their treatment approach (Shearsmith-Farthing, 2001). Patients need to be reassured that the hair loss is temporary. Patients may also experience nail damage secondary to chemotherapy and must be aware of the risk of nail-bed infections and potential link to lymphoedema (Chapter 11).

Menopausal symptoms

This includes flushes, weight gain and vaginal dryness as common side effects of adjuvant chemotherapy. Although drugs can be prescribed which may reduce the flushes, the effectiveness of these varies between individuals. Dietary advice, relaxation therapy and acupuncture may all be helpful in alleviating symptoms (Cancer Research Campaign, 2006).

AHP intervention for psychological sequelae of treatment

Sixty per cent of cancer patients suffer with psychological distress and experience a multitude of emotions ranging from shock, denial, anger, fear and guilt to anxiety and low mood (Zabora et al., 2001). These are all 'normal' responses to what is devastating news. This distress also involves their family and friends and can have an effect on the way they function daily. Some individuals may require assistance in helping to deal with these emotions which can manifest themselves physically as well as psychologically.

AHPs directly manage the treatment of anxiety and depression by relaxation therapy and cognitive therapy (Vockins, 2004) and it is essential that they are able to recognise their own limitations and utilise other appropriate resources (Cooper,

2006). Support and counselling for patients and their families can be accessed via many national and local support groups.

Some patients may require specialist intervention by a psychologist/psychiatrist and a knowledge of how to access these services is beneficial to staff and patients alike.

Group work and support sessions

Watson *et al.* (1996) and Hindley and Johnston (1999) state that group work can produce excellent results when it is well facilitated with clear guidelines and run by experienced AHPs. For example, Lewis (2006) demonstrated a significant improvement in quality of life and reduction in the incidence of lymphoedema with a 12-week rehabilitation and prevention of lymphoedema programme.

Watson *et al.* (1996) discussed a 6-week Breast Cancer Support Group using a CBT approach, in which the OT explored stress management and taught relaxation training at the end of each session. CBT has been shown to be effective in reducing anxiety and depression in cancer patients when provided within the context of individual sessions; this group successfully studied the application of CBT in a group setting. Hindley and Johnston (1999) reported how group sessions enabled patients to focus their thoughts in positive and constructive ways to cope successfully with their diagnosis and treatment.

Cancer patients and their significant others need information to understand events throughout the course of cancer (Grahn, 1996) and require support in mobilising coping strategies as situational demands exceed their personal resources.

Sexuality

The breast is an important aspect of a woman's femininity and sexuality (Young-McCaughan, 1996). Significant body image problems can occur following treatment for breast cancer, ranging from hair loss, change in weight, fatigue, mastectomy and sexual functioning (Shearsmith-Farthing, 2001). However, Shearsmith-Farthing (2001) emphasised that there is little evidence to suggest that this is an area actively pursued outside the realm of eating disorders.

Schover (1991) discusses the impact of breast cancer on intimate relationships in women who have received chemotherapy. The effects of aging and menopause complicate the assessment of sexual functioning in survivors of breast cancer, but a consistent pattern emerged in symptoms reported by them. Menopausal symptoms including weight change, hot flushes, mood swings and anxiety attacks were reported and symptoms of vaginal dryness, decreased libido and dissatisfaction with sexual activity.

AHPs develop a close therapeutic relationship with their patients and can allow the patient with breast cancer to discuss these difficulties (Shearsmith-Farthing, 2001) and seek help to overcome them. OTs, in particular, focus on change in occupational performance and should address altered body image concerns (Shearsmith-Farthing, 2001).

Sleep disturbances and anxiety management

These issues are covered in more detail in Chapter 15. Relaxation management, which promotes a client-centred and educational approach, facilitates the individual's recognition of potential stressors and equips them with the skills required to manage such stressors (Ewer-Smith & Patterson, 2002). This utilises the expert skills of trained, qualified and highly skilled staff to assess, analyse and select the most appropriate method of management. Although OTs and physiotherapists are trained in various forms of relaxation therapy, further courses may be advisable in dealing with oncology patients due to the complex nature of problems they may face (Vockins, 2004).

Leubbert *et al.* (2001) found that relaxation was effective in managing both distressing side effects of cancer treatment and consequently anxiety. Decker *et al.* investigated relaxation therapy as an adjunct with radiotherapy and concluded that it reduced anxiety and stress.

AHP palliative care intervention with patients with advanced breast cancer

Palliative care is more than symptom control and affirms life (National Council for Hospice and Specialist Palliative Care Services, 2000). Patients are classed as palliative when curative treatment is no longer an option. However, treatment of patients with advanced breast cancer may still include oncology cancer treatment to maintain and prolong life and may include all treatments previously mentioned (Tobias & Eaton, 2001).

AHPs have an important role to play with palliative patients and their carers. Their input can facilitate patients to live in their own home, maintain their independence for as long as possible and maximise quality of life before death. Vockins (2004) states that AHPs need to recognise that patients can present with complex functional problems, and require a multi-professional approach. Most palliative patients want to know what physical and emotional support can help them remain in their own homes for as long as possible (Kealey & McIntyre, 2005).

Kealey and McIntyre (2005) found that communication and the relationship with the therapist are highly valued by both patients and their carers. This was not simply provision of equipment by the OT, but included the therapeutic relationship which AHPs have with their patients, allowing ongoing issues to be addressed, including:

- Provision of equipment/adaptations
- Compensatory and rehabilitation techniques
- Range of movement and muscle strength
- Manual handling, transfers/mobility aids or hoists
- Advice regarding their medical condition
- Fatigue management
- Lymphoedema management

- Pain management
- Stress management
- Goal achievement
- Emotional support (Kealey & McIntyre, 2005)

Case study 1

Brenda, a 56-year-old married woman, worked full-time in the civil service, had two grown-up children and had an elderly dependent mother who lived locally. She had a supportive family and network of helpful friends. She was diagnosed with breast cancer 8 months prior to being seen by the AHPs, had a lumpectomy with level III axillary clearance, six cycles of chemotherapy and, at the time of referral to the AHPs, was just about to start 6 weeks of radiotherapy to the supraclavicular area.

Functional and psychological difficulties identified:

- Cording and shoulder stiffness
- Weight gain (from 72 to 84 kg in the last year) as well as hair loss (including eyelashes and eyebrows) resulting in low self-esteem
- Constantly feeling tired and having difficulties carrying out activities of daily living, resultant concern as to how she will manage returning to work
- Anxiety about the future and whether cancer will recur

Interventions:

A physiotherapy assessment was carried out pre- and post-operatively to establish a treatment programme in which shoulder mobilisation, soft tissue massage (quadrant and scars) and postural advice were carried out. Basic education regarding lymphoedema was provided, including prophylactic advice and the contact details for the local lymphoedema clinic. A home exercise programme also encouraged both active and passive stretching, strengthening exercises and self-massage. The aim was to resolve the cording and avoid further shoulder stiffness. Timely resolution of this problem was essential because Brenda had to be able to lie flat on her back, with her shoulder abducted and externally rotated to receive radiotherapy.

Occupational therapy assessment was carried out to assess how the limitations in Brenda's shoulder and arm affected any activities of daily living, including bathing and dressing, domestic activities of daily living, e.g. hanging out washing and carrying shopping. The physiotherapist and OT reinforced each other's information to emphasise the importance of skincare and minimal manual handling with the affected arm to avoid lymphatic damage.

Brenda also attended the 6-week Breast Cancer Support Group run by the OT, clinical psychologist and clinical nurse specialist in which a CBT approach was used and the OT taught a range of relaxation exercises. The group covered coping strategies for communication with the family and partners, coping with the overwhelming feeling of fatigue and how to plan for the future. Brenda found it very difficult to imagine coping with a future in which the thought of the cancer returning was hanging over her, but this was addressed by CBT, which looked at challenging negative thoughts. Energy conservation techniques of pacing and planning ahead were also taught and, although Brenda still had her concerns, she felt better equipped to take control of her life again.

The dietitian carried out a nutritional and dietetic assessment, discussed possible changes in Brenda's diet to help her with her weight gain and reassured her of the principles of healthy eating. Brenda reported that she was terrified of all the articles she had read in the media about specific diets to help in the treatment of cancer and the dietitian was able to address all her queries with evidence-based information.

Brenda felt more confident about wearing scarves and headwear as well as her wig to manage her hair loss until it grew back in approximately 4-month post-chemotherapy. Her hospital ran a 'look good, feel better' service in which local beauty therapists, funded by cosmetics companies, provided a makeover with a bag of cosmetics, which also boosted her confidence.

Although Brenda admitted that the worry of the cancer returning would always be with her, she was able to cope with the anxiety and focus more on gaining control of her life again. Every time she had followed up at the hospital, the worries would resurface, but Brenda felt better equipped to deal with them as time progressed.

Case study 2

Shirley is a 63-year-old woman; she is married and retired. Her daughter and son both have children and Shirley enjoys being able to look after the grandchildren, aged 8 and 10, after school until their parents return from work. Shirley's husband is 68; he has a cardiac condition which limits his physical exercise, but both of them are still driving and are active in their local church and community.

Shirley had been treated for breast cancer 16 years ago, had a mastectomy, axillary clearance, chemotherapy and radiotherapy, but had presented recently with ulnar nerve problems, i.e. numbness affecting the little and ring fingers of her right (dominant) hand. Her GP initially suggested gentle exercises with a rubber ball to maintain strength but the hand muscles have atrophied over 18 months and she was referred to the hospital for investigations, which confirmed not only RIBP but also recurrence of her cancer in the left lung. The metastatic lung cancer was asymptomatic at the time of her referral to physiotherapy for hand and arm exercises.

Functional and psychological problems:

- Mixture of numbness, pain and tingling in her right hand, which progressed over several months to the whole arm
- Lack of sensation in the hand put Shirley at risk of injury
- The deterioration over the course of several months resulted in complete lack of function in the right arm
- Anxiety and concern about herself, but mainly about her family as the disease progression became more symptomatic

Interventions:
Physiotherapy assessed her posture, pain and function (range of movement, strength, sensation and perception), identified atrophy of the brachial plexus, shoulder, arm and hand and provided a treatment programme. She also benefited from a walking stick as she was leaning towards right side. The physiotherapist gently introduced the fact that, whilst Shirley had a degenerative and irreversible condition, compensatory and coping strategies could be explored and referral was made to the OT.

The OT assessed her transfers in and out of the bath as Shirley felt unsteady doing this. She was shown the range of equipment to help with transfers and activities of daily living so that she was aware of what was available. This proved to be useful in the near future as her functional independence deteriorated and she was able to refer herself back to the AHPs, whom she knew and trusted, as felt comfortable in asking for more help. This enabled Shirley to be able to control when she accepted the interventions.

The physiotherapist and OT both reinforced the principles of energy conservation and discussed her lifestyle in detail to establish coping strategies that suited her individual needs. Shirley was able to share her worries and concerns with them, and they were able to liaise with the hospital's counselling service which was available to Shirley, but she preferred to use her local church.

To avoid overburdening Shirley with hospital visits, her care was transferred to the community services. The domiciliary physiotherapist was able to ensure that gait, general mobility and posture were monitored. Shirley was provided with a sling to avoid discomfort and prevent trauma of the shoulder as the arm became increasingly more weak and heavy. The community OT was able to monitor functional activities and provide appropriate equipment around the house as required, including an intercom service to enable Shirley to open the door, a perching stool in the kitchen for meal preparation, a trolley for carrying items around safely, grab and banister rails, bathing and toilet aids. These were introduced gradually without overwhelming the family and were viewed as a positive means of maintaining her independence rather than a symbol of deterioration and dependence.

As Shirley's condition progressed, she was transferred to the care of the local hospice who offered a day hospital as well as symptom management. Continuity of care from the hospital to the community to the hospice palliative care AHPs enabled Shirley to be comfortable with those who were treating her. Close liaison between services prevented Shirley having to repeat her story to everyone who treated her, though she was happy to share her narrative and was able to discuss her thoughts openly.

At the day hospital, as well as at her church, Shirley was able to take part in activities which reinforced that she was still able to be creative, sociable and productive. She reported that she always felt valued and this had been a worry for her that she would be a burden on her family and husband. Even though she was unable to look after the grandchildren, she was able to create a diary and leave mementos for them and her children.

Conclusion

The physical, functional and psychosocial sequelae of breast cancer and/or its treatments may include:

- Decreased range of movement
- Pain
- Fatigue
- Peripheral neuropathy
- Radiation-induced brachial plexopathy
- Body image problems, including scar management, skin changes, weight gain/loss, hair loss and postural adaptations
- Lymphoedema
- Nausea
- Menopausal symptoms
- Sexuality
- Sleep disturbances and anxiety management

Functional difficulties can be addressed by the multi-professional team allowing patients with breast cancer to receive interventions to maintain their independence and autonomy and have the support required to cope with practical and psychosocial problems (Vockins, 2004). This is true of all interventions from home assessments to physical and psychological treatment programmes whether at an acute or late stage of treatment, and illustrates the multi-professional approach required throughout the breast cancer journey.

Key learning points

- Breast cancer is the most common cancer in women with 44 000 being diagnosed every year.
- Survival rates are improving with 60% expected to live 20 years.
- Treatment can be very intensive but may result in comorbid conditions which decrease quality of life.
- AHPs have an important role in the management of breast cancer patients, addressing physical, functional and psychosocial needs.
- Management must be proactive and holistic to avoid potentially debilitating, costly side effects of cancer and its treatment.

References

Burnet, K. (2003). Radiotherapy as a treatment for breast cancer. Chapter 9 in: V. Harmer (Ed.), *Breast cancer nursing care and management*. London: Whurr.

Cancer Research UK (2006). *Breast cancer*. Retrieved 5 February 2007 from www.cancerreseachuk.org/breastcancer/breast_cancer/

Clodius, L. (2001). Minimizing secondary arm lymphoedema from axillary dissection. *Lymphology*, *34* (3), 106–110.

Coleman, M. P., Ratchet, B., Woods, L. M., Mitry, E., Riga, M., Cooper, N., Quinn, M. J., Brenner, H. & Esteve, J. (2004). Trends and socioeconomic inequalities in cancer survival in England and Wales up to 2001. *British Journal of Cancer*, *90* (7), 1367–1373.

Cook, A. & Burkhardt, A. (1994). The effect of cancer diagnosis and treatment onhand function. *American Journal of Occupational Therapy*, *48* (9), 836–839.

Cooper, J. (1998). Occupational therapy intervention with radiation-induced brachial plexopathy. *European Journal of Cancer Care*, *7* (2), 88–92.

Cooper, J. (2006). *Occupational therapy in oncology and palliative care*. Chichester: Wiley.

Davis, C. (1995). *Guidelines on the management of women with adverse effects following breast radiotherapy*. London: Royal College Radiologists.

Ewer-Smith, C. & Patterson, S. (2002). The use of an occupational therapy programme within a palliative care setting. *European Journal of Palliative Care*, *9* (1), 30–33.

Ferlay, J., Bray, F., Pisani, P. & Parkin, D. M. (2002). *Cancer incidence, mortality and prevalence worldwide (Version 2.0 IARC CancerBase no 5)*. Lyon: IARC Press.

Fourie, W. J. (2006). Chartered Society of Physiotherapy – Congress Presentation. (Unpublished).

Fourie, W. J. & Robb, K. A. (2008). Physiotherapy management of axillary web syndrome following breast cancer treatment: discussing the use of soft tissue techniques. *Physical Therapy*. (Submitted)

Futter, C. M., Webster, M. H. C., Hagen, S. & Mitchell, S. L. (2002). A retrospective comparison of abdominal muscle strength following breast reconstruction with a free TRAM or DIEP flap. *British Journal of Plastic Surgery*, *53* (7), 578–583.

Genetics Home Reference (2007) *Breast cancer*. Retrieved 7 February 2007 from www.ghr.nlm.nih.gov/condition=breastcancer;jsessionid=D8E79B73BE8C3023E1DD

Grahn, G. (1996). Coping with the cancer experience. I. Developing an education and support programme for cancer patients and their significant others. *European Journal of Cancer Care*, 5, 176–181.

Harmer, V. (2003). *Breast cancer nursing care and management.* London: Whurr.

Hindley, M. & Johnston, S. (1999). Stress management for breast cancer patients: service development. *International Journal of Palliative Nursing*, 5(3), 135–141.

Holden, S. & Felde, G. (1987). Nursing care of patients experiencing cisplatin-related peripheral neuropathy. *Oncology Nursing Forum*, 14 (1), 13–19.

Johansson, K., Ingvar, C., Albertsson, M. & Ekdahl, C. (2001). Arm lymphoedema, shoulder mobility and muscle strength after breast cancer treatment – a prospective 2 year study. *Advances in Physiotherapy*, 3 (2), 55–66.

Jung, B. F., Ahrendt, G. M., Oaklander, A. L. & Dworkin, R. H. (2003). Neuropathic pain following breast cancer surgery: proposed classification and research update. *Pain*, 104 (1), 1–13.

Karki, A., Simeonen, R., Malkia, E. & James, S. (2005). Impairments, activity limitations and participation restrictions 6 and 12 months after breast cancer operation. *Journal of Rehabilitation Medicine*, 37 (3), 180–188.

Kealey, P. & McIntyre, I. (2005). An evaluation of the domiciliary occupational therapy service in palliative cancer care in a community trust: a patient and carers perspective. *European Journal of Cancer Care*, 14 (3), 232–242.

Leidenius, M., Leppanen, E., Krogerus, L. & von Smitten K. (2003). Motion restriction and axillary web syndrome after sentinel node biopsy and axillary clearance in breast cancer. *American Journal of surgery*, 185 (2), 127–130.

Leubbert, K., Dahme, B. & Hasenbring, M. (2001). The effectiveness of relaxation training in reducing treatment-related symptoms and improving emotional adjustment in acute non-surgical cancer treatment: a met-analytical review. *Psycho-Oncology*, 10 (6), 490–502.

Lewis, M. (2006). Review of the breast cancer rehabilitation & prevention of lymphoedema scheme. *British Lymphology Society Newsletter, Sevenoaks, Kent, UK*, 54(May/June), 6–7.

Macleod, H. & Koelliing, P. (2003). Physiotherapy for patients with breast cancer. In: V. Harmer (Ed.), *Breast cancer nursing care and management.* London: Whurr.

Molassiotis, A. (2000). A pilot study of the use of progressive muscular relaxation training in the management of post-chemotherapy nausea and vomiting. *European Journal of Cancer Care*, 9 (4), 230–234.

Moskovitz, A., Anderson, B., Yeung, R., Byrd, D. R., Lawton, T. J. & Moe, R. C. (2001). Axillary web syndrome after axillary dissection. *American Journal of Surgery*, 181 (5), 434–439.

Mustoe, T., Cooter, R. D., Gold, M. H. & Hobbs, F. D. (2002). International clinical recommendations on scar management. *Plastic Reconstructive Surgery*, 110 (2), 560–571.

Naylor, W., Laverty, D. & Mallet, J. (2001). *Handbook of wound management in cancer care* (pp. 973–122). London: Blackwell Science Ltd.

National Council for Hospice and Specialist Palliative Care Services [NCHSPCS] (2000). *Fulfilling lives: rehabilitation in palliative care.* London: National Council for Hospice and Specialist Palliative Care Services.

National Institute for Clinical Excellence [NICE] (2002). *Guidance on cancer services improving outcomes in breast cancer.* London: National Institute for Clinical Excellence.

Office for National Statistics (2004). *Mortality statistics: cause. England and Wales 2004.* London: TSO.

Richardson, A. (2004). A critical appraisal of the factors associated with fatigue. Chapter 2 in: J. Armes, M. Krishnasamy & I. Higginson (Eds.), *Fatigue in cancer.* Oxford: Oxford University Press.

Robb, K. A., Williams, J. E., Duvivier, V. & Newham, D. J. (2006). A pain management program for chronic cancer treatment related pain: a preliminary study. *The Journal of Pain*, 7 (2), 82–90.

Roberts, S., Livingston, P., White, V. & Gibbs, A. (2003). External breast prosthesis use. *Cancer Nursing*, 26 (3), 179–186.

Ronka, R., Smitten, K., Sintonen, H., Kotomaki, T., Krogerus, L., Lappanen, E. & Leidenus, M. (2004). The impact of sentinel node biopsy and axillary staging strategy on hospital costs. *Annals of Oncology*, 15 (1), 88–94.

Royal College of Radiologists [RCR] (1995). *Management of adverse effects following breast radiotherapy*. London: Royal College of Radiologists.

Schover, L. R. (1991). The impact of breast cancer on sexuality, body image and intimate relationships. *CA A Cancer Journal for Clinicians*, 41 (2), 112–120.

Schultz, I., Barholm, M. & Grondal, S. (1997). Delayed shoulder exercises in reducing seroma frequency after modified radical mastectomy. *Annals of Surgical Oncology*, 4 (4), 293–297.

Shearsmith-Farthing, K. (2001). The management of altered body image: a role for occupational therapy. *British Journal of Occupational Therapy*, 64 (8), 387–392.

Silva, O. & Zurrida, S. (2005). *Breast cancer, a practical guide* (3rd ed.). Philadelphia: Elsevier/Saunders.

Skalla, K. A., Bakitas, M., Furstenberg, C. T., Ahles, T. & Henerson, J. V. (2004). Patients's needs for information on cancer therapy. *Oncology Nursing Forum*, 31 (2), 313–319.

Tobias, J. & Eaton, K. (2001). *Living with cancer*. London: Bloomsbury.

Ververs, J. M., Roumen, R. M., Vingerhoets, A. J. J. M., Vreugdenhil, G. Coebergh, J. W., Crommelin, M. A., Luiten, E. J., Repelaer van Driel, O. J., Schijven, M. Wissing, J. C. & Voogd, A. C. (2001). Risk, severity and predictors of physical and psychological morbidity after axillary lymph node dissection for breast cancer. *European Journal of Cancer*, 37 (8), 991–999.

Vockins, H. (2004). Occupational therapy intervention with patients with breast cancer: a survey. *European Journal of Cancer Care*, 13 (1), 45–52.

Watson, M., Fenlon, D., McVey, G. & Fernandez-Marcos, M. (1996). A support group for breast cancer patients: development of a cognitive-behavioural approach. *Behavioural and Cognitive Psychotherapy*, 24 (1), 73–81.

Worthington, H. V. & Clarkson, J. E. (2002). Prevention of oral mucositis and oral candidiasis for patients with cancer treated with chemotherapy: Cochrane systematic review. *Journal of Dental Education*, 66 (8), 903–911.

Young-McCaughan, S. (1996). Sexual functioning in women with breast cancer after treatment with adjuvant therapy. *Cancer Nursing*, 19 (4), 308–319.

Zabora, J., Brintzenhofeszoc, H., Curbow, B., Hooker, C. & Piantodosi, S. (2001). The prevalence of psychological distress by cancer site. *Psycho-Oncology*, 10 (1), 19–28.

Ziegler, R. G., Hoover, R. N., Pike, M. C., Hildesheim, A., Nomura, A. M., West, D. W., Wu-Williams, A. H., Kolonel, L. N., Horn-Ross, P. L., Rosenthal, J. F., Hyer, M. B. (1993). Migration patterns and breast cancer risk in Asian-American women. *Journal of National Cancer Institute*, 85 (22), 1819–1827.

Chapter 4

MULTI-PROFESSIONAL MANAGEMENT OF LUNG CANCER AND ASSOCIATED CONDITIONS

Debbie McKinney, Daniel Lowrie and Mandy Hamilton

Learning outcomes

After reading this section the reader should be able to:

- Discuss the cause and characteristic features of lung cancer, metastases secondary to lung cancer and superior vena cava obstruction
- Discuss the role of allied health professionals (AHPs) in providing support to lung cancer patients
- Discuss the different treatment options available
- Discuss related supportive and palliative care for patients with lung cancer and the implications for AHP intervention

---

Lung cancer is the most common cancer worldwide and is the leading cause of cancer death in both men and women in the United Kingdom (UK) (Matakidou *et al.*, 2005). The disease is associated with distress and a loss of functional independence, thus having a considerable impact on quality of life (QOL). As such, the support of individuals with lung cancer constitutes a major challenge for allied health professionals (AHPs). It is therefore essential that AHPs working in cancer care have a sound understanding of lung cancer and its associated conditions, and are confident when working with this patient group in order to help them manage their disease experience.

Lung cancer

Lung cancer results from a series of genetic mutations in cells within the lung epithelium (usually in the bronchi), which allow them to proliferate rapidly, avoid apoptosis, invade surrounding tissue and metastasise to distant regions of the body

(Franklin & Hirsch, 2004). Genetic mutations are caused by prolonged chronic exposure of the lung epithelium to irritant, carcinogenic substances, such as cigarette smoke.

Based on their histological characteristics lung cancers are broadly categorised within two main groups.

Non-small-cell lung cancer (NSCLC) is the most common and includes:

- Squamous cell carcinomas
- Adenocarcinomas
- Large-cell carcinomas (Souhami & Tobias, 2003)

Small-cell lung cancers (SCLCs) are aggressive tumours that:

- Arise in the large central airways and typically present in the main stem or lobular bronchi
- Frequently metastasise to hilar, mediastinal and distal sites occurring in approximately 20% of patients
- Often manifest with extensive disease and, consequently, a poor prognosis (Ross, 2003)

Mesothelioma is another form of cancer which begins in the mesothelium and incidence increases with asbestos exposure. Pleural mesothelioma is the most common form (www.mesotheliomainternational.org).

Incidence and prevalence

Recent data indicate that lung cancer comprises approximately 24% and 18% of cancer deaths for UK men and women respectively (Cancer Research UK, 2006). Relative risk increases with age, with a peak incidence between the ages of 75 and 84 years. Within the UK, men continue to develop lung cancer more frequently than women. This difference has changed dramatically over time from a 6:1 ratio (men:women) in the 1950s to a 3:2 ratio in 2002 (Cancer Research UK, 2006); much of this is attributable to increasing numbers of women who have taken up smoking. Women who experience the same lifetime exposure to tobacco smoke as men are one and a half times as likely to develop lung cancer as men (Zang & Wynder, 1996). Similarly, familial patterns of lung cancer have also been reported, and genetic factors may both act as an independent risk factor for lung cancer and increase the risk associated with environmental or behavioural factors, such as smoking (Nitadori *et al.*, 2006). Within the UK incidence varies regionally. Socioeconomic and ethnic backgrounds, alongside lifestyle and environmental factors, can account for these differences (Cancer Research UK, 2006; Quinn *et al.*, 2001).

Aetiology

Prolonged exposure to tobacco smoke is recognised as the most significant risk factor for lung cancer (Dineen & Silvestri, 2004). Once an individual stops smoking, his or her risk of developing lung cancer diminishes over time (Tyczynski *et al.*, 2003).

AHPs can contribute to lung cancer prevention through support for smoking cessation and also through advice regarding diet and exercise. Evidence suggests that both dietary factors and a lack of physical exercise can contribute to the development of lung cancer, an example being the existence of an inverse relationship between the development of lung cancer and high fruit and vegetable intake (Feskanich *et al.*, 2000; World Cancer Research Fund, 1997).

A number of environmental and/or occupational hazards have also been identified as increasing the likelihood of developing lung cancer. Examples of these potential hazards include exposure to radiation, pollution, asbestos, coal tar, asphalt, soot, creosote, chromium, ether, nickel or vinyl chloride (Cancer Research UK, 2006).

Screening and diagnosis

Routine screening for lung cancer is not currently carried out in the UK. To date, no firm evidence exists to indicate that screening using chest radiography or sputum cytology is effective in reducing mortality (Armstrong, 2005; Haas, 2003). Recent guidance published by the National Collaborating Centre for Acute Care (2005) recommends that urgent chest X-rays are carried out on any individual who presents with signs and symptoms characteristic of lung cancer (see Table 4.1).

A number of diagnostic tests have been developed that can contribute to the identification and staging of lung cancer (see Table 4.2). Each of these tests has advantages and disadvantages in terms of sensitivity, specificity, burden on the patient and financial cost.

Staging

Staging of lung cancer is an important process as it assists the decision-making process regarding the most appropriate medical management options for individuals that present with the disease. Two main classifications are used for the staging of lung cancers. The International Staging System, known as the TNM (tumour, nodes,

Table 4.1 Signs and symptoms of lung cancer.

Haemoptysis, or any of the following unexplained or persistent (>3 weeks) symptoms or signs:	Cough Chest/shoulder pain Dyspnoea Weight loss Chest signs Hoarseness Finger clubbing Features suggestive of metastasis from a lung cancer (e.g. in brain, bone, liver or skin) Cervical/supraclavicular lymphadenopathy

National Collaborating Centre for Acute Care (2005 p. 28).

Table 4.2 Identification and staging of lung cancer.

Imaging techniques	• Chest X-ray is typically used as the first-line assessment tool to assess for lung cancer • Computerised tomography (CT) is used to assist in the identification, location and staging of lung cancers • Positron emission tomography (PET) is used to detect groups of cells that are rapidly dividing. Integrated PET–CT scanners are also being introduced to improve diagnostic accuracy
Tissue confirmation	• Sputum cytology: This involves the examination of sputum under a microscope to identify abnormal cells • Bronchoscopy: It is used to facilitate confirmation of a diagnosis of lung cancer following a CT scan and has been found to be reasonably effective at identifying centrally located cancers. However it has poorer sensitivity for peripheral tumours • Percutaneous transthoracic needle aspiration/biopsy is used in the detection of peripherally located tumours or suspected metastases • Surgical techniques for diagnosis and staging include anterior mediastinotomy and surgical thoracoscopy

metastases) staging system (Mountain *et al.*, 1999), is used for NSCLC. SCLC is described as either limited-stage or extensive-stage disease. This is because 90% of patients with SCLC have locally advanced or metastatic disease at presentation and surgery does not tend to be a primary management approach (Joyce, 2004).

Medical management of lung cancer

After a process of investigations, specialist diagnosis, multidisciplinary cancer team (MDT) assessment and staging, a patient with lung cancer will commence cancer treatment. The decision regarding the appropriate treatment regime and intent is complex and is based on individual diagnosis, performance status and the presence or absence of metastases. The following section will highlight the treatment options for NSCLC and SCLC.

Medical management of NSCLC

Surgery
The most effective treatment for the survival of NSCLC is surgery, including wedge resection, segmentectomy, lobectomy, bilobectomy and pneumonectomy. Surgery is only recommended for those in early disease stages (stage I–IIIA) (NICE, 2004), who are medically and physically able to withstand and recover from surgery. Decision to proceed with surgery is based on examination of existing comorbid conditions, the results of pre-operative tests such as exercise testing and detailed discussion with each patient regarding risks and benefits (Martinolich & Rivera, 2001). Less than a third

of patients are eligible for surgery as most present in late stages. Palliative procedures can include pleurodesis and endobronchial stenting (Webber & Pryor, 1996).

Radiotherapy

Radical radiotherapy is given in early stage lung cancer, either as a stand alone or adjuvant or as high dose, i.e. up to 60 gray given daily for 5–6 weeks (Souhami and Tobias, 2003). Side effects include dysphagia, pericarditis and skin erythema.

Continuous hyperfractionated accelerated radiation therapy (CHART) demonstrates improvements in local tumour control (Saunders *et al.*, 1997). It is given in fractions three times a day for 12 consecutive days and is recommended for radical treatment to inoperable stage I and II patients or those who do not want chemotherapy (NICE, 2004).

Chemotherapy

Chemotherapy was previously considered unsuitable for NSCLC treatment. Recently, combinations of cytotoxic drugs have been found to have both survival and QOL benefits as adjuvant, neoadjuvant or first- and second-line palliative treatments. It can be used alone to treat patients in stage III and IV to improve tumour control, or in combination with radiotherapy (NICE, 2004).

Medical management of SCLC

As SCLC is usually widespread at presentation, radiotherapy is often unsuitable and surgery is rarely considered.

Treatment is based on likely prognosis, which is gauged from factors such as disease extent, stage, performance status, serum sodium and liver function tests. Chemotherapy can provide rapid palliation (Simmonds, 1999) and improve survival, but recurrence rates are high. NICE (2004) recommends multi-drug platinum-based chemotherapy, with no more than four cycles for palliative patients and up to six for curative, depending on patient condition and disease response. If there is a good response, consolidation thoracic radiotherapy should be offered during or after treatment.

To reduce the risk of cerebral metastases and to improve survival, prophylactic cranial irradiation can be offered to those with limited-stage disease and good response to primary treatment. If relapse occurs, second-line platinum-based chemotherapy can be offered; however, it is less beneficial.

Research into new drugs and radiotherapy methodology aims to improve cancer treatment and overall survival.

The role of AHPs in the management of lung cancer

People with lung cancer frequently experience a wide range of difficulties through the course of their disease. These may relate to physical symptoms, psychological distress, spiritual concerns and practical (household, self-care or financial) needs (Davies, 2003).

It has been proposed that lung cancer and its treatment cause a greater degree of symptom distress than any other type of cancer (Cooley, 2000). Numerous symptoms including breathlessness, cough, fatigue, pain, weakness, weight loss, appetite loss, nausea, vomiting, altered taste, anxiety and depression have been identified (Chan et al., 2005; Cooley et al., 2003; Gift et al., 2003; Okuyama et al., 2001). These symptoms have been shown to have a negative impact on activities of daily living (ADLs), relationships, mood and QOL (Tanaka et al., 2002). Distress associated with these symptoms increases as the disease progresses (Degner & Sloan, 1995).

It is therefore important that AHPs working with lung cancer patients conduct a thorough and holistic assessment reviewing the range and nature of symptoms experienced as evidence suggests that health care professionals tend to underestimate the symptom needs of these patients (Krishnasamy et al., 2001). Furthermore, as different symptoms can have a synergistic effect on each other, attempting to manage individual symptoms in isolation is likely to prove fruitless (Chan et al., 2005). Patients must be given the opportunity to discuss their own symptom experience and the personal meaning they attribute to their symptoms. This will enable them to come to terms with, and manage, their symptoms. Symptoms will vary depending on the disease stage and treatments provided.

Managing distress and facilitating good communication

Support should also be provided regarding the management of the psychological distress that accompanies the condition. Lung cancer is a disease that frequently results in feelings of uncertainty, loss of hope and fear for the future. Honest, empathetic communication between health care professionals and patients can significantly reduce the fear and distress associated with the disease (Moore, 2003). It is therefore vital that therapists facilitate good communication through being approachable, open, honest and ready to listen at all times.

Therapists can help patients to manage distress by assisting the development of personalised relaxation and anxiety management strategies (Cooper, 2006). This includes the use of relaxation techniques such as guided visualisation, progressive muscular relaxation (Salt & Kerr, 1997; Sloman, 2002), breathing control (Webber & Pryor, 1996) and autogenic training (Wright et al., 2002). This will be discussed in detail in Chapter 15.

Management of the patient throughout the cancer journey

A patient may require AHP involvement at any point of their pathway, depending on the outcome of the medical management design. For example, patients may present for supportive and palliative care from the pre-diagnosis stage onwards. The nature of disease and treatments also means that the care setting is likely to vary throughout the full patient journey. The AHP intervention is therefore designed to be flexible and adaptive to each individual's needs and should not represent the standard medical model format.

Pre-diagnosis/diagnosis phase

Prior to definitive medical diagnosis patients may be referred to AHPs with associated symptoms. It is important to recognise that this period of care is a vital opportunity for early intervention with symptoms which could affect lung cancer patients and discuss the AHP support throughout various stages and treatments.

Nutritional support

Between 46 and 61% of patients with lung cancer and mesothelioma experience weight loss before diagnosis and treatment (Brown & Radke, 1998). This can lead to clinical symptoms of weakness, fatigue, anorexia, muscle wasting, decreased functional ability and depression, as well as increased treatment toxicity and shorter survival.

Goals of nutritional support include preserving physical strength, optimising rehabilitation, enhancing QOL, reducing hospital stay and improving clinical outcome (Shaw, 2000). Weight stabilisation may lead to improved outcome in NSCLC but this is less likely in SCLC (Ross & Ashley, 2004).

Approximately 80% of patients in advanced stages have cancer cachexia (Goo & Hill, 2003), where metabolism is altered and resting energy expenditure is elevated due to tumour-related factors. This results in progressive weight loss (enhanced by early satiety), decreased food intake and nutrient malabsorption. Some short-term success has been achieved in promoting appetite and weight gain with pharmacological agents, such as corticosteroids and megesterol acetate (McMillan *et al.*, 1997), but they are not suitable for all patients. The effects of dietary counselling and conventional nutritional supplementation are limited in cachexia (Ockenga & Valentini, 2005). There is potential that a specialised supplement enriched with eicosapentaenoic acid (EPA) and high in protein and calories may promote weight stabilisation, leading to improved QOL and survival (Fearon *et al.*, 2003). Until evidence is further substantiated, oncology dietitians must question their use, with individual patients, over conventional supplements.

Other symptoms which can directly affect the appetite of a lung cancer patient at any stage include nausea, vomiting, constipation, diarrhoea, taste changes, mucositis, stomatitis, xerostomia, dysphagia, oesophagitis, fatigue, depression and breathlessness.

Psychological and physical support

Referral to physiotherapy for baseline assessment can be carried out in the community or local hospital. Cancer medical management is dependent on fitness levels and it is, therefore, important to assess fitness for cancer treatment at this stage. Breathlessness education may also be introduced to promote independent management and delay hospital admissions as treatment progresses and symptoms develop. Outcome measures include modified Rivermead Index, Borg level of breathlessness, fatigue scales and visual analogue scale for pain.

A baseline assessment from occupational therapy (OT) determines the social situation, previous functional ability and the level of intervention required, such as approaching activities differently to conserve energy, provision of equipment and/or home adaptations and lifestyle management.

Pre-surgery/surgery/post-surgery phase

Nutritional support

Many patients present with weight loss pre-surgery, and due to periods of fasting followed by recovery from the procedure, further malnutrition is possible. Weight loss predicts higher mortality, morbidity, increased post-operative complications and longer hospital stays. It is important to optimise nutritional status pre-surgery in order to promote recovery, wound healing and improved functional status. Commonly, nutritional intervention takes the form of oral nutritional support, which involves education for patients and carers on food fortification and preparation of nutrient-dense meals and snacks. For those with early satiety and breathlessness, it may be helpful to eat small, frequent portions throughout the day rather than three large meals. If the patient is unable to meet nutritional requirements, a variety of specialised nutrient-enhanced drinks or puddings can be taken along with the diet (Shaw, 2000). In a few cases it may be necessary to consider enteral tube feeding, but only if the patient is not able to maintain his or her nutritional status through oral intake alone and/or has lost significant weight.

Psychological and physical support

Individuals should be referred for pre- and post-operative physiotherapy assessment, education and treatment to include respiratory and rehabilitation needs. It is important to ensure that the patient is aware and understands the agreed goals of the physiotherapy intervention and participating activity. The therapist must also identify any risk factors, e.g. smoking and obesity, which may have an effect on the patient's post-operative recovery and discharge planning.

It is important to review blood counts particularly if there is a raised white cell count, indicating infection or a reduced red cell count, which may affect breathlessness. Low platelet counts will signify risks to exercise prescription and also the intensity of activity recommended.

Interventions vary depending on the type of procedure and the status of the patient, e.g. the presence of chest drains. Respiratory care can include positioning, breathing exercises and chest clearance techniques with supported cough. Early ambulation and functional independence is recommended. A person with circulatory problems or limited mobility should have anti-embolism stockings applied. Post-surgery, patients can have reduced shoulder range of movement and therefore prescribed exercise programmes may be necessary.

Pain control should be frequently reviewed as this can affect compliance.

These patients may also require education and advice on breathlessness (see Chapter 14), cancer-related fatigue management (see Chapter 12) and exercise for tolerance promotion.

Activities of daily living

The OT aims to maximise patients' functional potential within activities that are important to them. This can assist in fostering feelings of normality and hope (Lindsell, 2006) and can be achieved through graded support and practice of ADL chosen collaboratively by the patient and therapist.

As lung cancer patients will often be faced with deteriorating health and a poor prognosis, a compensatory approach to rehabilitation may need to be adopted. This will entail the use of activity analysis to devise strategies regarding alternative methods of enabling patients to achieve their goals, such as:

- Provision of wheelchairs
- Adaptive equipment
- Home modifications
- Education regarding energy conservation strategies to enable self-care
- Household or leisure-based tasks

Discharge planning

This is an integral part of care. It is important that the physiotherapist reviews the overall respiratory and rehabilitation status of the patient and organises any ongoing interventions as necessary. This may include provision of appropriate walking aids, nebulisers, home oxygen/compressors and individual exercise and strengthening programmes. Pulmonary rehabilitation classes may be offered 6 weeks post-operatively, depending on each individual patient's need.

The occupational therapist assesses how any change in exercise tolerance affects functional independence, including all self-care, domestic and work activities and others needed in daily life. A home visit might be indicated regarding coping at home, including necessary adaptations.

Written information, including contact details, should be issued to each patient. Assessment for community management should be identified during hospital admission with established communication links between AHPs in all care settings.

All interventions can be provided in any of the care settings and may depend on various factors, including:

- Patient choice
- Availability of AHP services
- Location of medical treatment, e.g. chemotherapy
- Individuals receiving their hospital-based cancer treatments as an out-patient and therefore travelling daily from a hospice, local hospital or home

Supportive and palliative care of lung cancer

Patients may attend follow-up clinics, which are usually coordinated by doctors, specialist radiographers and nurses. New referrals may arise at these reviews due to disease recurrence, continued weight loss or new rehabilitation problems, and should be forwarded to the relevant AHP in the most appropriate care setting.

The majority of lung cancer patients present with advanced disease at diagnosis (CRUK, 2006). Despite timely medical intervention this can progress locally; therefore, palliative care and symptom control play an integral role. This should be provided by general and specialist palliative care providers. All patients should have access to multidisciplinary non-drug intervention in all care settings (NICE, 2004), and AHPs are skilled to provide a variety of supportive approaches. The National Health Service document 'Improving Outcomes in Cancer Care' (2004) recommends that patients receive optimal symptom control, incorporating psychological, social, spiritual care and carer support.

Throughout the cancer journey, the patient's condition can fluctuate daily and a flexible approach is necessary. Goals must be realistic according to each individual's needs and wishes; for example, the aim of nutritional support can change from achieving calculated nutritional requirements and weight gain to providing support and advice depending on symptoms in order to minimise weight loss and improve QOL (Brown & Radke, 1998). Optimising nutrition may also help. Certain palliative patients benefit from physiotherapy, cope and continue with cancer treatments and maintain independence, ideally in the home environment. Before initiating any form of intervention, the patient's life expectancy should be considered and QOL must remain paramount.

When the patient enters end-of-life care, good cross-sector, multi-professional team working is essential to provide the necessary care in a timely and efficient manner.

Associated conditions

Over time, additional symptoms may develop due to advancing local disease and metastases. In advanced lung cancer the associated conditions of superior vena cava obstruction (SVCO), bone pain, malignant spinal cord compression (MSCC), neurological difficulties and higher rates of cachexia may be identified.

Metastases secondary to lung cancer

Lung cancer can spread locally or by lymphatic and haematogenous routes (Souhami and Tobias, 2003). Metastases can be identified by computed tomography (CT)/positron emission tomography (PET) scans, bone scans and magnetic resonance imaging (MRI). Chapter 5 describes brain metastases and MSCC.

In NSCLC, the most common sites of metastatic spread are to the brain, bone, liver and adrenal glands, followed by the local invasion to the lung, pleura and subcutaneous tissue. The incidence of metastases is higher in advanced stages of NSCLC. In SCLC, there may be lower occurrence of brain and adrenal metastases, but otherwise the sites are similar, and may also involve pancreas, abdominal lymph nodes or bone marrow (Detterbeck *et al.*, 2001). Metastases can occur in up to 80% of SCLC patients at diagnosis (Bamford & Kunkler, 2003).

Adrenal metastases are generally asymptomatic but can cause pain in the flank (Glisson *et al.*, 2004 p. 110). Other symptoms indicative of metastases are anorexia, weight loss and jaundice, which may indicate liver metastases.

AHP involvement for these patients with metastases is paramount as normal daily activities can be severely hindered by debilitating pain, fatigue and loss of function. A holistic patient-centred approach to assessment is required from all health care professionals involved, as discussed in Chapters 12 and 13.

Superior vena cava obstruction

SVCO is an uncommon manifestation of carcinoma of the bronchus (both SCLC and NSCLC), affecting a minority of patients at some point of their illness (Rowell & Gleeson, 2001). Malignant causes now account for over 90% cases of SVCO (Ostler *et al.*, 1997). In the majority, this is due to carcinoma of the bronchus, but less commonly lymphoma, metastatic disease and intrathoracic tumours, such as mesothelioma and thymoma, may be responsible. SVCO occurs when tumour compresses the superior vena cava in its course through the upper mediastinum to the right of the trachea. This is characterised by the presence of neck swelling and distended veins over the chest and swelling of one or both arms (Rosenbloom, 1949; Souhami & Tobias, 1998) (see Figure 4.1). Dyspnoea, hoarse voice, stridor and headache may

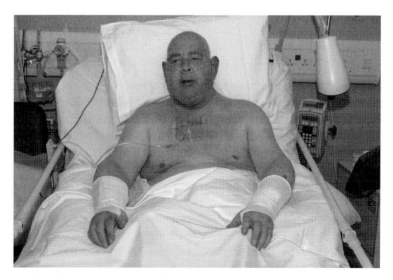

Figure 4.1 Superior vena cava obstruction presentation.

also be caused, although these symptoms may also arise from other manifestations of lung cancer.

Clinical investigations

- Chest X-ray usually depicts tumour or lymph nodes in the right paratracheal area (Macbeth *et al.*, 1996).
- CT or MRI can define the extent of tumour to assist with radiotherapy planning, act as a baseline for assessment of response to chemotherapy or identify impending SVCO prior to symptoms developing (Bechtold *et al.*, 1985).
- Venography can be carried out to determine the presence of the stenosis or occlusion and the extent of any thrombus formation.

Acute SVCO is a medical emergency requiring immediate treatment. Risk of death may be increased by airway obstruction from laryngeal or bronchial oedema or coma from cerebral oedema.

Medical interventions

- Steroids and diuretics
- Surgery (stenting)
- Chemotherapy
- Radiotherapy

The rates of relief are similar for chemotherapy and radiotherapy in both cell types: 76.9 and 77.6% in SCLC and 59.0 and 63.0% in NSCLC respectively (Coin, 1999; Rowell & Gleeson, 2001). Treatment options are evolving and continued evidence-based research is required to determine which modality will provide the greatest relief of symptoms and improved QOL.

AHP interventions

Holistic AHP assessments are vital given the clinical presentation of SVCO. A consistent approach is used in lung cancer presentation whether NSCLC, SCLC or SVCO. Evidence-based treatment plans with agreed goals should be discussed with the patient and his or her family.

In acute SVCO, the main symptoms concerning AHPs include:

- Dyspnoea/breathlessness leading to increased work of breathing/increased respiratory rate
- Overuse of accessory muscles with associated tension around neck and shoulders
- Retention of secretions
- Swelling of face, neck and one or both arms

- Fatigue due to increased respiratory rate over prolonged period
- Fear (not being able to get a breath)
- Panic (breathing being out of control)
- Dysphagia
- Lack of sleep/exhaustion

Cancer-related fatigue and breathlessness management are discussed in detail in Chapters 12 and 14 respectively.

In acute stages of SVCO, medical management is required to relieve the initial symptoms. Physiotherapy and OT interventions tend to relate to progressive lung cancer symptoms rather than those of SVCO, so the specific interventions may not always be clearly defined. In the acute stages, they focus initially on education of breathing control techniques, including positions of ease, diaphragmatic breathing exercises and relaxation. These may be modified depending on the position of the tumour; for example, the patient may not be able to sit leaning forward.

Oxygen therapy may be appropriate to reduce respiratory rate, optimise lung ventilation/perfusion and reduce anxiety. If there is retention of secretions, the physiotherapist will carry out modified chest clearance techniques such as active cycle of breathing or autogenic drainage. It is important to note that certain treatments may be contraindicated, e.g. chest percussion, vibrations and suction, depending on the individual case. Nebuliser therapy is useful for decreasing respiratory drive in an acute episode and also for assisting expectoration of secretions (Webber & Pryor, 1996). A portable device may be needed for discharge.

Transcutaneous electric nerve stimulation for pain control can be provided (see Chapter 13) and the patient advised in verbal and written format regarding positioning of the electrodes and frequency settings. Compression therapy should be avoided in upper limbs as this could increase obstruction. Walking aids can reduce oxygen demand whilst mobilising and facilitate diaphragmatic breathing through the forward leaning position. Inactivity, fatigue and generalised muscle weakness may be apparent; therefore, increased support via mobility aids will optimise functional independence.

Individual exercise programmes for muscle weakness and general deconditioning may be prescribed. Exercise tolerance will be monitored and pacing strategies will be adopted.

These patients can present with difficulty swallowing and/or difficulty eating, secondary dyspnoea and obstruction. The dietitian has a role in assessing dietary needs and individualised dietary programmes can be calculated with supplements to maintain or improve calorie intake.

The occupational therapist assesses and analyses functional ability of the patient, particularly with regard to ADL, and can provide aids and equipment to conserve energy both at ward level and on discharge. The occupational therapist works on programmes to teach compensatory techniques to cope with decreased abilities, energy conservation strategies and pacing activities to allow improved functional ADL. For some patients with lung cancer communicating about personal issues such as their desires, hopes, fears and ambitions may seem to be a challenging process. Occupational therapists can assist such patients to feel safe in sharing their thoughts and feelings through the development of a therapeutic relationship founded on shared involvement in carefully chosen, meaningful activities. The use of creative media such as art or narratives can be a powerful tool in enabling non-verbal expression. Involvement in such activities can prove to be a cathartic experience for many patients, allowing them to release previously withheld emotions. For other patients the use of creative media may facilitate them to 'tell their stories', thereby reaffirming their sense of self-worth or perhaps leave a lasting memory for those they leave behind (Boog, 2006).

Many of these patients will present with fear and anxiety due to their symptoms and an inability to cope. Listening skills, empathy, behavioural approaches and anxiety management can help overcome some of these distressing symptoms (Keable, 1997).

Managing breathlessness is discussed in Chapter 14, particularly prioritising, planning and pacing activities and considering physical positioning and giving oneself permission to take time to do so (Cooper, 2006).

If patients are stabilised and appropriate resources are available, referral to local dyspnoea clinics may optimise management of their symptoms and prevent early hospital readmission.

In addition, it is essential to introduce social work involvement from the outset in order to establish links with the family and address their ever-changing needs throughout the disease process, particularly with regard to financial support guidance. There is a fundamental requirement to provide close working relationships between all team members and recognise the importance of continuing care throughout the illness. This is especially the case should physical treatment techniques no longer be appropriate, particularly in the end-of-life stages. Close links should be established between community/hospice settings from an early stage to provide seamless discharge planning and continuity of care. Overall team working from all professionals will optimise continued education and advice to the patient, carer and health care worker throughout the cancer journey.

Case study: SVCO

Bill, a 67-year-old man, initially presented to Accident & Emergency with haemoptysis. He was previously treated for a chest infection. Following investigations and diagnosis of SVCO, he was referred to a cancer centre for four cycles of chemotherapy and subsequent radiotherapy to the right upper lobe lesion on completion.

Bill had worked in a shipyard for 30 years. He previously smoked 20 cigarettes per day and stopped in the 1950s. He lived with his wife in a two-storey house with bannister rails on both sides of the stairs. His family was very supportive, but his wife suffered from epilepsy and arthritis. Bill had recently been using long-term oxygen therapy at home (2 L/min via facemask).

Initial investigations carried out included a chest X-ray showing consolidation without cavitations in right upper lobe. A CT scan depicted a right upper lobe mass and early evidence of SVCO, enlarged mediastinal nodes and subcarinal nodes. Bronchoscopy showed a visible, necrotic, bleeding tumour totally occluding the upper lobe. Primary diagnosis was SCLC.

His presenting symptoms were shortness of breath (SOB), decreased mobility and marked arm and facial swelling. He was commenced on steroids and chemotherapy. A physiotherapy referral was received and both respiratory and rehabilitation assessments completed. Bill was recommended oxygen therapy for mobilising as he had significant shortness of breath on exertion with reduced oxygen saturations. An appropriate wheeled walking aid was supplied to conserve energy and improve support on mobilising. Daily breathing exercises and positions of ease were carried out by the physiotherapist.

The occupational therapist assessed his functional difficulties in personal and domestic ADLs and provided intervention to teach easier techniques. This included provision of a perching stool and showering equipment. They emphasised that they did not want to overwhelm him as this would add to his difficulties in adjusting to the recent diagnosis and disability.

Prior to discharge home, Bill completed a stair assessment. The physiotherapist taught the correct breathing and stepping techniques to control his symptoms. Home oxygen and concentrators were ordered via the general practitioner.

A community physiotherapy referral was made to continue his respiratory care and also to optimise functional mobility and community occupational therapy was involved in assessing needs following discharge. The dietitian had limited input as his dietary intake and appetite were normal.

Bill's next admission was 2 weeks later for his second cycle of chemotherapy. Clinical presentation had improved with a decrease in arm and facial swelling. SOB had also improved. The main problem was increasing weakness in both lower limbs and hence increased difficulty with mobilising. The community physiotherapist contacted the ward physiotherapist to update interventions and status. Bill continued to mobilise with an aid and used oxygen constantly. He started to require more help with transfers due to this weakness. The physiotherapist tested the muscle strength and there was a significant weakness particularly in the hip flexor muscles. Outcome measures had deteriorated. It was assumed that the high steroid dose was partially responsible for this deterioration. Simple lower limb strengthening exercises were performed by the physiotherapist and encouraged independently. The multi-professional team was made aware of his increasing needs. As the steroid dose was reduced, an improvement in his functional mobility and strength was identified. Level of assistance was reduced to one person within a few days. The occupational therapist carried out a further home visit and, having liaised with the multi-professional team, he agreed to a downstairs arrangement with all appropriate equipment in situ, e.g. hospital bed, mattress and a riser recliner chair. Portable oxygen was also ordered for outdoor use. On discharge, community links were resumed to provide continuity of care.

He was readmitted to the cancer centre 3 months later for emergency palliative radiotherapy following increased SOB and increased bilateral arm swelling. On assessment his functional status was significantly restricted. At best he was able to transfer out to a chair. Bill also found it very difficult to sleep and relax. The AHP input at this stage included physiotherapy to review oxygen requirements, reinforce and carry out breathing exercises and ensure effective nebuliser administration. The occupational therapist ensured that all necessary equipment was in place at home to support him and his family in independence. However, the clinical presentation continued to deteriorate further with increased respiratory distress. The palliative care teams were involved in symptom control and breathlessness management. Bill also required light sedation as he became more distressed. The grave outlook was discussed with the family circle by the consultant. Intervention continued to provide comfort and symptom relief. Bill's condition deteriorated further and he passed away in the early hours of the morning. Following his death the community teams were also informed. A postmortem was required due to asbestos exposure. The family was made aware of counselling services available to them within the hospital and also the close links with pastoral support. This had been present throughout the cancer journey along with close links with palliative care.

Key learning points

- The medical management of lung cancer, including the decision-making process regarding actual treatment and intent, is complex. It is based on individual diagnosis (including the presence of metastases) and performance status. Assessment following clinical presentation will determine the optimum approach to patient care.
- The role of AHPs in the management of lung cancer is paramount as patients experience a wide range of difficulties throughout the disease trajectory, e.g. physical, psychological, spiritual and practical.
- AHP intervention must be flexible and adaptive and not follow the standard medical model format. The nature of the disease and treatments means that the care setting is likely to vary greatly from diagnosis to end of care, necessitating excellent communication pathways and practice.

References

Armstrong, P. (2005). Population screening for lung cancer using computed tomography. Chapter 2 in: M. Muers, K. O'Byren, F. Wells & A. Miles (Eds.), *The effective management of lung cancer* (3rd ed.). London: Aesculapius Medical Press.

Bamford, C. K. & Kunkler, I. H. (2003). Oesophagus, gastrointestinal tract, lung, thymus, pancreas, liver. Chapter 12 in: *Walter and miller's textbook of radiotherapy* (6th ed.). Edinburgh: Churchill Livingstone.

Bechtold, R. E., Wolfman, N. T., Karstaedt, N. & Choplin, R. H. (1985). Superior vena cava obstruction: detection using CT. *Radiology, 157,* 485–487.

Boog, K. (2006). The use of creativity as a psychodynamic activity. Chapter 12 in: J. Cooper (Ed.), *Occupational therapy in oncology and palliative care.* Chichester: Wiley

Brown, J. K. & Radke, K. J. (1998). Nutritional assessment, intervention and evaluation of weight loss in patients with non-small cell lung cancer. *Oncology Nursing Forum, 25,* 547–553.

Cancer Research UK (2006). *UK lung cancer incidence statistics* [Online]. Retrieved 10 December 2006 from http://info.cancerresearchuk.org/cancerstats/types/lung/incidence/

Chan, C. W. H., Richardson, A. & Richardson, J. (2005). A study to assess the existence of the symptom cluster of breathlessness, fatigue and anxiety in patients with advanced lung cancer. *European Journal of Oncology Nursing, 9,* 325–333.

Cooley, M. E. (2000). Symptoms in adults with lung cancer: a systematic research review. *Journal of Pain and Symptom Management, 19* (2), 137–153.

Cooley, M. E., Short, T. H. & Moriarty, H. J. (2003). Symptom prevalence, distress, and change over time in adults receiving treatment for lung cancer. *Psycho-Oncology, 12,* 694–708.

Cooper, J. (2006). *Occupational therapy in oncology and palliative care* (2nd ed.). Chichester: John Wiley & Sons Ltd.

Davies, M. J. (2003). Multidisciplinary clinic approach to lung cancer. Chapter 7 in: M. L. Haas (Ed.), *Contemporary issues in lung cancer: a nursing perspective.* Boston: Jones and Bartlett Publishers.

Degner, L. & Sloan, J. (1995). Symptom distress in newly diagnosed ambulatory cancer patients and as a predictor of survival in lung cancer. *Journal of Pain and Symptom Management, 10* (6), 423–431.

Detterbeck, F. C., Jones, D. R. & Molina, P. L. (2001). Extrathoracic staging. Chapter 6 in: F. C. Detterbeck, M. P. Rivera, M. D. Socinki & J. G. Rosenman (Eds.), *Diagnosis and treatment of lung cancer. An evidence-based guide for the practicing clinician.* Philadelphia: W.B. Saunders Company.

Dineen, K. M. & Silvestri, G. A. (2004). The epidemiology of lung cancer. Chapter 4 in: J. P. Sculier & W. A. Fry (Eds.), *Malignant tumours of the lung.* Berlin: Springer.

Fearon, K. C. H., Von Meyerfelt, M. F., Moses, A. G. W. & Geenan, R. (2003). Effect of a protein and energy dense n-3 fatty acid enriched oral supplement on loss of weight and lean tissue in cancer cachexia: a randomised double blind trial. *Gut, 52,* 1479–1486.

Feskanich, D., Ziegler, R. G., Michaud, D. S., Giavunnucci, E. L., Speizer, F. E., Willett, W. C. & Colditz, G. A. (2000). Prospective study of fruit and vegetable consumption and risk of lung cancer among men and women. *Journal of the National Cancer Institute, 92* (22), 1812–1823.

Franklin, W. A. & Hirsch, F. R. (2004). Molecular and cell biology of lung carcinoma. Chapter 1 in: J. P. Sculier & W. A. Fry (Eds.), *Malignant tumours of the lung.* Berlin: Springer.

Gift, A. G., Stommel, M., Jablonski, A. & Given, W. (2003). A cluster of symptoms over time in patients with lung cancer. *Nursing Research, 52* (6), 393–400.

Glisson, S. G., McKenna, R. J. & Movsas, B. (2004). *Cancer management: a multidisciplinary approach. Medical, surgical and radiation oncology* (8th ed.). New York: CMP Healthcare Media.

Goo, C. & Hill, D. (2003). Nutritional support in cancer. *Clinical Nutrition Update, 8,* 3–5.

Haas, M. L. (2003). *Contemporary issues in lung cancer: a nursing perspective.* Boston: Jones and Bartlett Publishers.

Joyce, M. (2004). Small cell lung cancer. Chapter 7 in: N. G. Houlihan (Ed.), *Lung cancer.* Pittsburgh: Oncology Nursing Society.

Keable, D. (1997). *The management of anxiety – client packs.* Edinburgh: Churchill Livingstone

Krishnasamy, M., Wilkie, E. & Haviland, J. (2001). Lung cancer health care needs assessment: patients' and informal carers' responses to a National Mail Questionnaire Survey. *Palliative Medicine, 15,* 213–227.

Lindsell, G. (2006). Client-centred approach of occupational therapy programme – case study. Chapter 7 in: J. Cooper (Ed.), *Occupational therapy in oncology and palliative care–* (2nd ed.). Chichester: John Wiley & Sons Ltd.

Macbeth, F., Milroy, R., Steward, W. & Burnett, R. (1996). Lung cancer a practical guide to management. *Management of advanced symptomatic disease* (pp. 102–112). New Jersey: Harwood Academic Publishers.

Martinolich, K. & Rivera, M. P. (2001). Pulmonary assessment and treatment. In: F. C. Detterbeck, M. P. Rivera, M. D. Socinki & J. G. Rosenman (Eds.), *Diagnosis and treatment of lung cancer. An evidence-based guide for the practicing clinician.* Sidcup: W.B. Saunders Company.

Matakidou, A., Houlston, R. & Eisen, T. (2005). Genetics of lung cancer: current thinking on the nature and assessment of genetic predisposition to the disease. Chapter 1 in: M. Muers, K. O'Byrne, F. Wells & A. Miles (Eds.), *The effective management of lung cancer* (3rd ed.). London: Aesculapius Medical Press.

McMillan, D. C., Gorman, P. O., Fearon, K. C. H. & McArdle, C. S. (1997). A pilot study of megestrol acetate and ibuprofen treatment of cachexia in gastrointestinal cancer patients. *British Journal of Cancer, 76,* 788–790.

Moore, K. (2003). Living with hope with lung cancer. Chapter 13 in: M. L. Haas (Ed.), *Contemporary issues in lung cancer: a nursing perspective.* Boston: Jones and Bartlett Publishers.

Mountain, C. F., Libshitz, H. I. & Hermes, K. E. (1999). *Lung cancer: a handbook for staging, imaging and lymph node classification.* Retrieved 10 October 2006 from http:www.ctsnet.org

National Collaborating Centre for Acute Care (2005). *Diagnosis and treatment of lung cancer*. London: National Collaborating Centre for Acute Care.

National Institute for Clinical Excellence (NICE) (2004). *Lung cancer: the diagnosis and treatment of lung cancer*. London: National Institute for Clinical Excellence.

Nitadori, J., Inoue, M., Iwasake, M., Otani, T., Sasazuki, S., Nagai, K. & Tsugane, S. (2006). Association between lung cancer incidence and family history of lung cancer. *Chest, 130*, 968–975.

Ockenga, J. & Valentini, L. (2005). Review article: anorexia and cachexia in gastrointestinal cancer. *Alimentary Pharmacology & Therapeutics, 22*, 583–594.

Okuyama, T., Tanaka, K., Akechi, T., Kugaya, A., Okamura, H., Nishiwaki, Y., Hosaka, T. & Uchitomi, Y. (2001). Fatigue in ambulatory patients with advanced lung cancer: prevalence, correlated factors and screening. *Journal of Pain and Symptom Management, 22* (1), 554–564.

Ostler, P. J., Clarke, D. P., Watkinson, A. F. & Gaze, M. N. (1997). Superior vena cava obstruction: a modern management strategy. *Clinical Oncology, 9*, 83–89.

Quinn, M., Babb, P., Brock, A., Kirby, L. & Jones, J. (2001). *Cancer trends in England and Wales 1950–1999: studies on medical and population subjects No. 66*. London: The Stationery Office.

Rosenbloom, S. E. (1949). Superior vena cava obstruction in primary cancer of the lung. *Annals of Internal Medicine, 31*, 470–478.

Ross, E. (2003). Biology of lung cancer. Chapter 2 in: L. Haas (Ed.), *Contemporary issues in lung cancer. A nursing perspective*. Boston: Jones and Bartlett Publishers.

Ross, P. J. & Ashley, S. (2004). Do patients with weight loss have a worse outcome when undergoing chemotherapy for lung cancers? *British Journal of Cancer, 90*, 1905–1911.

Rowell, N. P. & Gleeson, F. V. (2001). Steroids, radiotherapy, chemotherapy and stents for superior vena caval obstruction in carcinoma of the bronchus. *Cochrane Database of Systematic Reviews*, Issue 4, Art. no. CD001316. DOI: 10.1002/14651858.CD001316.

Royal College of Radiologists Clinical Oncology Information Network (COIN) (1999). Guidelines on the non-surgical management of lung cancer. *Clinical Oncology, 11*, S1–S53.

Salt, V. L. & Kerr, K. M. (1997). Mitchell's simple physiological relaxation and Jacobson's progressive relaxation techniques: a comparison. *Physiotherapy, 83* (4), 200–207.

Saunders, M., Dische, S., Barrett, A., Harvey, A., Gibson, D. & Mahesh, P. (1997). Continuous hyperfractioned accelerated radiotherapy (CHART) versus conventional radiotherapy in non-small-cell lung cancer: a randomised multicentre trial. *Lancet, 35*, 161–165.

Schraufnagel, D. E., Hill, R., Leech, J. A. & Pare, J. A. P. (1981). Superior vena caval obstruction. Is it a medical emergency? *American Journal of Medicine, 70*, 1169–1174.

Simmonds, P. (1999). Managing patients with lung cancer. *British Medical Journal, 319*, 527–528.

Shaw, C. (2000). *Current thinking: nutrition and cancer interpreting the scientific evidence behind nutritional practice*. Retrieved 15 November 2006 from http://www.novartis.co.uk/index.shtml

Sloman, R. (2002). Relaxation and imagery for anxiety and depression control in community patients with advanced cancer. *Cancer Nursing, 25* (6), 432–435.

Souhami, R. & Tobias, J. (1998) *Cancer and its management* (1st ed.). Malden: Blackwell Publishing.

Souhami, R. & Tobias, J. (2003). *Cancer and its management* (4th ed.). Malden: Blackwell Publishing.

Tanaka, K., Tatsuo, A., Okuyama, T., Nishiwaki, Y. & Uchitomi, Y. (2002). Impact of dypnea, pain and fatigue on daily life activities in ambulatory patients with advanced lung cancer. *Journal of Pain and Symptom Management, 23* (5), 417–423.

Tyczynski, J. E., Bray, F. & Parkin, M. D. (2003). Lung cancer in Europe 2000: epidemiology, prevention and early detection. *The Lancet Oncology*, 4 (1), 45–55.

Webber, B. A. & Pryor, J. A. (1996). *Physiotherapy for respiratory and cardiac problems, 1993*. Edinburgh: Churchill Livingstone.

World Cancer Research Fund (1997). *Food, nutrition and the prevention of cancer: a global perspective*. Washington: American Institute for Cancer Research.

Wright, S., Courtney, U. & Crowther, D. (2002). A quantitative and qualitative pilot study of the perceived benefits of autogenic training for a group of people with cancer. *European Journal of Cancer Care*, 11, 122–130.

Zang, E. A. & Wynder, E. L. (1996). Differences in lung cancer risk between men and women: examination of the evidence. *Journal of the National Cancer Institute*, 88 (3/4), 183–192.

Further reading

Rice, T. W., Rodriguez, R. M. & Light, R. W. (January 2006). The superior vena cava syndrome: clinical characteristics and evolving etiology. *Medicine [Baltimore]*, 85 (1), 37–42.

Spiro, S. G., Shah, S., Harper, P. G., Tobias, J. S., Geddes, D. M. & Souhami, R. L. (July 1983). Treatment of obstruction of the superior vena cava by combination chemotherapy with and without irradiation in small-cell carcinoma of the bronchus. *Thorax*, 38 (7), 501–505.

Tan, E. H. & Ang, P. T. (November 1995). Resolution of superior vena cava obstruction in small cell lung cancer patients treated with chemotherapy. *Annales Academiae Medicae Singapore*, 24 (6), 812–815.

www.cancerbacup.org.uk (retrieved 23 November 2006).

www.macmillan.org.uk (retrieved 23 November 2006).

www.mesotheliomainternational.com (retrieved 23 November 2006).

Chapter 5

MULTI-PROFESSIONAL MANAGEMENT OF PATIENTS WITH NEUROLOGICAL TUMOURS AND ASSOCIATED CONDITIONS

Joanne Carr, Paula Finlay, Debbie Pearson, Kathy Thompson and Helen White

---

Learning outcomes

After studying this chapter the reader should be able to:

- Describe the classification, presentation, diagnosis, staging and medical management of primary and secondary neurological tumours
- Identify the complex nature of signs and symptoms associated with neurological malignancy
- Discuss the importance of multi-professional collaboration in the management of patients with tumours affecting the central nervous system
- Incorporate knowledge of neurological tumours into clinical reasoning when devising rehabilitation programmes for patients with neurological tumours

---

Introduction

Tumours of the central nervous system (CNS) can have catastrophic consequences for the patient and present many challenges to the medical professionals. While primary CNS tumours are rare, accounting for less than 2% of all cancers (Bell *et al.*, 1998), brain metastases and malignant spinal cord compression are more prevalent amongst the cancer population. As treatments for systemic disease improve and survival figures are lengthened, incidences of these secondary CNS complications are likely to increase. Throughout this chapter we aim to give an introduction to brain tumours, spinal tumours and malignant spinal cord compression and the consequences for rehabilitation professionals when dealing with patients with these diseases. A collection of associated neurological conditions will also be discussed.

Brain tumours

The diagnosis of a brain tumour can have a devastating effect on patients and their carers. Patients with CNS tumours present with many complex and varied signs and symptoms which often result in profound physical, functional, cognitive, psychological and social problems. Patients with aggressive disease often experience a dramatic change in their physical and cognitive function over a short period of time. Those with more dormant disease may experience similar problems in the face of an uncertain future as the disease trajectory can be unpredictable and erratic.

Brain tumours may be of primary or secondary origin, with metastatic lesions accounting for up to half of all intercranial tumours (Bell *et al.*, 1998). The most frequently occurring primary CNS tumours are those of glial origin – the gliomas. Of these, the glioblastoma multiforme (GBM) is the most rapidly advancing and aggressive and unfortunately the most common. Meningiomas are the second most common primary CNS tumour (Kirshblum *et al.*, 2001) and although they are often referred to as 'benign' tumours, they can be responsible for the presentation of debilitating symptoms and may be ultimately fatal if they cannot be resected in their entirety.

Table 5.1 describes the characteristics of the commonly encountered types of brain tumours.

The incidence of brain disease in the cancer population has been shown to have gradually increased in recent years (Kirshblum *et al.*, 2001). This is thought, likely, to be contributable to the aging population, advancements in treatments of systemic cancers and improved imaging and diagnostic techniques.

Clinical presentation, signs and symptoms

Primary brain tumours most commonly occur in the elderly, adolescents and young children. They are the most common solid tumour in children and second only to leukaemia as a cause of death from cancer in the young age group. In adulthood, males have a slightly higher incidence as do those in higher socioeconomic groups (Quinn *et al.*, 2001). Their aetiology is largely unknown. The only established causative factors are ionising radiation – usually in the case of patients treated with cranial radiation as a child who later go on to develop a brain tumour and immune suppression – with a raised risk of CNS lymphoma in AIDS patients. Some genetic conditions, e.g. neurofibromatosis, von Hippel–Lindau syndrome, Li–Fraumeni and Turcot's syndrome, also predispose to development of brain tumours.

Patients with brain tumours present with a variety of complex physical, cognitive and psychosocial symptoms. Initially symptoms are often vague and nebulous. Determining a diagnosis may take months or even years resulting in additional anxiety and frustration for the patient as a number of differential diagnoses may be made before reaching a definitive conclusion. Symptoms occur for a number of reasons: increased intercranial pressure, local tumour invasion, hydrocephalus and cerebral ischaemia and may be focal or diffuse in origin. Non-specific headache is the most common

Table 5.1 Common brain tumours and their characteristics

Astrocytomas

Tend to be invasive, infiltrating tumour masses; therefore, difficult to remove

Arise in the scaffolding cells which hold the neurones together

Grade I/II – low-grade, slow-growing, 'good' prognosis. Median survival 7–10 years, usually referred to as 'benign', though may change over time and become higher grade. May undergo surgery. Usually 'watch and wait' approach

Grade III – 'Anaplastic' growth rate increasing. Median survival 2 years. Appears on scan with surrounding oedema. Usually undergo surgery, radical radiotherapy and chemotherapy

Grade IV – (GBM) Highly malignant, rapid growing. Median survival less than 1 year. Unfortunately, GBM is the most common primary brain tumour. Large tumour >3cm, usually has necrotic core on scan. Increased vascularity and oedema in surrounding tissues, 3-month survival without treatment

Brain metastases

More common than primary brain tumours (approx 50% of intercranial lesions)

Twenty per cent of autopsies show evidence of brain metastases

Common sites – lung, breast, testicular, melanoma and renal cancers

Multiple metastases in 50% cases

One in four will develop brain metastases, average survival 3–4 months

Symptomatic management mainly – steroids palliative radiotherapy, chemotherapy for chemosensitive tumours

Solitary lesions may be resected – allows biopsy and chance for primary to be identified

Meningiomas

Arise from arachnoid cells

Second most common primary brain tumour

Occur mainly in elderly

Slow growing, well circumscribed

Usually benign – though cause symptoms by compression of brain tissue

Cure can be achieved through complete resection, though this is rare as often in high risk, surgically inaccessible areas

Oligodendrogliomas

Arise in the cells responsible for the production of myelin sheath surrounding the axon of CNS

Account for 6% of primary brain tumours

Generally well-defined encapsulated lesions

Found in cerebral cortex, typically frontal

Potential for drop metastases in spine

Better prognosis than astrocytoma. High grade – 4 years, low grade – 15 years.

Possibly due to increased sensitivity to chemo- and radiotherapy

Ependymomas

Arise from the ependymal cells (cells lining the ventricles)

Account for 5% of primary brain tumours, more common in spine

Most common in adolescents and young children

High-grade infratentorial tumours have high propensity to seed into CSF

Surgery, possible for complete resection but highly unlikely

Table 5.1 *(continued)*

Primary CNS lymphoma

Account for 2% of primary brain tumours

Associated with high-grade non-Hodgkin's disease (+immunosuppression, i.e. HIV, following transplant)

Prognosis usually poor as poor systemic status

Solitary lesion may respond to aggressive systemic chemotherapy and give prolonged remission

Medulloblastomas

Arise from primitive neuroepithelial cells in the fourth ventricle

Common in children age 5–15

Posterior fossa tumours – visual problems, ataxia and cranial nerve palsies

Good 5-year survival (60%) with surgery/craniospinal radiotherapy, poorer in very young (<3 years)

Pituitary tumours

Account for 6–10% of primary brain tumours

Usually slow-growing adenomas

Most common in 40–50 age group

Can cause endocrine imbalance (small tumours) or mass effects (larger tumours)

---

symptom. Typical features of a tumour-related headache are daily headache worse on waking, exacerbation of pain on coughing, sneezing or bending and headache associated with vomiting and other neurological signs. Headache is also one of the most common complaints in the non-cancer general population. It is not unusual for tumour patients to have been given a diagnosis of 'stress' or 'depression' at early presentation. It is only when symptoms progress that investigations may be sought.

The site of the lesion has an impact on symptoms. Supratentorial tumours typically present with focal neurological symptoms and seizures. Patients may complain of weakness, hemiparesis, hemiplegia, dysphasia, mental deterioration, intellectual impairment or mood disturbance, while infratentorial tumours result in ataxia, incoordination and cranial nerve deficits. Size is also an important factor. A small tumour occupying the cerebellum may present early as ataxia and dysarthria – signs that would prompt urgent investigation. In contrast, a fairly large tumour growing in the frontal lobe may have been producing subtle personality and cognitive changes for a while, which may have wrongly been attributed to other factors such as stress and depression.

Investigations and staging

It is likely that investigations are not performed until focal physical signs are elicited. Epilepsy is present as the initial symptom in up to 40% of patients, and 20% of adults who present with new-onset seizures will have a brain tumour (Snyder *et al.*, 1993). The appearance of epilepsy in adulthood should trigger immediate investigation as to the cause and hence this group of patients has a slightly better prognosis as their tumours are usually detected at an earlier stage.

Determining a diagnosis of brain tumour is fraught with difficulties which result in frustration for both patients and professionals. When considering that a general practitioner can expect only five new cases in his or her entire working lifetime (Grant, 2004), it is perhaps understandable that recognition of signs and symptoms is problematic in the primary care setting. Once suspicion of a tumour is raised, diagnosis is confirmed by imaging and if possible by a biopsy. Magnetic resonance imaging (MRI) is the scan of choice as it gives the clearest image of all of the brain structures. Computerised tomography (CT) is also used, though evidence suggests that 10% of glioma patients may have a negative CT scan (Grant, 2004). Once the scan has been performed, an interim diagnosis of 'space-occupying lesion' is given. All patients with a positive scan should be referred to a neurosurgical unit in order to establish a tissue diagnosis. Tumours situated in the pons and brain stem are generally surgically inaccessible. It is likely that these tumours will have only a radiologically confirmed diagnosis. All brain surgery carries significant risks to morbidity and mortality. At the time of surgery the neurosurgeon will aim to gather tissue in order to achieve a pathological specimen and remove as much of the tumour mass as is possible without causing further problems for the patient. Surgical procedures include open biopsy with resection and/or debulking, stereotactically guided biopsy and decompression techniques (e.g. ventriculostomy and shunt insertion). Examination of the cerebrospinal fluid (CSF) via a lumbar puncture, together with a full biochemical and endocrine assessment, adds to the clinical picture. If the scan and histological appearance are suggestive of brain metastases, investigations to discover the origin of the primary disease may be performed, e.g. full-body CT scan, mammography and chest X-ray.

Brain tumours are classified according to the World Health Organization (WHO) (Kleihues & Cavanee, 2000), which describes the tumour according to its cell of origin, e.g. glioma, menigioma and metastases. Gliomas are the most common type of primary brain tumour. They arise in the neuroepithelial cells – the astrocytes, oligodendrocites and ependymal cells that, respectively, provide a scaffolding network for neural cells, nourish the myelin sheath and line the ventricles. Tumours arising in these cells are distinctly different, though they share some sinister characteristics. Their intrinsic, interweaving nature means complete resection and hence cure is impossible; they all demonstrate increased rate of growth and malignancy over time and the likelihood of local recurrence is high. Astrocytomas are further subdivided. Low-grade (WHO grade I/II) tumours have a very slow growth rate. They carry a median prognosis of 7–10 years. These tumours are often referred to as 'benign', although over time they can exhibit faster growth rates and change to a higher grade. High-grade tumours (WHO grade III/IV) are more worrying. Median survival for grade III is in the region of 24 months; this drops dramatically to 9 months (with treatment) for the GBM grade IV tumour (Bell et al., 1998).

Following biopsy a heterogeneous sample is often obtained and accurate grading and classification is therefore difficult. Tumour masses may contain a mixture of malignant cells of differing tissue origin and growth rates. At worst, a patient may be told that he or she has a low-grade tumour as this is what the sample reflected, although the residual tumour may contain cells of a higher grade and so deterioration of symptoms may occur earlier than anticipated or expected.

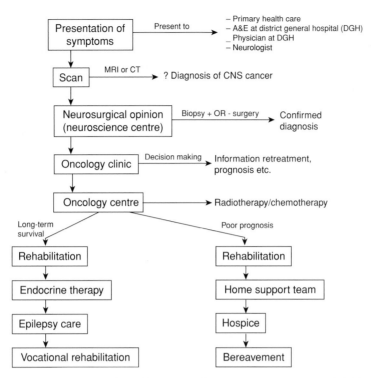

Figure 5.1 Typical neuro-oncological patient pathway (Carr, 2002, personal slide).

Medical management of brain tumours

Treatment options depend on a number of factors, including classification, stage and grade of tumour, the patient's symptoms, performance status and their treatment preference. Figure 5.1 shows a typical patient pathway. The main aims of medical treatment are to alleviate and relieve symptoms, to optimise quality of life and to offer increased survival where possible. Surgery, radiotherapy and chemotherapy are the main arms of treatment with steroids, anticoagulants and antiepileptics prescribed as supportive therapies.

Surgery

When considering surgery the risks versus benefits have to be carefully assessed and discussed with the patient. Patients with low-grade tumours who have no physical symptoms may opt to defer any surgical intervention until such symptoms appear, whilst others may prefer elective surgery to minimise the 'ticking time bomb' they perceive to have in their head. Intraoperative cortical monitoring is utilised to minimise surgical damage to vital functional areas of the brain.

Patients with high-grade tumours may have rapidly deteriorating symptoms. Emergency surgery, e.g. decompression, may need to be performed to prevent further neurological damage, with the surgeon attempting as much resection as is possible to offer relief of symptoms.

Radiotherapy

Radiotherapy is used as an adjuvant treatment for inoperable tumours. The aim is to facilitate maximum tumour kill without causing excessive complications. Radical radiotherapy may be given over a course of 30 days, with palliative treatments being reduced to 16 fractions or less. External beam radiation is delivered in a limited defined field to a primary brain tumour and to the whole brain for brain metastases or a diffuse GBM. Treatment fields and dose depend on the physical state of the patient and their presenting symptoms. Stereotactic radiotherapy, or 'gamma knife surgery', uses a fine beam of radiation targeted directly onto the tumour through a frame secured to the patient's skull. It is a successful treatment for tumours less than 3 cm in diameter and reduces the risk of radiation-induced necrosis to surrounding normal brain tissue (Grant, 2004). Radiation offers good relief of symptoms and, in some cases, prolonged survival but is not without its side effects, which can be categorised into short and long term. Short-term effects include alopecia, skin reactions, tinnitus and exacerbation of symptoms as the radiation causes local oedema, which will raise intercranial pressure. The patient may suffer worsening headaches, nausea and vomiting with deterioration of physical symptoms. It is difficult to distinguish this radiation-induced encephalopathy from tumour progression and high-dose steroids are given to reduce the swelling. Symptoms should start to improve as the steroids take effect. Patients and carers get increasingly distressed as their hope of successful treatment is replaced by fear of failure. It is unfortunate that in a few cases a highly aggressive tumour will progress through the treatment and supportive measures are then taken to ensure the patient is kept as comfortable as possible. Somnolence syndrome is the specific overwhelming exhaustion felt by patients undergoing radiotherapy to the brain. It may be caused by the temporary inability of the oligodendrocytes to maintain the myelin sheaths. It commonly starts about half way through the course of radiotherapy and can reappear about 5–6 weeks after the completion of treatment. The severe fatigue and lethargy can adversely affect the patient's ability to cope with the demands of daily living and participate in rehabilitation activity. Radiation-induced necrosis can occur years after radiotherapy to the brain. In limited-field radiation a defined area similar to the site and size of the original tumour will appear on a scan as an 'space-occupying lesion' and may cause focal problems. The patient will worry that the original tumour has recurred and only a biopsy will confirm or allay his or her suspicions. If problematic, the necrotic scar can be resected. Diffuse radiation necrosis resulting from cortical atrophy occurs after whole-brain radiation. This may present as early onset cerebrovascular disease, dementia and psychomotor retardation. Symptoms may be alleviated by the use of steroids.

Chemotherapy

Chemotherapy has limited use in the management of primary brain tumours due to difficulties posed by the blood–brain and blood–tumour barriers. It is largely a palliative treatment with an aim to control tumour growth and prolong survival. It has little effect on symptoms and is generally only offered to patients who are 'well' with a good performance status. Patients presenting with brain metastases may derive some benefit from systemic chemotherapy.

Steroid treatment

Patients with brain tumours are often prescribed high-dose steroids for short periods or low-dose steroids over a longer time frame in order to combat cerebral oedema and control associated symptoms. Steroid myopathy, steroid-induced psychoses, weight gain and diabetes are frequent side effects. Patients who have taken steroids for longer than 3 weeks are more likely to present with secondary problems (Batchelor & DeAngelis, 1996). Reducing regimens are attempted; however, for many patients with high-grade tumours, a low level of steroids may be necessary to relieve symptoms for the remainder of their lives. Immobility, weakness and a hypercoagulable state significantly increase the risk of a brain tumour patient developing a deep vein thrombosis (DVT) or pulmonary embolism (PE) with estimates of up to 45% of patients being affected (Kirshblum *et al.*, 2001). Anticoagulant therapy, compression stockings and intermittent pneumatic compression are used to reduce this risk.

Rehabilitation of the patient with a brain tumour

I feel like my whole life has been thrown up into the air, chopped into a million pieces and is now on the floor in front of me. How do I make sense of this? Where do I start?

(Newly diagnosed brain tumour patient)

CNS tumour patients present with a variety of complex physical, cognitive and psychological problems that may be related to both their disease and the treatments they have received (Table 5.2).

Their disease trajectory may be varied and complex and symptoms can change dramatically over a short period of time. Functional impairment, loss of independence and severe disability will have devastating consequences for patients and their families.

Brain tumours present challenging problems particularly for rehabilitation professionals. As well as dealing with difficult neurological disorders, the added complication of an often relentlessly deteriorating disease means that treatment aims and goals are based on managing fluctuating abilities and a gradual decline of the patient's physical, psychological and cognitive state in an attempt to optimise independence and maximise the quality of life. Studies comparing rehabilitation of brain tumour patients with stroke or traumatic brain injury patients reveal favourable evidence in terms of achievement of comparable functional gains, shorter hospital lengths of stay and successful discharge outcomes (Huang *et al.*, 1998, 2000; O'Dell *et al.*, 1998). Despite this, access to specialist neurorehabilitation programmes remains problematic for brain tumour patients. In 2006, the National Institute for Health and Clinical Excellence published its *Improving Outcomes for People with Brain and Other CNS Tumours* guidance. This document stresses the need for a standardised approach to the medical management of this patient group and emphasises the importance of provision of rehabilitation and supportive therapies.

Whilst similarities arise with the symptoms and management of brain tumours and other neurological conditions, distinct differences mean that rehabilitation

Table 5.2 Common problems experienced by brain tumour patients.

Physical	Psychosocial
Motor loss/weakness	Personality change
Sensory changes	Cognitive difficulties
Dysphasia	Problems with executive functioning
Communication difficulties	Poor concentration
Decreased bladder/bowel function	Alteration of mood
Decreased function	Impaired memory
Increased dependence on others	Fear, anxiety and uncertainty
Dyspraxia	Body image issues
Ataxia	Sexuality issues
Headache/vomiting	Relationship problems
Epilepsy	Altered family dynamics
Cranial nerve palsies	Financial problems
Visual disturbance	Loss of control
Cranial scar	Loss of career/role in family/society
Alopecia	Increased dependence on others
Cushing syndrome	Loss of dignity
Somnolence syndrome	
Radiotherapy reactions	
Mucositis	
Nausea	
Weight gain	
Sleep disturbance	
Risk of DVT/PE	
Steroid-induced diabetes	

professionals have to tailor their approach to be timely, responsive and adaptable to the specific needs of the brain tumour patient. Progressive and fluctuating levels of functional decline, difficult psychological adjustment, fatigue, depression, uncertainty and medical fragility are described by Kirshblum *et al.* (2001) as factors which impact on rehabilitation. The effects of steroids, somnolence syndrome, epilepsy and side effects of treatments also need to be considered.

Patients with high-grade gliomas have a poor prognosis and their care and support needs differ from those with a longer life expectancy. Patients with high-grade tumours require urgent rehabilitation aimed at optimising function to allow maximum quality of life. This may involve pre-empting and preventing further problems or carefully managing the decline of the patient's physical, cognitive and psychological state. Patients with low-grade tumours may also need rapid access to rehabilitation professionals, though their treatment aims and goals should be geared appropriately towards the longer term and involve activities which aim to reintegrate the individual into their social roles. They may have rehabilitation needs for a prolonged period of time, possibly years after their initial diagnosis. In all cases a person-centred approach to practice enables the therapists to identify with the patient those activities which are important to them and their way of living. Rehabilitation goals are tailored to reflect patients' and carers' individual needs and cover a broad spectrum reflecting the diversity of occupations of daily life and the complex interplay of symptoms which can arise from a brain tumour. Ongoing assessment of patients' and carers' needs is pivotal to the holistic management of patients with brain and CNS tumours.

In order for effective rehabilitation programmes to be implemented, realistic, attainable goals should be discussed with the patient and carer and they must be included in all decisions concerning the rehabilitation process. Multidisciplinary working is essential to achieve the patient's goals. Whilst it is necessary for each therapist to have his or her own treatment aims and objectives, it is vital to understand that the problems experienced by the patients are often interconnected and that the expertise required for effective intervention may elude a single profession (Fisher, 1998). Interplay and collaboration between team members is essential. For example, the profoundly disabled patient presenting with a dense hemiplegia and poor balance may have a goal to feed him- or herself independently. The physiotherapist would be concerned with facilitating sitting balance and improving sitting posture, the occupational therapist (OT) would then work in the sitting position on the retraining of the functional task using equipment if necessary. If language is impaired, the speech and language therapist (SLT) may be concerned with identifying the barriers to effective communication and providing strategies to support both patients, their relatives or carers or other health care professionals involved in their treatment. If swallowing is impaired, a clinical swallow examination by the SLT helps identify any necessary swallow manoeuvres or strategies. They work closely with the dietitians to recommend appropriate food consistencies and the dietitian advises on food fortification or modification to ensure nutritional status is maintained.

Brain tumour patients are likely to encounter 'specialist' palliative care/oncology AHPs (National Institute for Clinical Excellence [NICE], 2004). Professionals working outside of the specialist centres may be unfamiliar with the pathology, disease trajectory and treatments for CNS cancers and, as a result, may require support, education and advice from the specialists in order for them to continue to meet the needs of the patient in a primary care setting. This is of particular importance at the point of discharge of the patient from hospital.

Primary aims of physiotherapy are to maintain or improve mobility, function, strength and range of movement, prevent contractures and deformities and optimise safety in all aspects of patient mobility and in their handling by carers. Treatment techniques include progressive exercise programmes, eutrophic electrical stimulation, balance retraining, modified 'normal movement' techniques, gait re-education, transfer practice and wheelchair education if necessary. Advice and information regarding fatigue management and pacing of activities will be reinforced by other professionals. Exercise advice to combat the debilitating effects of steroids is beneficial for all patients.

OT interventions include, for example, work rehabilitation, cognitive skills retraining, risk assessment and management, facilitating engagement in leisure, personal and domestic activities, identifying environmental adaptations and assistive equipment to enable the patient to be as independent as possible. The Canadian Occupational Performance Measure is a good starting point for assessment. The OT aims to enable patients to make their own decisions, regain control and become more empowered, throughout all stages of the disease.

Speaking and eating are fundamental to quality of life. Patients may present with communication and swallowing difficulties. These impairments can be deeply distressing for the patient and their carers and adding to the social exclusion patients may already be feeling as a result of their illness. Aphasia is a complex disorder of language processing and may affect one or all modalities. When you combine a diagnosis of a malignant brain tumour with an acquired communication problem, the effect is often described as devastating (White, 2004). The SLT may work to improve or enhance communication or to augment communication skills in carers through a variety of techniques.

Another key role for the SLT is an advocate for the patient. If the patient has dysphasia, it is the language that is impaired. So, they are trying to make sense of their disease and their treatment options using the very medium that is damaged. If their speech is dysarthric, exercises to maintain, improve or compensate oral muscle activity might be beneficial. As previously mentioned, a clinical swallow examination will facilitate appropriate swallow management, i.e. positioning and manoeuvres to assist an effective swallow and allow a patient to continue safe feeding.

Assessment by a dietitian is important in the holistic management of the CNS tumour patient. Patients with swallowing difficulties and at risk of aspiration may have a compromised nutritional status. Dietitians are able to offer individualised advice and support on diet modification and food fortification to combat these problems. Many patients experience significant weight gain or diabetes in response to steroid medication and the dietitian provides specific dietary intervention and education for both of these conditions. Patients undergoing chemotherapy need to avoid certain foods for the duration of their treatment, the dietitian is able to tailor an appropriate nutritional programme for each patient.

Case study 1: Patient with a high-grade tumour

Mrs M, a 55-year-old teacher, was discharged from hospital following surgery and radiotherapy for a GBM. She was fatigued, lethargic and had a slight weakness affecting her left side. On discharge from hospital, Mrs M had declined input from community rehabilitation services as she felt she was able to manage with support of her husband Mr M. The diagnosis of GBM had devastated the couple; however, for the sake of their teenage children they were determined to maintain a degree of 'normality' at home. Over a period of a few weeks, Mrs M's symptoms began to deteriorate. She attended her general practitioner and subsequently agreed to see the community-based OT and physiotherapist.

The therapists completed a joint assessment. Mrs M had lost the vision in her left eye and progression of the left-sided weakness had impacted on all aspects of mobility, transfers and daily living tasks. She had limited movement but no functional use of her left arm. Sensory awareness of her left side was impaired. Her gait was compromised by lack of control of the left hip and knee and poor pelvic stability; however, she had continued to mobilise unsteadily around the house and was climbing the stairs with physical assistance from her husband. Significant safety risks were identified. Whilst uncomplaining, Mr M looked tired and during an opportunity for a private discussion he was tearful, fearful of the future and admitted the burden of care was 'draining'.

A rehabilitation programme was established with Mr and Mrs M, which reflected their priorities:

• Mrs M's goal was to remain mobile for as long as possible. She was issued with an ankle-foot orthosis and a walking stick to aid balance. Discussions were held between the couple and the therapists regarding the potential safety risks, and advice and demonstration of appropriate handling techniques were given. A stair lift was installed, which improved safety on the stairs and had the added benefit of helping the patient to conserve energy for other activities.

- The couple worked with the therapists on balance, hip and knee control and practised transfers to and from the bed, chair and toilet.
- Mrs M learned how to maintain midline position in sitting and lying.
- Principles of normal movement patterns were integrated during therapy sessions and practice of functional activities, e.g. washing, dressing and showering.
- Mrs M was taught how to compensate for the loss of sensation of her left side and how to position her limbs.
- A programme to facilitate upper-limb function and maintenance of range of movement with passive exercise was established.
- Equipment to help function and independence including a chair-raising unit, a shower chair, a plate guard, a helping hand, a freestanding toilet frame and a transit wheelchair were provided.
- Ways to manage fatigue by planning, pacing and prioritising activities were identified.
- Mrs M also agreed to attend a local day hospice; this was not an easy decision, but she realised that it would provide respite for herself and her husband and an opportunity for counselling and support for all the family, and allow for the introduction of hospice care in anticipation of her ultimate decline and possible need for admission as her condition deteriorated.

Mrs M made some progress through a difficult period. Establishing achievable goals, improving safety and functional performance and offering support with regard to the psychological impact of their situation were important. Combining physiotherapy and occupational therapy approaches ensured a coordinated service which enabled Mrs M to function in her own home until she decided to go to the hospice, her preferred place of care at the end of her life. The therapists maintained contact with the couple and offered bereavement support for the family after her death.

Primary spinal tumours

Intradural spinal tumours are extremely rare. Within the dura tumours are classified as either extramedullary (arising inside the dura but outside the spinal cord) or intramedullary (originating in the spinal cord itself). Typical extramedullary tumours are schwannomas and meningiomas, gliomas (ependymomas and astrocytomas) arisen from the cord tissue itself. Very rare extramedullary tumours include primary lymphoma.

Spinal tumours usually present with a protracted history of primary pain with associated neurological dysfunction below the level of the tumour as the mass grows and causes destruction of the spinal cord. High-grade tumours within the spinal cord carry a poor prognosis with an average life expectancy of between 6 and 12 months (NICE, 2006).

MRI plays a large part in the diagnosis of primary spinal tumours with occasionally spinal angiography adding to the clinical picture. Whole-brain and spinal cord scans allow for a thorough assessment of the CNS and any distant growths will be seen. While metastases from primary CNS tumours to systemic organs is extremely rare, tumours arising in CNS tissue can spread via the cerebrospinal fluid to other areas of the CNS causing secondary tumour masses.

Decompression of the spine together with excision of as much tumour bulk as possible is the primary aim of surgery. Radiotherapy will usually follow in order to treat any residual high-grade tumours. Patients with low-grade tumours, who have a longer life expectancy, may be advised to defer radiotherapy in order to minimise radiation-induced spinal damage. Chemotherapy plays a minor role in the management of primary spinal tumours, tending to be offered at disease recurrence when the maximum cord-tolerant dose of radiotherapy has been administered and hence no more can be given.

Rehabilitation of the patient with a low-grade primary spinal tumour closely mimics that of any patient with a spinal injury. These patients may have a good outlook in terms of longevity, though they may have functional problems that require the ongoing input from a range of rehabilitation professionals in the long term. Patients with high-grade tumours may deteriorate rapidly and so need immediate intervention.

Malignant spinal cord compression

Malignant spinal cord compression (MSCC) is a manifestation of advanced malignant disease. It occurs whenever an extradural tumour mass impinges on the spinal canal and causes compression of the spinal cord or cauda equina. A positive diagnosis is made when a clear indentation of the theca, corresponding to the level of symptoms, can be seen on imaging (Loblaw & Laperriere, 1998). In the majority of cancer patients, invasion of the epidural space by vertebral body metastases is the most common presentation; however, bony collapse and soft-tissue masses, e.g. lymphoma, may also result in compression. The consequences are often devastating for patients and their carers. A complex array of psychosocial problems, relating to the loss of their normal level of function and movement, and the realisation that their disease has 'spread' may further exacerbate the physical consequences of the compression. MSCC is an oncological emergency, requiring precise assessment of symptoms, urgent investigation and immediate treatment. The presentation of MSCC presents many challenges to the medical profession with respect to aspects of its diagnosis and treatment. Once a diagnosis of MSCC has been made, the majority of patients will die within 12 months (Hacking et al., 1993). Appropriate rehabilitation of these patients is crucial to ensure that they achieve their optimum level of function to enable their maximum quality of life.

Clinical presentation, signs and symptoms

Bone metastases are found in up to 60% of cancer patients; of these it can be expected that 10% will develop neurological problems as a result of MSCC (Huddart et al., 1997). Evidence suggests that 10% of patients, who had no prior malignant diagnosis, will present with MSCC as their first manifestation of cancer (Perrin et al., 1997).

Any primary cancer, with the exception of the primary CNS tumours, can metastasise to the skeleton. The diseases that are most likely to result in bone metastases can however be classified into those of high to low risk, although it should always

High:	Lung, breast, prostate disease
Medium:	Kidney, melanoma, sarcoma, myeloma, lymphoma
Low:	Colorectal, gynaecological disease

Figure 5.2 Relative risk for MSCC. N.B. Breast, lung and prostate diseases account for 50% of all MSCC (Bucholtz, 1999).

be borne in mind that *any* type of malignant disease can result in MSCC. Figure 5.2 shows the high-to-low categories.

In 70% of cases compression occurs in the thoracic spine, with 20% in the lumbar spine and 10% in the cervical region (Perrin *et al.*, 1997). In many cases patients will have disease throughout the spinal column and may have several sites of compression – a factor which has a strong influence on treatment choice. Neurological dysfunction occurs as a result of direct trauma of the neural tissues as the mass causes distortion of the cord and interruption of the ascending and descending tracts. Spinal shock – the acute inflammatory response to injury – will cause further injury, while interruption of blood flow to the cord may cause areas of ischaemia and hence neurological damage.

The four cardinal symptoms of MSCC are pain, motor dysfunction, sensory disturbance and bladder or bowel dysfunction. Pain is usually the earliest symptom of MSCC and may have been present for some time in the absence of other symptoms. Pain usually originates in the centre of the back and radiates like a 'tight band' around the trunk and may extend into the lower limbs. Patients may be able to describe quite focally where their pain originates – this will usually correspond to the level of the compression. The pain often has a mechanical element, worsened by movements such as coughing, sneezing and bending. The use of escalating doses of analgesia with little relief from pain would strongly suggest MSCC.

Motor dysfunction such as weakness or tonal changes may have a slow or rapid onset. Patients may experience a sudden weakness or inability to stand and bear weight – an extremely frightening event which is often the trigger for acute investigations. A more gradual onset may cause ambiguity in establishing a diagnosis as many cancer patients experience pain, lethargy, fatigue and weakness for a myriad of reasons. Weakness associated with MSCC is however always progressive and, depending on the extent of the compression, may present as a symmetrical or asymmetrical pattern. Complaints of heavy limbs and stiff muscles may be reported subjectively. Compromise of the autonomic nervous system may result in disruption of bowel or bladder control. Initially this will present as constipation and urinary retention; as the compression advances, complete loss of sphincter control will occur.

Sensory disturbance happens as a result of interruption of the ascending tracts. It always occurs below the level of the compression. Patients may describe the presence of 'tingling', 'pins and needles' or 'electric-shock'-type sensations or may have a complete numbness or paraesthesia, hypersensitivity and proprioception deficit. It is of worthy note that some patients with an established or impending MSCC may in fact have intact sensory awareness. This was highlighted in a study by Levack *et al.* (2002), who concluded – 'Don't wait for a sensory level!' – when the presence of severe back pain and motor dysfunction occurs against a history of malignant disease, imaging of the spine should be performed immediately to confirm or rule out a diagnosis of MSCC. They also reported patients with selective proprioceptive and sensory loss and no motor dysfunction, which highlights how a variety of symptoms may occur.

Accurate and precise history taking is vital in establishing a suspicion of MSCC, which will then instigate appropriate clinical imaging. Problems with early recognition of signs and symptoms and delaying of investigation and treatment can adversely affect the outcome for the patients. Evidence suggests that functional outcome depends very much on the degree of neurological impairment at the time of diagnosis (Husband, 1998). Those patients who have severe neurological dysfunction, i.e. have complete paraplegia at diagnosis of MSCC, have a very slim chance of recovering any motor function. Patients who have some leg power but are unable to walk have a 50% chance of recovering their mobility, whilst patients who are ambulant at diagnosis are likely to retain their mobility.

Medical management of MSCC

The principle aims of treatment are to relieve pain and to preserve or restore neurological function. Accurate history taking of signs and symptoms is essential. A detailed clinical investigation should follow, which should include a full neurological assessment of muscle tone and power, sensation testing, proprioception testing and upper- and lower-motor neurone testing. Once a suspicion of MSCC is raised, urgent imaging is required. MRI is the investigation of choice (Husband *et al.*, 2001). Plain X-rays will only pick up on actual bony destruction of the spinal column and hence may present a false negative result. An MRI of the whole spine is often performed. This will identify other areas of impending or actual compression and will provide valuable information for treatment planning.

The stability of the spine is a key factor in the management of MSCC. An assessment needs to be made to determine the risk of causing further compression and deterioration of symptoms through movement and function. On suspicion of MSCC and in the absence of definitive evidence, good practice advocates that it should always be assumed that *the spine is unstable unless clinical features or radiological findings suggest otherwise* (Pease *et al.*, 2004). A scan which shows the complete destruction of a vertebral body with displacement of an adjacent vertebral body would be highly suggestive of an unstable spine. In reality, however, interpretation of scans may not be so clear-cut and an element of uncertainty regarding spinal stability is very realistic. It is then that clinical signs and symptoms need to be closely observed and monitored. Any complaint of pain on movement or exacerbated by movement would indicate pain of mechanical, potentially unstable origin. Likewise, if movement results in an increase in sensory symptoms, instability should be assumed. When instability is suspected, the patient should be kept on strict bed rest, catheterised and log rolled for all nursing needs. In the case of a cervical compression, a hard collar should be applied. At all times the patient needs to be informed of the reasoning behind these measures and made aware of the importance of reporting any changes in their symptoms immediately.

The first step to take when MSCC is suspected in a patient is the commencement of high-dose steroids. This is usually in the form of dexamethasone and loading doses of 16–100 mg are advocated with a reducing regimen to follow (Husband *et al.*, 2001). The steroids will start to reduce the oedema at the site of the compression and may be enough to allow relief of pain and symptoms. Gastric protection is usually prescribed alongside steroids in order to reduce the risk of gastric complications. Due to the reduced mobility and enforced bed rest of many MSCC patients anticoagulant therapy should be administered to minimise the risk of DVT and PE.

In the unstable spine, surgery to decompress the tumour and stabilise the spine is the treatment of choice. It is useful when a tissue diagnosis is needed in the case of an 'unknown primary' and is also advocated when the patient has undergone previous radiotherapy to the same area of the spine (Case study 2). Evidence suggests that surgical techniques that both decompress and stabilise the spine offer better outcomes for the patients (Klimo *et al.*, 2003). The main limitation to surgery is the performance status of the patient. Spinal surgery is major surgery with significant risks and potential problems post-operatively. Therefore, the patient has to be fit enough to undergo such invasive treatment. The majority of patients unfortunately are deemed to be unfit for surgery. External beam radiotherapy then becomes the treatment of choice. It is non-invasive and can be performed (if services allow) immediately. It is used in the treatment of radiosensitive tumours (e.g. lymphoma and multiple myeloma) with good result (Huddart *et al.*, 1997). If prognosis is expected to be less than 4 months, radiotherapy is a convenient, effective way of providing symptom relief and has been shown to be comparable to a surgical decompression. Treatment regimens vary from single fractions to a course of treatment over a week or two. Side effects of treatment include oesophagitis, nausea and vomiting and diarrhoea as the radiation beam passes through the gastrointestinal tract. The role of chemotherapy in the management of MSCC is limited and is often used as an adjunct to surgery or radiotherapy in order to treat the primary malignancy. It may have particular benefit in the management of chemosensitive tumours.

Bisphophonates are a family of drugs that are used in widespread skeletal metastatic disease. They aim to regulate osteoclast activity, which is increased in bone metastases, to reduce loss of calcium from the bones, relieving pain and promoting bone strength. They are typically given to patients with metastatic breast and prostate disease to protect the skeleton.

Rehabilitation of the patient with MSCC

Early referral to rehabilitation professionals is of paramount importance in the management of the MSCC patient. Referral to the physiotherapist should be made as soon as a suspicion of MSCC arises. In addition to a holistic assessment of the patient including his or her psychosocial status and home circumstances, the physiotherapist and occupational therapist (OT) is able to perform a 'baseline' assessment of the patient's neurological function through a structured objective evaluation of muscle power according to muscle group, muscle tone, sensory awareness according to dermatome and proprioception. Use of a structured assessment tool such as the American Spinal Injury Association tool (American Spinal Injury Association [ASIA], 1996) will aid documentation of this. When a patient has to be immobilised to reduce the risk of causing further spinal damage, the physiotherapist plays an important role in educating patients, carers and health care staff regarding the need for such measures and can advise regarding appropriate handling and positioning of the patient. When a cervical collar has to be fitted it is usually the physiotherapist who would do this, although any suitably trained multi-professional team member would be appropriate.

Prevention of further medical complications and the consequences of prolonged bed rest would be one of the early aims of physiotherapy. Respiratory function may need to be closely monitored, particularly in a patient with a high cervical lesion or in a patient with pre-existing lung pathology. The use of deep breathing exercises and chest clearance techniques such as the active cycle of breathing may prevent chest complications, e.g. chest infection or pneumonia. The use of compression antiembolism stockings (TEDs) together with passive movements and calf massage is important in the prevention of circulatory complications. Where possible the patient should be encouraged to perform his or her own 'toes, ankles and quads' exercises to aid maintenance of circulation and maintain any muscle activity he or she might have. Passive movements will also aim to minimise the effects of any muscle shortening and joint stiffness – factors which can adversely affect rehabilitation further down the line. Techniques such as transcutaneous electrical nerve stimulation (TENS), heat and positioning and support may aid pain relief.

Active rehabilitation should only commence once the multidisciplinary team has discussed the patient and all members are satisfied that to embark on a rehabilitation programme will not result in further neurological damage. If a patient has undergone surgery, this is usually a straightforward decision taken after surgery when the surgeon is happy with the outcome of the procedure and clinical signs and symptoms have been relieved. In the case of radiotherapy however the decision is not so easy to make. As there is no standardised radiotherapy management protocol in the case of MSCC, there follows that there is also no standardised rehabilitation protocol. Improving Outcomes Guidance, currently in development by NICE, will aim to inform management of this patient group. Again best practice (Pease *et al.*, 2004) advocates that the decision to mobilise and commence a rehabilitation programme should be based on a bedside assessment of the patient's clinical symptoms. Some doctors prefer their patients to wait until radiotherapy has completed before rehabilitation commences, whilst others may proceed before the course of treatment has finished. The physiotherapist plays an important role in this assessment. A fundamental assessment of spinal stability would be to monitor any signs and symptoms whilst the patient's legs are being passively moved in the bed, including a degree of hip and knee flexion, or the response of the patient to gentle rolling. If these movements increase or cause pain then the patient would remain on flat bed rest until further multiprofessional team discussion or a review of analgesia has been performed. Pease *et al.* (2004) recommend that the patient should be supervised through a gradual increase of incline of the head of the bed with symptoms being closely monitored.

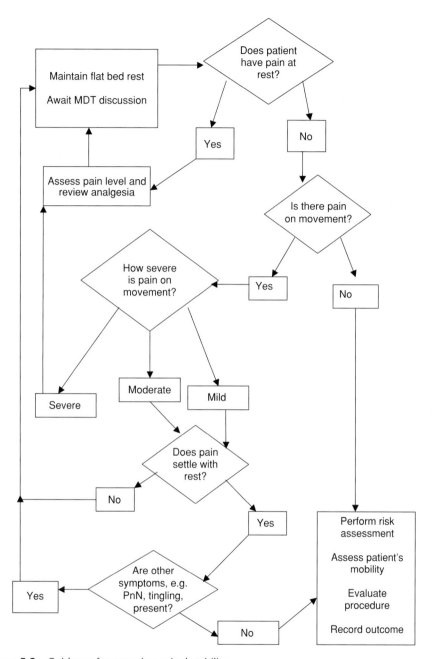

Figure 5.3 Guidance for assessing spinal stability.

Some patients may be able to progress from supine, through 45° up into long sitting in a short space of time, while others may take a little longer. Once the patient is able to sit up in bed with no increase in symptoms then active rehabilitation can begin. Figure 5.3 shows a typical flow chart regarding the assessment of spinal stability.

Table 5.3 Key aims of rehabilitation with MSCC patient

Pre-treatment stage
  Immobilisation of spine
    Flat bed rest
    Hard collar/sand bags for cervical lesion
  Baseline assessment of neurological function
  Prevention of respiratory/circulatory problems (e.g. chest infect immuno suppression on and DVT)
  Pain relief
  Maintenance of muscle strength and joint ROM
  Education, information and support

Post-treatment (depending on stability of spine and response to treatment)
  Education, information and support
  Improve muscle power/strength
  Facilitate progression from flat bed rest to 45° position
  Facilitate bed mobility, transfer out of bed – suitable seating and appropriate pressure relief
  Facilitate independent transfers where possible with use of equipment if necessary
  Assessment of home and provision of equipment/assistive devices
  Improve sitting/standing balance
  Gait re-education
  Progression of functional activity to maximise independence
  Educate the patient in use of wheelchair if necessary
  Encourage independence in activities of daily living/recreational activities
  Improve exercise tolerance
  Facilitate management of anxiety and relaxation
  Educate and support regarding fatigue management and pacing of activities
  Education and support regarding long-term use of collar/brace if required

---

Most patients will be able to start a structured rehabilitation programme once their medical treatment has commenced. It is unfortunate, however, that a small number of patients will continue to have distressing symptoms or will continue to deteriorate in terms of function despite medical treatment. Their prognosis is extremely poor. These patients usually require input from the specialist palliative care team for symptom control. Rehabilitation should be focused on achieving an appropriate discharge plan in accordance with the patient and their carer's wishes with prompt provision of equipment and care services to facilitate a timely discharge.

Each patient will require an individualised rehabilitation programme tailored to his or her own level of function and capabilities. The principles of assessing spinal stability and response to treatment should be integral to all therapy sessions. Key aims of therapy are listed in Table 5.3.

Early involvement of the OT is also important. During the early 'flat bed rest' stage, advice regarding positioning of the patient and items in his or her environment will aim to minimise the risk of excessive reaching and movement. It will also limit the isolation the patient might be feeling as a result of the enforced immobility. The dietitian advises on coping with difficulties eating whilst lying flat and may work with the OT regarding the use of adaptive cutlery to cut up food and eat it safely.

Once active rehabilitation has begun, work on transfers and mobility with appropriate equipment is usually done in combination with the physiotherapist, giving toileting transfers a priority in order to regain a degree of normality for the patient. A problem-solving approach to washing and dressing, bathing and domestic skills with the teaching of coping mechanisms and compensation strategies can greatly improve a patient's level of function. Discharge planning, assessment of the home environment, provision of equipment and liaison with community colleagues will facilitate discharge from hospital.

Referral to a specialist spinal rehabilitation may be appropriate and has been proved to be effective for MSCC patients (McKinley *et al.*, 1999).

Case study 2: MSCC

Mr D was a 49-year-old civil servant admitted to hospital in May with a 1-month history of progressively worsening back pain, lower-limb weakness, reduced mobility and, on the day of admission, numbness distal to the umbilicus. On admission he was found to have a broad-based ataxic gait. Muscle power of right and left hip flexors and knee extensors was 4/5 with full power at both ankle joints. Reflexes were brisk, planters were down going and sensation was diminished below the level of T9. Joint position sense was assessed as normal.

An MRI scan revealed a solitary lesion at the level of the T7–T8 vertebrae with pedicle involvement and cord compression. He was immediately commenced on high-dose steroids, anticoagulant therapy and put on strict bed rest. The next day he underwent emergency radiotherapy, receiving a course of 5 fractions with a total dose of 20 Gy. On completion of radiotherapy, the neurosurgeon recommended the use of a hyperextension brace to limit spinal movement – this was to be worn at all times. Investigations were performed in order to provide a tissue diagnosis; a biopsy revealed that the mass was metastatic disease from a primary renal tumour. Mr D began chemotherapy 1 month after admission. He was assessed by the physiotherapist on completion of his radiotherapy treatment and was given an individualised muscle-strengthening programme for the lower limbs and began to work on gait re-education. At the time of initial assessment he was independently mobile with the use of a rollator frame. The OT worked on functional tasks and discussed with Mr D about his home environment and any equipment that may be needed. He was unable to go upstairs and downstairs and so following a goal-setting session, adaptation to downstairs living was being planned for. After a period of weekend leave from the ward Mr D complained to the physiotherapist of acute severe back pain in the night 'like it was before I had my treatment' and an inability to get out of bed. Reassessment of muscle power revealed that the left hip flexors were reduced to 2/5, the right hip flexors 3/5 and bilateral knee extensors 3/5. Proprioception was severely compromised. Immediately the findings were reported to the medical team that ordered an urgent rescan. This scan showed progression of the spinal mass. As Mr D had received a maximum cord-tolerant dose of radiotherapy previously, he underwent an emergency laminectomy and transpedicular approach to decompress the tumour mass with immediate reconstruction via fusion and instrumentation. Following the surgery Mr D began to make gradual recovery and improvement with rehabilitation. His hip and knee strength improved to allow facilitated standing in parallel bars. Reduced truncal control and impaired sensation meant that his balance in both sitting and standing was poor. He was able to transfer out of bed to a wheelchair with assistance of one person and a transfer board. Therapy sessions consisted of a mixture of intensive lower-limb muscle-strengthening exercises, balance re-education in sitting, functional activity in sitting, transfer practice and gait re-education. As his sitting balance improved, so too his ability to transfer – achieving independent transfers in 2 weeks. Proprioception and sensation remained poor; however, compensation strategies improved functional activity and gait. Three weeks after surgery he started to work on 'stepping up' on to a 2-in block;

by the end of 5 weeks he was able to climb a mini set of stairs in the gym. Mr D was transferred from the acute hospital to a regional rehabilitation hospital where his rehabilitation continued. Six months after his admission with MSCC Mr D was discharged home fully mobile with a rollator frame, able to climb stairs and was completely independent in all activities of daily living.

Other neurological conditions associated with malignant disease

Peripheral neuropathy

The appearance of a distal, symmetrical neuropathy affecting sensory, motor and autonomic peripheral neurons in chemotherapy patients is well documented in the literature (Visovsky & Daly, 2004). Vinca alkaloids, platinum-based compounds and taxols are the cytotoxic drugs most commonly associated. The extent of neurological damage depends on the drug used, the duration of treatment and the cumulative dose applied (Quasthoff & Hartung, 2002). Consequences for the patient can be distressing and can severely impact on function and quality of life. The exact mechanism of injury is unknown; however, alteration of conductivity of the axon and effect on the Schwann cells are potential causes. Recovery is possible only if the peripheral nervous system has sufficient time to regenerate and repair; often radical chemotherapy regimens do not allow such time and in many cases the neuropathy is only partly reversible. The neuropathy is viewed as an unfortunate but tolerated side effect of radical anticancer treatment. In the palliative situation the detriment to function and quality of life becomes paramount and dose alteration, drug change or cessation of treatment may happen.

Patients may complain of distal paraesthesia, allodynia, hypersensitivity and muscle cramps and weakness as the condition advances. Analgesics such as gabapentin, carbamazepine and amitriptyline may be effective in relieving neuropathic pain. Massage, relaxation and guided imagery techniques may provide relief from uncomfortable sensory disturbance. Rehabilitation aims to relieve pain, strengthen weak muscles, promote movement and function and maximise independence by the provision of adaptive equipment and assistive devices. In addition patients need to be educated about the potential safety risks associated with sensory dysfunction.

Peripheral nervous system metastases

Peripheral nerve involvement of tumour cells can present functional problems for patients. Common sites of peripheral nervous system (PNS) metastases are the cranial nerves, nerve roots and plexi, with problems resulting from direct invasion from local tumour cells, lymphadenopathy and secondary masses. Pain is the predominant complaint with associated weakness and sensory symptoms as the condition deteriorates. In the cervical region pain presents in the neck, shoulders and throat and is exacerbated by movement, coughing or swallowing. Weakness of the neck musculature and related poor posture may add to the patient's problems. Phrenic nerve involvement may result in a paralysed hemidiaphragm causing distressing dyspnoea (Ramchandren & Dalmau, 2005). If the brachial plexus is involved, pain around the neck, shoulder and arm and sensory deficit in the hands can have a significant effect on function. Radiating limb pain, sphincter and leg weakness are characteristic of lumbosacral plexus metastases. Mobility and movement often provoke intense pain.

Metastatic involvement of plexi usually signifies a poor prognosis. Treatment usually involves radiotherapy or chemotherapy to reduce the tumour and relieve pain and multi-modality analgesia, including opiates, regional nerve blocks and non-pharmacological interventions (Ramchandren & Dalmau, 2005). Rehabilitation aimed at relieving pain and maximising functional independence may enhance quality of life.

Leptomeningeal carcinomatosis

This occurs when malignant cells circulating in the CSF lodge in the leptomeninges of the CNS. It can occur whenever CNS metastases are present, though it is more prevalent in breast and lung disease and melanoma. Symptoms include headache, spinal or limb pain, weakness, sensory disturbance and altered mental status (Carmadella, 2002). Once diagnosed, prognosis is poor with death expected within 6 weeks if no treatment is given. The use of radiotherapy and intrathecal chemotherapy offers a prolonged survival of a median 6 months (Carmadella, 2002). Rehabilitation interventions should aim to maximise patient comfort and quality of life by relieving pain and optimising function and mobility, advise and educate carers regarding handling and support of the patient and facilitate discharge to preferred place of care.

Paraneoplastic syndromes

Neurological paraneoplastic syndromes (PNS) are rare, occurring in less than 1% of all cancer patients (Vedeler et al., 2006). They can however cause a variety of cognitive, sensory and motor deficits which can be extremely distressing for the patient and may require input from a variety of AHPs. Their exact cause is unknown, though scientific theories suggest that they are likely to be a consequence of an immune-mediated response to tumour cells resulting in disruption of nerve conduction and motor end-plate function, cellular degeneration and alteration of neurotransmitters (Das et al., 1999). They are most commonly associated with small-cell carcinoma of the lung. Unlike most other complications of cancer, they tend to occur early in the course of the illness and may be the first presentation of malignancy. Management involves identification and treatment of the primary malignancy, intravenous immunoglobulins, plasma exchange and steroids.

As with any neurological condition rehabilitation professionals need to employ a problem-solving approach – identifying patient problems, setting realistic goals and implementing an appropriate treatment plan.

Key learning points

- Neurological malignant diseases have devastating consequences for the patients and their families, resulting in complex physical, functional and cognitive problems, together with profound psychological and emotional distress.
- Many of the problems associated with neurological malignancy are respondent to appropriate rehabilitative intervention, leading to optimised patient performance and maximum quality of life.
- The majority of patients with neuro-oncological disease will have a poor prognosis. In order to maximise outcome, rehabilitation needs to be implemented as a matter of urgency. Continual assessment of the patient is required to adapt and modify rehabilitation programmes to be appropriate to the patients condition.
- The management of physical, functional, cognitive and psychosocial decline and the planning for this decline when working with patients is an important aspect of any therapy programme.

References

American Spinal Injury Association [ASIA] (1996). *International standards for neurological and functional classification of spinal cord injury.* Chicago: American Spinal Injury Association.

Batchelor, T. & DeAngelis, L. M. (1996). Medical management of cerebral metastases. *Neurosurgical Clinics, 7,* 435–436.

Bell, K. R., O'Dell, M. W., Barr, K. & Yablon, S. A. (1998). Rehabilitation of the patient with brain tumour. *Archives of Physical Medicine and Rehabilitation, 1* (79), s37–s46.

Bucholtz, J. D. (1999). Metastatic epidural spinal cord compression. *Seminars in Oncology Nursing, 15* (3), 150–159.

Carmadella, D. (2002). Leptomeningeal carcinomatosis. *Rehabilitation Oncology, 20* (2), 18–19.

Carr, J. (2002). *Metastatic spinal cord compression guidelines* (unpublished). Manchester: Christie Hospital.

Das, A., Hochberg, F. H. & McNelis, S. (1999). A review of the therapy of paraneoplastic neurologic syndromes. *Journal of Neuro-Oncology, 41,* 181–194.

Fisher, S. N. (1998). Multidisciplinary teamwork. In: D. Guerrero (Ed.), *Neuro-oncology for nurses* (pp. 221–252). London: Whurr.

Grant, R. (2004). Overview: brain tumour diagnosis and management/Royal College of Physicians guidelines. *Journal of Neurology Neurosurgery and Psychiatry, 75,* 18–23.

Hacking, H. G. A., Van As, H. H. J. & Lankhorst, G. J. (1993). Factors related to the outcome of inpatient rehabilitation in patients with neoplastic epidural spinal cord compression. *Paraplegia, 31,* 367–374.

Huang, M. E., Cifu, D. X. & Keyser-Marcus, L. (1998). Functional outcome after brain tumour and acute stroke: a comparative analysis. *Archives of Physical Medicine and Rehabilitation, 79,* 1386–1390.

Huang, M. E., Cifu, D. X. & Keyser-Marcus, L. (2000). Functional outcomes in patients with brain tumour after inpatient rehabilitation: comparison with traumatic brain injury. *American Journal of Physical Medicine and Rehabilitation, 79* (4), 327–335.

Huddart, R. A., Rajan, B., Law, M., Meyer, L. & Dearnaley, D. P. (1997). Spinal cord compression in prostate cancer: treatment outcome and prognostic factors. *Radiotherapy and Oncology*, *44*, 229–236.

Husband, D. J. (1998). Malignant spinal cord compression: prospective study of delays in referral and treatment. *British Medical Journal*, *317*, 18–21.

Husband, D. J., Grant, K. A. & Romaniuk, C. S. (2001). MRI in the diagnosis and treatment of suspected malignant spinal cord compression. *British Journal of Radiology*, *74*, 15–23.

Kleihues, P. & Cavanee, W. K. (2000). *World Health Organisation classification of tumours: tumours of the nervous system – pathology and genetics*. Lyon, France: IRAC Press.

Klimo, P., Kestle, J. R. W. & Schmidt, M. H. (2003). Treatment of metastatic spinal epidural disease: a review of the literature. *Neurosurgical Focus*, *15* (5), 1–9.

Kirshblum, S., O'Dell, M. W., Ho, C. & Barr, K. (2001). Rehabilitation of persons with central nervous system tumours. *Cancer*, *92* (4 Suppl), 1029–1038.

Levack, P., Graham, J., Collie, D., Grant, R., Kidd, J., Kunkler, I., Gibson, A., Hurman, D., McMillan, N., Rampling, R., Slider, L., Statham, P. & Summers, D. (2002). Don't wait for a sensory level – listen to the symptoms: a prospective audit of the delays in diagnosis of malignant cord compression. *Clinical Oncology*, *14*, 472–480.

Loblaw, D. A. & Laperriere, N. (1998). Emergency treatment of malignant extra-dural spinal cord compression: evidence-based guideline. *Journal of Clinical Oncology*, *16* (4), 1613–1624.

Mckinley, W. O., Huang, M. E. & Brunsvold, K. T. (1999). Neoplastic versus traumatic spinal cord injury: an outcome comparison after inpatient rehabilitation. *Archives of Physical Medicine and Rehabilitation*, *80* (10), 1253–1257.

National Institute for Clinical Excellence [NICE] (2004). *Improving supportive and palliative care for adults with cancer*. London: National Institute for Clinical Excellence.

National Institute for Health and Clinical Excellence [NICE] (2006). *Improving outcomes for people with brain and other CNS tumours*. London: National Institute for Clinical Excellence.

O'Dell, M. W., Barr, K., Spanier, D. & Warnick, R. (1998). Functional outcome of inpatient rehabilitation in persons with brain tumours. *Archives of Physical Medicine and Rehabilitation*, *79*, 1530–1534.

Pease, N. J., Harris, R. J. & Finlay, I. G. (2004). Development and audit of a care pathway for the management of patients with suspected malignant spinal cord compression. *Physiotherapy*, *90*, 27–34.

Perrin, R. G., Janjan, N. A. & Langford, L. A. (1997). Spinal axis metastases. In: P. Levin (Ed.), *Cancer of the nervous system*. New York: Churchill Livingston

Ramchandren, S. & Dalmau, J. (2005). Metastases to the peripheral nervous system. *Journal of Neuro-Oncology*, *75*, 101–110.

Quasthoff, S. & Hartung, H. P. (2002). Chemotherapy-induced peripheral neuropathy. *Journal of Neurology*, *249*, 9–17.

Quinn, M., Babb, P., Brock, A., Kirby, L. & Jones, J. (2001). *Brain cancer trends in England and Wales 1950–1999: studies on medical and population subjects*, No. 66. London: The Stationary Office.

Snyder, H., Robinson, K., Shah, D., Brennan, R. & Handrigan, M. (1993). Signs and symptoms of patients with brain tumours presenting to the emergency department. *Journal of Emergency Medicine*, *11*, 253–258.

Vedeler, C. A., Antoine, J. C., Giometto, B., Graus, F., Grisold, W., Hart, I. K., Honnorat, J., Sillevis Smitt, P. A. E., Verschuuren, J. J. G. M. & Voltz, R. (2006). Management of paraneoplastic neurological syndromes: report of an EFNS task force. *European Journal of Neurology*, *13*, 682–690.

Visovsky, C. & Daly, B. (2004). Clinical evaluation and patterns of chemotherapy-induced peripheral neuropathy. *Journal of the American Academy of Nurse Practitioners*, *16* (8), 353–359.

White, H. (2004). Acquired communication and swallowing difficulties in patients with primary brain tumours. In: S. Booth & E. Bruera (Eds.), *Palliative care consultations primary and metastatic brain tumours* (pp. 117–134). Oxford: Oxford University Press.

Chapter 6

MULTI-PROFESSIONAL MANAGEMENT WITHIN HAEMATO-ONCOLOGY

Jennifer Miller, Rachel Barrett, Philomena Canning, Sarah Taggart and Val Young

---

Learning outcomes

After studying this chapter, the reader should be able to:

- Discuss the clinical presentation and grading of haemato-oncological malignancies
- Describe the medical management of such malignancies
- Identify the role of each allied health professional within the patient's individual journey
- Implement an evidence-based approach to the therapeutic management of haematological malignancies

---

Introduction

Haemato-oncology is concerned with the diagnosis and treatment of cancers of the blood and lymphatic system, examples of which include myeloma, leukaemia and lymphoma, which collectively account for 8% of cancer diagnoses per annum in the UK (Cancer Research UK, 2006a).

Main types of haemato-oncological conditions

Leukaemia

The four main types of leukaemia are acute myeloid (AML), acute lymphoblastic (ALL), chronic myeloid (CML) and chronic lymphocytic (CLL). In acute leukaemias, the abnormal cells, also referred to as abnormal blasts, are immature and continue to divide after the normal cells have stopped. Whereas in chronic leukaemia, the more mature cells are affected and, due to their abnormality, have a longer lifespan and hence build up to excessively large numbers. Classification of myeloid or lymphocytic leukaemia is determined by cell origin. Myeloid leukaemia, also referred to as myelocytic or myelogenous, originates from myeloid cells, whereas lymphocytic leukaemia develops from lymphocytes or lymphoblasts in the bone marrow (Cancerbackup, 2006).

Lymphoma

Essentially, lymphoma is cancer of the lymphatic system occurring as a result of rapidly multiplying cells within organs such as the spleen, bone marrow, lymph nodes and thymus (Cancer Research UK, 2006b). There are two main types of lymphoma, Hodgkin's and non-Hodgkin's (NHL), which are differentiated by the type of cell that multiplies and how it presents itself (Cancerbackup, 2006).

Myeloma

Myeloma, also known as multiple myeloma or myelomatosis, occurs as a result of abnormal plasma cells being produced in great quantities and therefore impacting on production of platelets, red and white cells within the bone marrow. In addition, myeloma cell proliferation can manifest itself as osteolytic lesions within the skeleton. Solitary lesions, known as plasmacytomas, can require radiotherapy and monitoring, as there is potential for these lesions to progress to multiple myeloma (Cancerbackup, 2006).

Clinical presentation

A variety of signs and symptoms may occur in haemato-oncology to indicate the need for diagnostic tests, including:

- Unusual bleeding, which is due to a reduction in the number of platelets, manifested in bruising, bleeding gums, nose bleeds and heavy periods
- Longevity in healing
- Itching
- Anaemia, which is caused by reduced red blood cells, with the patient presenting as easily fatigued, breathless, tired and pale
- Repeated infections, which are due to a lack of healthy white blood cells resulting in impaired antibody production
- Aching joints and bones
- Weight loss
- Sweating, particularly night sweats
- Pyrexia

- Swollen lymph glands within the neck, armpits and/or groin
- Enlarged spleen

(Cancerbackup, 2006.)

Diagnostic testing

There are a number of investigations within haemato-oncology following presentation of one or more of the previously mentioned symptoms. Blood tests and bone marrow aspirations are routine to confirm the presence of abnormal white blood cells, disease-specific cells as in the cases of myeloma and lymphoma or the Philadelphia chromosome in CML, which is a non-inherited genetic abnormality in most people (Cancerbackup, 2006). In AML, ALL and myeloma, cytogenetic testing may be performed to determine structural changes to the chromosomes of the diseased cells in order to predict prognosis and ensure that the most appropriate course of treatment is given. Additionally, in lymphoma, a lymph node biopsy can be used to confirm diagnosis and in myeloma, urine tests are used to measure kidney function and identify the presence of paraproteins, which are abnormal antibodies that limit production of normal antibodies.

Imaging is commonly used to establish specific location of the disease and metastases. This may include computerised tomography (CT), positron emission tomography (PET), magnetic resonance imaging (MRI) and ultrasound.

Staging/grading

Leukaemia

Each leukaemic disease is classified based on different characteristics and presentation features. For AML, the *French–American–British* (FAB) system is used to grade leukaemia according to the type of cell that has proliferated and its stage of maturation on a scale of 0–7.

In ALL, classification is based on whether the leukaemia is of B or T lymphocyte lineage. Indicators of B lineage will be exhibited as 'B symptoms', which commonly include night sweats, weight loss and unexplained fevers. Additionally, within ALL, grading occurs through using the FAB system whereby L1–3 indicates the maturation of the lymphoblasts.

CML is challenging to stage due to the widespread nature of the disease, although it is still necessary for the purpose of treatment planning to determine which one of three phases the patient is in: chronic, accelerated or blast. The amount of blast cells in the bone marrow and blood are measured and their appearance analysed to establish the phase.

CLL is commonly classified using one of two systems. The Rai staging system stages the disease on a scale of 0–4, depending on involvement of the nodes, liver and spleen, with stage 0 having the greater median survival. The Binet system uses the letters A–C, again depending on the number of enlarged lymph nodes and platelet level (Leukaemia Research Foundation, 2007).

Lymphoma

The World Health Organization (WHO) system classifies lymphoma dependent on:

- Morphology, which is the appearance of the cells under the microscope.
- Immunohistochemistry, the use of stains to identify the presence of certain substances.
- Whether the lymphoma is of B or T lymphocyte lineage. Indicators of B lineage will be exhibited as 'B symptoms', which commonly include night sweats, weight loss and unexplained fevers.

Hodgkin's lymphoma is further classified as:

- Stage I – one group of lymph nodes affected
- Stage II – two or more groups of lymph nodes affected on the same side of the diaphragm
- Stage III – nodes on both sides of the diaphragm affected
- Stage IV – other parts of the body, outside of the lymphatic system, affected

NHL is graded as high or low grade, with high-grade lymphoma requiring prompt treatment due to the rapid speed at which it grows (Cancer Research UK, 2006b).

Myeloma

Myeloma is commonly staged using the *Durie–Salmon system*, which considers bone structure, calcium levels, haemoglobin (Hb), monoclonal proteins and paraproteins. Stages 1–3 indicate that the myeloma is at an early, intermediate or advanced stage, respectively, and the disease is further classified by normal (A) or abnormal (B) renal kidney function (Cancer Research UK, 2006b).

Treatment

Conventional treatment needs to be aggressive in order to achieve remission. Single-agent or combination chemotherapy is generally the main form of treatment alongside steroids and, less frequently, radiotherapy. For some patients a bone marrow transplant (BMT) or peripheral blood stem cell transplant (PBSCT) involving high-dose chemotherapy and, at times, total body irradiation (TBI) is used (Cancer Research UK, 2006b).

The aim of treatment is dependent on the type and stage of the disease, ranging from cure in leukaemia to maximising quality of life during a disease-free period of time

Table 6.1 Side effects of treatment modalities impacting on physical abilities, nutritional status, and psychosocial well-being (Cancer backup 2006).

Poor appetite
Anorexia
Weight loss
Nausea and vomiting
Early satiety (feeling of fullness)
Abdominal pain/cramping
Profuse watery diarrhoea
Constipation
Hyposmia/dysosmia (loss, or distorted sense, of smell)
Dry mouth
Salivary changes
Taste changes
Bleeding – oral cavity
Respiratory infections, i.e. para-influenza, cytomegalovirus (CMV)
Oral infections, i.e. candida
Oesophagitis
Gastritis
Severe mucositis (mouth – anus)
Dysphagia
Odnophagia (pain on swallowing)
Neutropenia (±infection, sepsis)
Multiple oral medications
Prolonged isolation – low mood
Food aversions
Extreme fatigue and lethargy
Graft-versus-host disease
Hepatic veno-occlusive disease
Atypical infections, i.e. tuberculosis, CMV and pneumonitis
Neutropenic sepsis
Pulmonary fibrosis

in myeloma. There are numerous disease- and treatment-related side effects that may exhibit themselves within haemato-oncology and this has implications for the individual's physical abilities, nutritional status and psychosocial well-being (Table 6.1).

Chemotherapy

Often referred to as the induction phase of treatment, chemotherapy is given in the majority of cases, with exception of those conditions such as low-grade lymphomas that may be monitored on a 'watchful waiting' basis. As treatment is commonly intensive, chemotherapy may be administered via a central line, e.g. a peripherally inserted central catheter , port-a-cath or Hickman line, and orally (Cancer Research UK, 2006b).

Radiotherapy

Radiotherapy may be a treatment option for those who exhibit areas of localised disease or require prophylactic radiotherapy secondary to chemotherapy, as the latter is unable to pass through the blood–brain barrier to the brain, spine or testes. TBI may also be used to destroy bone marrow cells. Radiotherapy may also be used to prevent or relieve symptoms of spinal cord compression or potential fractures (Cancer Research UK, 2006b).

Steroid treatment

Steroids can be given to enhance the effectiveness of chemotherapy and limit the proliferation of cancer cells through the steroid's ability to deceive the pituitary gland into switching off the adrenal glands, as it perceives enough hormones are being produced (Cancerbackup, 2006).

Biological therapy

Biological therapies, also known as immunotherapies, include monoclonal anti-bodies, e.g. rituximab, interferon and thalidomide. This group of drugs contains substances found naturally within the body, but the dosage amounts are greater. The purpose is to eliminate cancer cells by limiting their growth and differentiation (Cancer Research UK, 2006b).

Transplant

Stem cell transplants are performed to enable the use of higher doses of treatment (conditioning regimen), which may include both high-dose chemotherapy and/or TBI and are known as mini and full transplants respectively. There are two types of transplants: autologous or autograft, which is where the patient's own stem cells or bone marrow are used, and allogeneic or allograft, where stem cells or bone marrow are donated from another person, usually a sibling. If somebody other than a sibling donates, this is referred to as a matched unrelated donor (MUD). Patients undergoing high-dose chemotherapy will often be in isolation because of the risk of infection (Cancerbackup, 2006).

Graft-versus-host disease (GvHD) may develop post-allograft when the graft (new cells) reacts against the host (patient's tissue) (Cancerbackup, 2006). Severity of the GvHD is indicated by the extent to which the skin, liver and gut are affected and can occur acutely (within 100 days) or chronically (after 100 days post-transplant). Common symptoms of acute GvHD may include jaundice, skin blistering or rash and diarrhoea, while in the chronic stage stiff joints and dry mouth generally occur. Although at its most advanced it can cause irreversible damage to major organs and even death, GvHD is not necessarily a sign of a failed transplant and in some cases can instead be indicative of a graft-versus-leukaemic effect (GvL) whereby the patient's immune system attacks remaining cancer cells (Cancer Research UK, 2006b).

Surgery

Due to the nature of haemato-oncological malignancies, surgical options for treatment are extremely limited. Debulking surgery may occasionally be used in NHL if there is a tumour within the abdomen. Although other procedures such as lymph node biopsies are carried out, this is more for the purpose of diagnosis as opposed to treatment (Cancer Research UK, 2006b).

Supportive therapy

Supportive therapies assist in controlling the symptoms of haemato-oncological conditions; examples include blood transfusions, plasma exchange, platelet transfusions, donor lymphocyte infusions and the administration of growth factors. Additionally, electrolyte repletion, pain control and the management of gastrointestinal (GI) symptoms may be necessary. In some cases, patients may require admission to intensive care or the high-dependency unit to assist in the management of severe side effects such as GvHD, neutropenic sepsis and respiratory infections.

Allied health professionals' involvement in the management of the haemato-oncological patient

The availability of site-specific specialist allied health professionals (AHPs) in cancer care is often limited even in tertiary referral centres; however, this is changing. As the role of the multidisciplinary team continues to evolve beyond doctors and nurses to incorporate AHPs, the knowledge and expertise of such teams is invaluable to the both medical management and care of all patients, particularly in those with haemato-oncological malignancies.

Haemato-oncology patients benefit from early and continued input, ideally in the form of pre-assessment from the physiotherapist, dietitian and occupational therapist. The role of the psychologist, speech and language therapist and complementary therapists must also be recognised. It is also vital to consider the support needed by relatives, friends, especially sibling donors, as well as the patient throughout their journey. These interventions may also be available locally within both the health and voluntary sectors.

Interprofessional working significantly enhances the patient's experience and promotes quality patient care in an era of decreased resources and enhanced expectations (Lindeke & Sieckert, 2005). Of particular importance is the role of the key worker (often the clinical nurse specialist), who acts as a central point of contact for both the patient and their relatives during treatment.

Cognition

Cognitive deficits can occur both as a symptom of disease and as a potential treatment-related side effect, particularly during transplant (De Brabander *et al.*, 2000). They can be acute or chronic and require the interventions of the clinical psychologist, occupational therapist or speech and language therapist. Reduced attention span and a decline in speed of information processing may occur as a result of fatigue or lability (Wagner & Cella, 2004) and patients should be encouraged to minimise distractions when participating in their chosen activities.

Pathological fractures and spinal cord compression

In myeloma, plasma cells infiltrate the bone and bone marrow in a patchy manner, presenting as a focal tumour mass. These tumours have osteolytic properties and eventually erode the bone resulting in skeletal abnormalities (lytic lesions) in two-thirds of patients with resultant pain (Souhami & Tobias, 1998). Patients are then predisposed to pathological fractures or vertebral collapse (with loss of height) and these are often the first noticeable symptoms of multiple myeloma (Claytor, 1999).

Pathological fractures can be debilitating for patients and are generally immobilised or surgically fixed. These patients require advice on gentle mobilisation (as permitted by the orthopaedic consultant) and will need exercises to increase muscle strength in the affected area and/or rehabilitation. They may also require advice on adaptive techniques, equipment or specialist seating and positioning. Spinal cord compression can be a distressing consequence of vertebral collapse in myeloma and requires specialist management (see Chapter 5).

Nutritional management

Although patients with haemato-oncological malignancies rarely present with malnutrition and cachexia, the onset of high-intensity treatments often means that nutritional status is easily compromised at the early stages of treatment (Table 6.1). Those patients likely to need early and more frequent dietetic input include those diagnoses where medical management is more intensive, such as ALL, AML, and high-grade lymphomas. Assessment and application of appropriate nutritional support is an important component of the overall treatment programme (Aldamiz-Echerarria *et al.*, 1996).

Unintentional weight loss of $\geq 10\%$ within the previous 6 months signifies a substantial nutritional deficit, and optimum nutrition improves tolerance to treatment and outcome in such patients (Arends *et al.*, 2006; Rivadeneira *et al.*, 1998). In addition, metabolic abnormalities, particularly during PBSCT, have been reported (Barerra, 2002).

Since the majority of patients diagnosed with haemato-oncological malignant disease will become immunocompromised, implementation of a neutropenic or 'clean diet' can assist in minimising the risk of infection during treatment (see Table 6.2).

Table 6.2 Recommended diet associated with grade of neutropenia (Rees, 2005).

Neutropenia
    Neutrophil count 2.0-0.5 $\times$ 10^9/L and other neutropenic at-risk groups
    Food safety and handling advice and avoidance of high-risk foods
Profound neutropenia
    Neutrophil count <0.5 $\times$ 10^9/L
    Food safety and handling advice and clean diet advice

Food-borne infection can be avoided by eliminating any potential source of bacteria or fungi by omitting those foods and drinks that are a potential source. Although the healthy immune system can manage a variety of bacteria, the compromised immune system cannot. Due to the high levels of bacterial and/or fungal contamination such as coliforms and listeria in commercially bottled mineral water (Hunter, 1993), freshly run tap water (Rees, 2005) or filtered water (Hall *et al.*, 2004) is the recommended fluid of choice.

To date there is no clear consensus on clean diets, and the lack of clinical evidence is demonstrated by implementation at different stages of treatment, varying levels of restriction and no standard of practice (Hartkopf Smith & Besser, 2000). Dietary restrictions in patients who are unwell will further compromise nutritional status and increase morbidity and mortality. Whilst the source of infections is often undetected in the septic neutropenic patient, these infections are considered to arise primarily from the GI tract, i.e. *Escherichia coli* and *Pseudomonas aeruginosa* (Hughes *et al.*, 2002; Risi & Tomascak, 1998). Bacterial translocation is of great importance, especially if peristaltic action is not maintained due to poor oral intake.

Consideration should be given to the relaxation of previous dietary advice, i.e. diabetes mellitus and lipid lowering, for this patient group. Food fortification should be considered where possible, as oral intake is often limited and taste changes apparent. Interference of normal foods and fluids should be limited to maximise palatability. Dietary advice to aid symptom control, such as nausea and dry mouth, is also of value alongside appropriate pharmacological interventions. Consistency modification to liquids, puree, soft or mashed foods can also benefit those with dry, sore mouths or mucositis.

With its associated GI complications, BMT may result in varying degrees of nutritional depletion (Papadopoulou *et al.*, 1996). Nutritional support is frequently delivered routinely after BMT to prevent malnutrition or to meet increased nutrient requirements (Muscaritoli *et al.*, 2002). Malnutrition may be either secondary to GI toxicity or related to the conditioning regimen. Recovery to full health and improved appetite can take up to a year, particularly in those who have undergone an allograft (Henry, 1997); therefore, comprehensive nutritional assessment is necessary to ensure early recognition of malnutrition and both appropriate and timely dietetic interventions.

The use of oral nutritional supplements (ONS) can be effective, although it is most useful in chemotherapy or in those undergoing autograft. Taste fatigue, secondary to long-term ONS use, along with the side effects of disease and/or treatment as discussed in Table 6.1 can impact on the ability to tolerate ONS.

There has been increasing use of enteral nutrition (EN) due to recent advances in BMT such as 'mini-allografting' and the use of PBSCTs, resulting in reduced duration of neutropenia and mucosal toxicity. Advantages include stimulation of intestinal recovery, reduction of cholestasis and bacteraemia by maintaining GI function (Papadopoulou *et al.*, 1997). Gastric stasis (delayed gastric emptying) can often occur and a nasojejunal (NJ) tube maybe preferable to a nasogastric (NG) tube.

Prophylactic NG or NJ tube placement from admission up until day +1 post-stem-cell return should be considered for allogeneic transplants and should ideally be placed no later than day +4 due to severity of mucositis and with platelets $>20 \times 10^9$/L, to reduce the risk of haemorrhage. Some centres are starting to use more long-term feeding tubes, i.e. percutaneous endoscopy gastrostomy/jejunostomy, particularly in paediatrics and young adults, but there is a clear need for early insertion prior to treatment to allow for adequate healing.

If EN is not possible or poorly tolerated, parenteral nutrition (PN) via a dedicated lumen is needed, although there is a paucity of evidence comparing the relative effectiveness of EN and PN (Murray & Pindoria, 2004). PN is easy to administer (central line in situ), provides a reliable delivery of nutrients and is easier to modulate fluid and electrolyte balance. A triple-lumen central line should be placed prophylactically in all patients undergoing full TBI-based and MUD transplants due to the increase risk and severity of mucositis. There is suggestion that PN delays resumption of oral intake in patients (Charuhas et al., 1997) and is associated with increases in cost, days of diuretic use, hyperglycaemia and sepsis (Szeluga et al., 1987).

Exercise and activity tolerance

Treatments used in the management of haemato-oncological conditions have been shown to reduce patients' exercise levels (Courneya & Friedenreich, 1999) and induce fatigue (National Institute for Clinical Excellence, 2003). Reduced physical performance is a universal problem (Dimeo et al., 1997a) and is mainly attributed to deconditioning due to lack of exercise whilst in isolation (Dimeo et al., 2003). Muscle wasting is common and steroid therapy further increases the risk of muscle weakness and osteoporosis (Coleman et al., 2003). Chemotherapy-induced peripheral neuropathy (Stillman & Cata, 2006) can affect functioning and may require a range of interventions to optimise independence. These symptoms can last for months or even years and can cause difficulty in resuming normal activity (Dimeo et al., 1997b) and work and family roles, ultimately affecting quality of life (Fobair et al., 1986).

Two evidence reviews have shown that exercise programmes can be beneficial in reducing fatigue, regaining physical function and improving quality of life (Galvao & Newton, 2005; Knols et al., 2005). Physiotherapists are well placed to prescribe individualised exercise which can often be the only activity that makes these patients feel 'normal' (James, 1987) and gives them back a sense of control (Holtzman, 1988). Decisions about the level of exercise in which the patient participates must be made using the results of laboratory blood tests and the patient's vital signs (Sayre & Marcoux, 1992). It is generally accepted that platelet levels should be above 20×10^9/L for gentle exercises on the ward and above 50×10^9/L for an increase in physical activity involving resistance, thus limiting the likelihood of bleeds, particularly cerebrally (Zavadsky, 2001). Before mobilising patients outside of their rooms, neutrophil levels should be greater than 0.5×10^9/L in order to avoid exposure to infection (Sayre & Marcoux, 1992). In addition, it is important to be aware of the patient's haemoglobin levels. If these levels are low, patients may be breathless, fatigued or dizzy and therefore they may need to be monitored more closely or may need their treatment modified. Normal values are 13.0–18.0 g/dL (male) and

Table 6.3 Summary of physiotherapy involvement during transplant or high-dose chemotherapy.

Platelets must be greater than $20 \times 10(9)/L$
Exercises for major muscle groups
Static bicycle in room
Mobilise out of room if neutrophils $>0.5 \times 10^9/L$

$11.5–16.5$ g/dL (female) (Provan & Krentz, 2004). Table 6.3 summarises the physiotherapy involvement during transplant and high-dose chemotherapy.

Following assessment, physiotherapists can begin the rehabilitation process by providing suitable exercises to improve strength, range of movement, flexibility and balance. In the initial stages the patient may be in isolation. Exercises will include strengthening of all major muscle groups and may include stretch bands to provide resistance to movement, marching on the spot and exercising on a static bicycle if possible. It is essential that a written sheet detailing the exercises be given to the patient in order to aid compliance.

When patients are allowed out of isolation they can be advised to walk for a set distance or time period with a mobility aid if necessary. This type of exercise is amenable to the majority of patients, is functional and can be administered as an inpatient or outpatient. Patients going home after lengthy admissions often find that they feel weak climbing stairs, and it is beneficial to practice stairs prior to discharge. It should be noted that all patients must be monitored regularly to ensure that their exercise level is still safe, appropriate and is achieving the desired effect. If discharged patients still find it difficult to return to their normal level of functioning, they should be referred to physiotherapy for advice and exercise.

Fatigue management

Fatigue is a significant side effect for the majority of oncology patients (Ahlberg *et al.*, 2003) and this is certainly the case specifically within haematology. The occupational therapist and physiotherapist can work with the patient to educate them on fatigue management techniques as a means of conserving energy and maximising participation in valued activities. The provision of equipment to eliminate excessive bending and twisting during personal and domestic activities of daily living may also be necessary (see Chapter 12 for further details).

Psychological support

The psychological impact of an extended period of time in isolation is well documented within the literature, which results in familial separation and role changes (Parkinson, 2006). Stress management techniques and psychological support can be particularly beneficial to patients at this time as they come to terms with their diagnosis and experience a variety of different emotions. This may be delivered in the forms of pastoral care, relaxation, art therapy and massage. Relaxation in particular has been shown to have a positive effect on the psychological experience of living with cancer, particularly relating to anxiety and stress management (Cheung *et al.*, 2003; Leubbert *et al.*, 2001) and decreasing depression (Sloman, 2002).

Discharge

Although patients will generally look forward to returning home, it can be an anxious time. Discharge home following an intensive admission can be destabilising for both patients and their families or carers, especially if the patient is unable to resume normal activities as quickly as expected. This can have an enormous impact on emotional well-being. It can also be a time of great concern as the patient's immunity to infection will still be compromised, and there is continued opportunity for side effects like GvHD to arise. Patients will be encouraged to use their key worker as a point of contact if any problems or concerns arise and the multidisciplinary team is likely to have continued involvement as described later on this chapter.

Sometimes, equipment or a package of care may be provided either on a temporary or permanent basis to facilitate optimal safety and independence in functional activities, mobility and transfers which may be compromised by muscle weakness, myelopathy or bone disease.

Post-transplant

Some centres are able to provide supervised circuit training for haemato-oncological patients, out patients once or twice a week. Regimes consist of a mixture of aerobic exercise and resisted exercise, with patients encouraged to improve performance by keeping a performance chart. Once patients have attended for a predetermined period of time, they are encouraged to return to their previous activity level and attend their local gyms. The aim of providing this type of service is to enable patients to have confidence in developing their own activity regime and to feel able to return to work. It also provides social contact and peer support. It should be noted that this type of intervention is not suitable for patients with anaemia, neutropenia, thrombocytopenia, metastatic bone and brain disease or other health problems preventing exercise. These patients should be assessed individually and provided with appropriate exercise advice.

Research following transplant has so far concentrated on the benefits of aerobic exercise (Dimeo *et al.*, 1997b), but reduced activity following cancer and its treatment can also result in muscle wasting, restricting the ability to perform aerobically. Hayes *et al.* (2004) examine the role of a mixed type of moderate intensity exercise programme in the recovery of patients after PBSCT using aerobic exercise together with a resistance exercise programme. Twelve participants were allocated to either a control group or an aerobic exercise group, and measurements of muscular strength and average peak aerobic capacity were used as outcome measures. Whilst the control group did not demonstrate any improvements in the outcome measures, the experimental group experienced significant improvements in aerobic capacity and body strength, which showed continual improvement when they were reassessed 3 months post-experiment. They concluded that participation in this type of exercise

Table 6.4 Main points for outpatient physiotherapy programme following transplant or high-dose chemotherapy

Platelets greater than 50×10^9/L
Neutrophil levels appropriate for mixing with public
Start with a warm-up and finish with cool down and stretches
Concentrate on aerobic and strengthening exercises
Keep a performance chart
Use a recommended outcome measure, e.g. 6-min walking test
Aim to return patients to previous activities or public leisure centre

programme can bridge the gap between the end of cancer treatment and a return to normal life.

Whilst evidence indicates that it would be appropriate to provide supervised exercise-based rehabilitation programmes for oncology patients (see Table 6.4), few hospitals are able to offer this. A postal survey by Stevinson and Fox (2005) found that 19 hospitals in the UK offered some kind of exercise programme or class for all oncology patients. A feasibility study found that group-based exercise rehabilitation intervention was feasible to operate and of benefit to patients (Stevinson & Fox, 2006).

In addition to the physical benefits of post-transplant rehabilitation, specific programmes incorporating the multidisciplinary team can provide the patient with peer support and the opportunity to discuss any concerns or problems that may arise post-discharge with the appropriate professional.

Returning to work and other chosen occupations

Demanding treatment regimes, regular hospital appointments, fatigue and low resistance to infection make it challenging for this patient group to continue with, or return to, either their paid employment or other chosen occupation. Practical solutions can include a referral to the social worker for advice on benefits, which is particularly helpful for those patients who are the main breadwinner. The occupational therapist can play a significant role in vocational rehabilitation by advising about work-life balance and assisting the patient in structuring a graded return to work in collaboration with the employer. Whilst work can help maintain a sense of normality, some patients may cease work either through personal choice or because of necessity and they should be made aware of support agencies to assist them in dealing with the emotional and financial implications that this may have.

Death and dying

Despite the advances in treatment options within haemato-oncology, there are still approximately 14 250 mortalities per annum in the UK (Cancer Research UK, 2006b). Although the preferred place of death for 56% of patients is home, in reality only 25% of cancer patients achieve this (Higginson, 2003). If discharge home for terminal care is feasible, there is a significant role for the discharge coordinator, occupational therapist and other members of the multidisciplinary team as appropriate, to organise essential equipment and liaise with community services to enable a smooth transition from hospital to home.

Case study 1: Mrs J

Age: 56
Diagnosis: Stage IIIB diffuse large B-cell lymphoma

Medical history
Mrs J presented to her general practitioner with backache, tiredness and weight loss. Blood tests indicated altered biochemistry, and Mrs J was referred to a haematologist, where further testing in the form of a CT scan showed lymphadenopathy in the para-aortic, mediastinal and celiac axis region, in addition to a right pleural effusion.

Social history
Mrs J is married with no children, and works as a shop assistant. She describes herself as leading an active lifestyle.

Treatment and multidisciplinary management
Mrs J commenced a combination of immunotherapy and chemotherapy. However, following the first cycle of chemotherapy she developed oedema to her lower abdomen and an increase in her right pleural effusion. On referral to physiotherapy and occupational therapy the problems highlighted were poor mobility, fatigue and shortness of breath on exertion. While physiotherapy focused on assessment of muscle strength, mobility and transfers, the occupational therapist completed a personal care assessment, encouraging Mrs J to use energy conservation techniques.

At this point, a CT scan showed a partial response of the lymphoma to chemotherapy.

After the second cycle of chemotherapy, Mrs J was transferred to the critical care unit (CCU) with acute pulmonary oedema, myocardial infarction and septicaemia, where she required ventilation and inotropic support. Multidisciplinary management included respiratory intervention by the physiotherapist and introduction of EN by the dietitian to maintain nutritional status.

Following discharge from CCU, Mrs J was referred to the occupational therapist for anxiety-related symptoms. Anxiety patterns were discussed with Mrs J, and techniques such as breathing control and challenging negative thoughts were identified as strategies, in addition to regular relaxation sessions. The clinical psychologist further supported this.

Mrs J was motivated to increase her levels of independence and so weekly goals were set. The aims underpinning treatment were:

• Fatigue management to optimise functional independence
• To increase stamina and strength, diminished as a result of prolonged bed rest
• Monitor and optimise nutritional needs
• Safe and optimally independent discharge

Following one further cycle of chemotherapy, Mrs J was discharged home. Despite ongoing fatigue, bilateral oedema and pleural effusion, she was independent with personal care, mobilising safely and independently on the level and upstairs/downstairs and was managing a good dietary intake.

Mrs J had two further cycles of chemotherapy after which a CT revealed progressive disease to such an extent that there were no further treatment options and a palliative approach was taken. Unfortunately, she was admitted to the palliative care ward with dyspnoea, which was controlled with the use of oxygen, medication and intervention from physiotherapy and occupational therapy, addressing mobility within the confines of breathlessness and increasing fatigue, positioning and facilitating discharge.

Discharge planning was lengthy and Mrs J was banded as requiring National Health Service's continuing care due to the complexity of her needs, limited prognosis and palliative nature of the disease. The occupational therapist undertook a joint access visit with the district nurse to assess the environment for provision of a hospital bed which was based on the ground floor of her house. She received four calls per day, in addition to ongoing support from the district and Macmillan nurses in the form of symptom control and emotional support for her husband and family as her needs changed.

Case study 2: Mr W

Age: 59
Diagnosis: AML

Medical history

Mr W was diagnosed with AML in March 2003. He presented to his general practitioner with unusual markings on his legs and feeling generally achy. The doctor initially diagnosed erythema nodosum, which he was confident would clear up without any treatment; however, a chest X-ray and blood tests were also requested. Unfortunately, these tests demonstrated depleted platelets and red and white blood cells, and a bone marrow confirmed a diagnosis of AML.

Social history

Mr W is a 59-year-old previously fit married man. He is married with three grown-up children and is a retired naval officer.

Treatment and multidisciplinary management

He was admitted for combination chemotherapy and suffered significant complications, including tuberculosis (TB). He continued to lose weight, struggling with both his chemotherapy and his TB treatment and was referred to both physiotherapy and dietetics for advice.

NJ feeding was commenced due to continued nausea, weight loss and poor oral intake. His mobility was assessed and he was unsteady on his feet, requiring a walking stick and general exercises to increase activity. He was encouraged to walk around the ward to maintain functional activity and developed a circuit using nearby corridors with support from his wife.

At this point he was in remission from AML; however, the treatment for TB took over 6 months to complete. He was eventually discharged home on overnight NJ feeding and continued walking regularly on the flat to build up stamina and strength. His appetite and strength improved over the following weeks, his feeding tube was removed and he was able to undertake normal daily activities.

In December 2004, after 15 months in remission, he relapsed with limited treatment options. A compassionate case was made for combination chemotherapy, which was on trial in America, and treatment with this resulted in remission. A matched unrelated donor PBSCT was planned; however, just before transplant he relapsed again, requiring further clofarabine, and was eventually admitted for transplant in January 2006.

During transplant both a physiotherapist and a dietitian assessed him. The physiotherapist provided a range of exercises to do whilst in isolation. These consisted of leg exercises, theraband for arm exercises and a static bicycle in the transplant room. He was encouraged to take control of these exercises himself.

Nutritional support during transplant was discussed at the multidisciplinary team meeting and it was agreed that the conditioning regimen, which consisted of busulphan, fludarabine and Campath, was unlikely to cause severe mucositis. In addition, the patient was very motivated to comply with dietetic advice, so an elective feeding tube was not placed. Despite high motivation and nutritional sip feeds, he lost 13% of his body weight over a month, reflecting both muscle and adipose tissue loss, which is clinically significant and required nutritional support. Contributing factors included nausea, fatigue, reduced activity and episodes of sepsis/infection.

Although his general condition was improving slowly, his mood remained low. It became clear that he had been thinking about his diagnosis and treatment in the isolation of his side room and was now becoming increasingly concerned about his family's finances. He was the sole breadwinner in the family and was missing seeing his family. Subsequently, he was referred to the social worker for benefits advice and a counsellor to discuss his feelings of anxiety.

The occupational therapist addressed fatigue management with Mr W in preparation for his discharge home. This focused specifically on prioritising the activities he enjoyed and also learning to pace himself during personal care activities as he has a tendency to rush them.

He was discharged in February 2006 and attempted to improve his stamina by walking on the flat and then gradually hills. Following discharge his weight remained stable, appetite improved and nutritional sip feeds were subsequently stopped.

Still experiencing difficulty in regaining fitness levels he was referred to physiotherapy for gym circuit sessions in May 2006. The circuit consists of a treadmill, static bicycle, workstation and step-ups. His goal was to achieve 10-min running on the treadmill. After 3 months of attending the gym, twice weekly, he achieved this and now attends his own gym, as he did prior to becoming ill.

Summary

In summary, the AHP plays an important role in the management of patients undergoing treatment for haemato-oncological malignancies, including assessment prior to, during and after all treatment modalities. It is vital to recognise the numerous factors that affect nutritional, physical and psychological status, particularly as a result of such treatments, and address them as appropriate, without disregarding the importance of the involvement of the patient's family, friends and carers, to ensure a holistic approach.

Key learning points

• The intensive medical management of haemato-oncological malignances means there is a real need for input from AHPs to optimise functional recovery.
• Input is appropriate from pre- to post-treatment due to the physical presentation and consequent functional deficits that this particular group of patients experiences.
• Complications as a result of the disease and treatment may result in changing needs of the patient, requiring flexibility.

References

Ahlberg, K. M., Ekman, T., Gaston-Johansson, F. & Mock, V. (2003). Assessment and management of cancer-related fatigue in adults. *Lancet, 362* (9384), 640–650.

Aldamiz-Echerarria, L., Bachiller, M. P., Ariz, M. C., Gimenez, A., Barcia, M. J. & Marin, M. (1996). Continuous versus cyclic parenteral nutrition during bone marrow transplantation: assessment and follow up. *Clinical Nutrition, 15*, 333–336.

Arends, J., Bodoky, G., Bozzetti, F., Fearon, K., Muscaritoli, M., Selga, G., van Bokhorst-de Van Der Schueren, M. A. E., von Meyenfeldt, M., Zurcher, G., Fietkau, R., Aulbert, E., Frick, B., Holm, M., Kneba, M., Mestrom, H. J. & Zander, A. (2006). ESPEN guidelines enteral nutrition: non-surgical oncology. *Clinical Nutrition, 25*, 245–259.

Barerra, R. (2002). Nutritional support in cancer patients. *JPEN, 26* (5), S63–S71.

Cancerbackup (2006). [Online]. Retrieved 7 November 2006 from http://www.cancerbackup.org.uk

Cancer Research UK (2006a). *Statistics on the most commonly diagnosed types of cancer in the UK* [online]. Retrieved 7 November 2006 from http://info.cancerresearchuk.org/cancerstats/types/? %20a=5441

Cancer Research UK (2006b). [Online]. Retrieved 15 November 2006 from http://www.cancerresearchuk.org

Charuhas, P. M., Fosberg, K. L., Bruemmer, B., Aker, S. N., Leisenring, W., Seidel, K. & Sullivan, K. M. (1997). A double-blind randomised trial comparing outpatient parenteral nutrition with intravenous hydration: effect on resumption of oral intake after marrow transplantation. *JPEN, 21* (3), 157–161.

Cheung, Y. L., Molassiotis, A. & Chang, A. M. (2003). The effect of progressive muscle relaxation training on anxiety and quality of life after stoma surgery in colorectal cancer patients. *Psychooncology, 12*, 254–266.

Claytor, R. (1999). Multiple myeloma. *Rehabilitation Oncology, 17* (2), 14–17.

Coleman, E. A., Coon, S., Hall-Barrow, J., Richards, K, Gaylor, D. & Stewart, B. (2003). Feasibility of exercise during treatment for multiple myeloma. *Cancer Nursing, 26* (5), 410–419.

Courneya, K. S. & Friedenreich, C. M. (1999). Physical exercise and quality of life following cancer diagnosis: a literature review. *Annals of Behavioral Medicine, 21*, 171–179.

De Brabander, C., Cornelissen, J., Sillevis Smitt, P. A., Vecht, M. J. & van den Bent, M. J. (2000). Increased incidence of neurological complications in patients receiving allogenic bone marrow transplantation from alternative donors. *Journal of Neurology, Neurosurgery and Psychiatry, 68*, 36–40.

Dimeo, F., Fetscher, S., Lange, W., Merterlsmann, R. & Keul, J. (1997a). Effects of aerobic exercise on the physical performance and incidence of treatment related complications after high dose chemotherapy. *Blood, 90*, 3390–3394.

Dimeo, F., Schwartz, S., Fietz, T., Wanjua, T., Boning, D. & Thiel, E. (2003). Effects of endurance training on the physical performance of patients with haematological malignancies during chemotherapy. *Support Care Cancer, 11*, 623–628.

Dimeo, F., Tilmann, M., Bertz, H., Kanz, L., Mertelsmann, R. & Keul, J. (1997b). Aerobic exercise in the rehabilitation of cancer patients after high dose chemotherapy and autologous peripheral stem cell transplantation. *Cancer, 79*, 1717–1722.

Fobair, P., Hoppe, R. T. & Bloom, J. (1986). Psychosocial problems among survivals of Hodgkin's disease. *Journal of Clinical Oncology, 4*, 805–814.

Galvao, D. A. & Newton, R. U. (2005). Review of exercise intervention studies in cancer patients. *Journal of Clinical Oncology, 23* (4), 899–909.

Hall, J., Hodgson, G. & Kerr, K. G. (2004). Provision of safe potable water for immunocompromised patients in hospital. *Hospital Infection, 58* (2), 155–158.

Hartkopf Smith, L. & Besser, S. (2000). Dietary restrictions for patients with neutropenia: a survey of institutional practices. *Oncology Nursing Forum, 27,* 515–520.

Hayes, S. C, Davies, P. S., Parker, T. W., Bashford, J. & Green, A. (2004). Role of a mixed type, moderate intensity exercise programme after peripheral blood stem cell transplantation. *British Journal of Sports Medicine, 38,* 304–309.

Henry, L. (1997). Immunocompromised patients and nutrition. *Professional Nurse, 12* (9), 655–659.

Higginson, I. (2003). *Priorities and preferences for end of life care.* London: National Council for Hospice and Specialist Palliative Care Settings.

Holtzman, L. S. (1988). Physical therapy intervention following bone marrow transplantation. *Clinical Management, 8* (2), 6–9.

Hughes, W. T., Armstrong, D., Bodey, G. P., Bow, E. J, Brown, A. E., Calandra, T., Field, R., Pizzo, P. A., Rolston K. V. I., Shenep, J. L. & Young L. S. (2002). Guidelines for the use of antimicrobial agents in neutropenic agents in neutropenic patients with cancer. *Clinical Infectious Diseases, 34,* 730–751.

Hunter, P. R. (1993). The microbiology of bottled natural mineral waters. *Journal of Applied Bacteriology, 74* (4), 345–352.

James, M. C. (1987). Physical therapy for patients after bone marrow transplantation. *Physical Therapy, 67* (6), 946–952.

Knols, R., Aaronson, N. K., Uebelhart, D., Fransen, J. & Aufdemkampe, G. (2005). Physical exercise in cancer patients during and after medical treatment: a systematic review of randomized and controlled trials. *Journal of Clinical Oncology, 23* (16), 3830–3842.

Leubbert, K., Dahme, B. & Hasenbring, M. (2001). The effectiveness of training in reducing treatment-related symptoms and improving emotional adjustment in acute non-surgical cancer treatment, a meta-analysis. *Psychooncology, 10,* 490–502.

Leukaemia Research Foundation (2007). Retrieved 21 August 2007 from http://www.lrf.org.uk/

Lindeke, L. L. & Sieckert, A. M. (2005). Nurse-physician workplace collaboration. *Online Journal of Issues in Nursing, 10* (1), 5.

Murray, S. M. & Pindoria, S. (2004). Nutrition support for bone marrow transplant patients. In: *The Cochrane library* (Issue 3). Chichester, UK: John Wiley and Sons, Ltd.

Muscaritoli, M., Grieco, G., Capria, S., Iori, A. P. & Fanelli, F. R. (2002). Nutritional and metabolic support in patients undergoing bone marrow transplantation. *American Journal of Clinical Nutrition, 75,* 183–190.

National Institute for Clinical Excellence (2003). *Guidance on cancer services – improving outcomes in haematological cancers – the manual.* London: National Institute for Clinical Excellence.

Papadopoulou, A., MacDonald, A., Williams, M. D., Darbyshire, P. J. & Booth, I. W. (1996). Gastrointestinal and nutritional sequelae of bone marrow transplantation. *Archives of Disease in Child, 75,* 208–213.

Papadopoulou, A., MacDonald, A., Williams, M. D., Darbyshire, P. J. & Booth, I. W. (1997). Enteral nutrition after bone marrow transplantation. *Archives of Disease in Child, 77,* 131–136.

Parkinson, J. (2006). Experiences of selves in isolation: a psychodynamic approach to the care of patients being treated in a specialized medical unit. *Psychodynamic Practice, 12* (2), 149–163.

Provan, D. & Krentz, R. J. (2004). *Oxford handbook of clinical and laboratory investigation.* Edinburgh: Churchill Livingstone.

Rees, W. (2005). Low microbial diets in immunocompromised patients. *British Journal of Cancer Management*, 2 (2), 21–23.

Risi, G. F. & Tomascak, V. (1998). Prevention of infection in the immunocompromised host. *American Journal of Infection Control*, 26, 594–604.

Rivadeneira, D. E., Evoy, D., Fahey, T. J., Lieberman, M. D. & Daly, J. M. (1998). Nutritional support of the cancer patient. *Clinical Journal of Cancer*, 48, 69–80.

Sayre, R. S. & Marcoux, B. C. (1992). Exercise and autologous bone marrow transplants. *Clinical Management*, 12 (4), 78–82.

Sloman, R. (2002). Relaxation and imagery for anxiety and depression control in community patients with advanced cancer. *Cancer Nursing*, 25, 432–435.

Souhami, R. L. & Tobias, J. S. (1998). Myeloma and other paraproteinaemias. In: R. L. Souhami & J. S. Tobias (Eds.), *Cancer and its management* (3rd ed., pp. 470–483). Oxford: Blackwell Science.

Stevinson, C. & Fox, K. R. (2005). Role of exercise for cancer rehabilitation in UK hospitals: a survey of oncology nurses. *European Journal of Cancer Care*, 14, 63–69.

Stevinson, C. & Fox, K. R. (2006). Feasibility of an exercise rehabilitation programme for cancer patients. *European Journal of Cancer Care*, 15 (4), 386–396.

Stillman, M. & Cata, J. P. (2006). Management of chemotherapy induced peripheral neuropathy. *Current Pain and Headache Reports*, 10 (4), 275–287.

Szeluga, D. J., Stuart, R. K., Brookmeyer, R., Utermohlen, V. & Santos, G. W. (1987). Nutritional support of bone marrow recipients: a prospective, randomized clinical trial comparing total parenteral nutrition to an enteral feeding program. *Cancer Research*, 47, 3309–3316.

Wagner, L. I. & Cella, D. (2004). Fatigue and cancer: causes, prevalence and treatment approaches. *British Journal of Cancer*, 91, 822–828.

Zavadsky, A. J. (2001). Platelet disorders and their implications on physical therapy intervention. *Rehabilitation Oncology*, 19 (3), 11–13.

Chapter 7

HEAD AND NECK CANCER

Brenda Nugent, Gillian Lusty, Lorraine Ashcroft
and Nicola Evans

Learning outcomes

Having read this chapter the reader will be able to:

- Describe the diagnosing procedures, staging process and treatments for the patient with head and neck cancer
- Describe the side effects from treatments and their management
- Discuss the role and benefits of multi-professional team working in the management of head and neck cancer

---

The term head and neck cancer is used to classify a variety of malignant tumours which can develop in a number of sites:

- Lip
- Tongue
- Floor of mouth
- Gum
- Salivary glands
- Oropharynx
- Nasopharynx
- Larynx
- Nose and sinuses
- Ear
- Thyroid

These are a complex group of cancers (Feber, 2000) which require multi-professional team working to ensure that complete holistic care is given to patients throughout the cancer journey. A multi-professional team approach allows different disciplines to apply their own professional perspectives to the problems experienced (Machin & Shaw, 1998). Optimum management requires multi-professional intervention to commence as early as possible. Ideally, this should be prior to the medical management, continue throughout the treatment period and on through any further rehabilitation that is required.

> *Realistically cancer care is incomplete unless rehabilitation is addressed. So that if only the cancer itself is treated and the patient is not offered rehabilitation there has been a failure to provide complete care*
>
> *(Watson, 1992, pp. 167–173)*

Aetiology

A number of risk factors for the development of head and neck cancer have been identified. One of the primary risk factors is tobacco. Daily consumption, duration of the habit, type and manner in which the tobacco is used will determine the cancer site, e.g.

- Cigarette smokers have a tendency towards laryngeal and lung cancer.
- Pipe smokers have an increased risk of lip and oral cavity cancers.
- Snuff users are at increased risk of cheek and gum malignancies.

Another major risk factor is alcohol consumption, especially spirits. If used together with tobacco then the risks increase in a synergistic way. For those who have a heavy alcohol consumption and are also heavy smokers, the risk of oral cancer is over 35 times greater than that for those who neither smoke nor drink (Sanderson & Ironside, 2002).

A number of other risk factors have also been identified:

- Occupational exposure to dust, fumes and chemicals (Feber, 2000).
- Consumption of salted fish particularly if this is during childhood, where there is an association with a higher risk of nasopharyngeal cancer. This has been observed amongst the Chinese population (Fee, 1998).
- Ionising radiation – the only clearly identified cause of thyroid cancer (Feber, 2000).
- Viruses; e.g. Epstein–Barr virus has been linked to nasopharyngeal cancer (Silverman, 2003).

Incidence

About 7800 people in the UK are diagnosed with cancer of the head and neck annually. Of these, about:

- 400 occur in the eye
- 360 in the lip
- 1400 in the mouth
- 400 in the nose

- 1650 in pharynx
- 500 in the salivary glands
- 1250 in the tongue

(Cancerbackup, 2005)

Signs and symptoms

Symptoms are often insidious and similar to those experiencing minor ailments. They should be investigated if they persist for more than 2 weeks. Common symptoms include:

- Persistent blocked nose or nose bleeds.
- Sore throat.
- Hoarse voice.
- Ear ache, ringing in the ear or difficulty in hearing.
- Mouth ulcers that do not heal within a few weeks.
- Swollen lymph glands.
- Difficulty in swallowing or pain when chewing or swallowing.
- Numbness in the mouth or lips.
- Unexplained loose tooth.
- Pain in the face or upper jaw.
- Leukoplakia (skin lesion usually on tongue or inside of cheeks. Usually white or grey and has a thick, slightly raised, hardened surface) or erythroplakia (flat red patch or lesion in the mouth – usually floor of mouth, tongue or soft palate, characterised by a soft, velvety texture) (Cancerbackup, 2006).
- Trismus (reduced jaw opening).

Investigations

Following referral by the general practitioner or dentist to the maxillofacial surgeon or ENT specialist, current symptoms and medical history will be recorded. The mouth and throat are examined clinically and then a number of investigations may be undertaken:

- Nasendoscopy.
- Biopsy – using fine needle of biopsy forceps. This may be done at the clinic or the patient can be admitted to allow detailed examination under general anaesthetic. A number of biopsies can then be taken from any areas thought to be suspicious.
- Fine-needle aspiration cytology (FNAC) – using a fine needle and syringe, a sample of cells from the suspicious lump is removed and sent for examination.
- Microcytoscopy – a new test still in research stages, which can be used with patients with pre-cancerous conditions who are being monitored through regular biopsies. In the procedure a small amount of blue dye is painted on to the abnormal area,

which is then examined under microscope. This replaces the need to take a biopsy (Cancerbackup, 2006).

- X-ray – of the face and neck to see the extent of the area affected by disease. An X-ray of the chest may be done to check general health or spread to the lungs.
- An orthopantomogram (OPG) to look at the jaw and teeth.
- Computerised tomography (CT) scan.
- Magnetic resonance imaging (MRI) scan – similar to CT, but uses magnetism instead of X-rays.
- Bone scan – cancers of the head and neck do not usually spread to other parts of the body, apart from the lymph glands in the neck. However, occasionally a bone scan is necessary to see if spread has occurred to nearby areas such as the jawbone. Bone scans are very sensitive and can detect cancer cells before they show up on X-ray.
- Ultrasound scanning.
- Positron emission tomography (PET) scan.

Pathology

The majority of head and neck tumours are squamous cell carcinomas (SCC). The cells most commonly involved within this site-specific group are squamous epithelial cells. Adenocarcinomas arise from glandular tissue and are the predominant type in the salivary glands and thyroid gland (Feber, 2000).

Treatments

Primary treatments are radiation therapy or surgery or a combination of both. Many patients are treated with radiotherapy alone, but more advanced disease may require both radiotherapy and surgery or combined chemotherapy and radiotherapy (chemoradiation). The interval between surgery and radiotherapy should be as short as possible, ideally less than 6 weeks (National Institute for Clinical Excellence [NICE], 2004). The optimal combination of treatments for the individual patient depends on the site and stage of the disease.

Surgery

It is generally recognised that the staging of the tumour will determine the type of surgery required (Haskins, 1998). The main aim is for maximal eradication of disease whilst restoring form and function and improving quality of life where possible. The type of surgery performed can be determined by:

- Site and size of the tumour
- Presence of metastases
- Requirement of reconstructive surgery

The surgery is complex due to the complicated anatomy of this area and the fact that the tumour is often in close proximity to delicate organs such as the eyes and spinal cord.

Radiotherapy

The aim is to target the primary tumour and the lymph nodes with apparent or suspected metastasis. This is made difficult by the complex anatomy of the head and neck region, with many critical and radiation-sensitive organs in close proximity to the target. Limiting the dose of ionising radiation to the non-cancerous tissues will offer the potential for therapeutic gains. The dose of ionising radiation delivered will be determined by the extent and location of the primary tumour.

Treatment regimes will vary depending on clinical staging and grading. Treatment dose (measured in gray, Gy) can vary from 40 to 70 Gy extending over 20 to 35 days (2 Gy being delivered daily on a 5-day week basis).

Chemotherapy

Chemotherapy may be used in conjunction with radiation therapy for advanced disease, or it may be used as an alternative to immediate surgery, e.g. avoid total laryngectomy for hypopharyngeal cancer. Chemotherapy may be administered prior to radiotherapy (induction) or in combination with radiotherapy (concurrent) (Lamont & Vokes, 2001).

Prognosis

Cancers of the head and neck are unusual in that there appears to have been little, if any, improvement in survival rates over recent decades (NICE, 2004). This may be attributable to the fact that many patients are lifelong smokers, which in itself leads to significant comorbidities such as cardiovascular disease.

As with any type of cancer, the prognosis for individual patients depends heavily on the cancer site:

- Oral cavity – including mouth and lip
  Five-year survival rate is over 80% for people with early stage localized disease. For those whose disease has spread to the neck survival is 40% and then falls below 20% where there is distant metastatic disease (NICE, 2004).
- Larynx
  Survival rates are better than for oral or pharyngeal cancer with nearly two-thirds of patients surviving for 5 years (NICE, 2004).

- Pharynx
  Cancer of the pharynx is less common and 5-year survival rates are estimated in the region of 40% for cancer of the oropharynx and 20% for the hypopharynx (NICE, 2004).
- Thyroid
  Survival rates for this type of cancer are regarded as excellent, with curative treatment intent. The main exception is anaplastic thyroid cancer for which the outlook is poor (NICE, 2004).

Medical treatment side effects and their management

The range and severity of side effects experienced by an individual will depend on tumour site and treatment(s) delivered. Due to the nature of the disease and types of treatment delivered, 'assessment and intervention are ongoing and may span a period of months or even years' (Machin & Shaw, 1998, p. 93). As the nature of the side effects is ongoing, there is a 'demonstrated need for longer-term support and follow-up assessment' (Rose & Yates, 2001, p. 262).

Post-operative period

Post-operative care needs to be individually tailored to each patient's specific needs. However, some general principles do apply.

It is essential to:

- Maintain the patient's airway.
- Monitor circulation (as hypertension can lead to bleeding and haematoma formation, whilst vasoconstriction can compromise flap survival) (Frank *et al.*, 1997, cited by Talmi, 1999).
- Prevent infection.
- Control pain. Not only does this improve well-being but also influences the patient's ability to clear lung secretions and mobilise, thus affecting overall recovery.

Care of drains and flaps in head and neck surgery

Since the 1980s, advances in microvascular surgery saw the development of 'free flaps'. Tissue can be taken from one body part and used to repair or replace other non-adjacent tissues. The flap should have the colour, thickness and general characteristics similar to that of the native tissue. Post-operative management of the flap is of vital importance for flap viability. It should be monitored initially every half hour and then gradually less often for 36 hours post-operatively (Feber, 2000).

The clinical signs used to assess flap viability are:

- Colour (should be pink)
- Temperature (warm to touch)

- Capillary refill (1–3 seconds post-blanching)
- Tissue turgor (soft to touch) (Feber, 2000)

Management of surgical drains includes ensuring the patency of the drain and monitoring colour, consistency and amount of fluid draining. Any deviation from normal should be noted immediately as it may indicate a problem which could lead to a difficulty with wound healing or loss of flap viability. Care of the donor site must also be taken into consideration. Often this area is very painful and slow to heal.

Grafted skin no longer produces oil or sweat as these glands are sacrificed during harvesting. Daily moisturising and massage of this area can prevent an increase in pain and hypertrophic scarring from occurring (Feber, 2000).

Surgery

Surgery to remove disease present in the cervical lymph nodes, or to prevent this from happening, can take the form of a radical neck dissection (RND) or modified neck dissection (MND) (Kuntz & Weymuller, 1999). An RND involves complete removal of all ipsilateral cervical lymph nodes, sternocleidomastoid, internal jugular vein and the spinal accessory nerve (Robbins, 1998). This can result in a 'shoulder syndrome', characterised by a dropped shoulder, winged scapula, reduced and weakened range of movement and localised pain (Kuntz & Weymuller, 1999). An MND removes all the lymph nodes but spares one or more of the features, normally the spinal accessory nerve. This eventually results in less pain, with increased shoulder function and improved quality of life (Feber, 2000).

Airway management and tracheostomy care

A tracheostomy may be temporary or permanent. The overall aims of care are to:

- Ensure a patent airway is maintained.
- Maintain comfort by excluding dyspnoea, cyanosis etc.
- Ensure respiratory rhythm, depth and breathing pattern are regular (Pryor & Prasad, 2002).

Complications can include:

- Haemorrhage
- Tracheoesophageal fistula
- Infection
- Obstruction/displacement of tracheostomy tube

Patients frequently experience retained secretions post-operatively and during radiotherapy. It is recommended that breathing exercises, cleaning of trache tubes and the clearance of secretions are carried out at least every 2–3 h initially or more if required. Suction is often required, but should be carried out only when needed and should be as aseptic as possible to prevent introducing infection into the lungs (Feber, 2000; Pryor & Prasad, 2002). It is also essential that humidification is used to prevent drying and crusting of secretions. Patients are also encouraged to become as independent as possible in all aspects of care, as such home nebulisers and suction units may be required.

Mucositis

Mucositis can be caused by radiation or chemotherapy. It occurs when there is a break down in the epithelial cells which line the gastrointestinal tract. This leaves the mucosal tissue open to ulceration and infections such as candidiasis. It can occur anywhere along the digestive tract but probably the most common is oral mucositis. It occurs in 40% of patients treated with chemotherapy alone and up to 100% of patients receiving combination radiation and chemotherapy (Agarwala & Sbeital, 1999). As chemo/radiotherapy can affect the ability of the cells to reproduce there is a slow healing of the oral mucosa. The severity depends on:

- Dental hygiene
- Treatment schedule, field and dose
- Age of patient

Mucositis associated with radiotherapy usually appears at the end of the second week of treatment and may last for 6–8 weeks (NHS Direct, 2004).

Skin reactions

The skin is composed of two main layers, the outer epidermis (comprised of five layers) and the underlying dermis. The superficial cells are shed through a normal process known as desquamation. The deeper layer contains blood vessels, glands, nerves and hair follicles. This is the supportive structure which is necessary for the epidermal layer to be renewed. When exposed to radiation the ability of the cells within the basal layer to reproduce is affected, thereby preventing the process of repopulation. Radical radiotherapy repeatedly impairs this cell division within the basal layer and leads to skin reactions, which can range from mild erythema (redness) to moist desquamation where the dermis is exposed and oozes serum (Parsons, 1994). At its most severe, skin reaction can sometimes be dose limiting. Other factors such as general skin condition and the nutritional status of the patient, their age, ethnicity, general health and any pre-existing diseases can all exert an influence. The degree of skin reaction will also be affected by the radiation dose, the energy and the fractionation regime. Reaction can be increased by the use of chemical irritants, e.g. perfume and aftershave. The rate of healing will be affected by the presence of infection – bacterial or fungal or can be delayed by friction, e.g. from clothing or shaving. Certain treatment techniques will also increase the likelihood of the skin receiving doses that will cause a visible reaction. Severity will also be affected by the use of chemotherapy as this will tend to exacerbate side effects of the radiation (O'Rouke, 1987; See *et al.*, 1998). Other influences include:

- If the area has been previously irradiated
- Site of treatment
- Smoking
- Thermal irritants
- Volume of tissue irradiated (Best Practice Statement, 2004)

Glean *et al.* (2001) and Best Practice Statement (2007) advocate the following for skin care during radiotherapy:

- Gentle washing using a mild unperfumed soap and warm water.
- Avoidance of friction, by patting the skin dry and wearing loose cotton clothing.
- Use of a simple moisturiser, e.g. aqueous cream.
- Avoiding perfumed skin products, deodorants, make up and talc.
- Use of mild, fragrance-free detergents for washing clothes.
- Avoiding wet shaving.
- Avoiding sun exposure during treatment and using at least SPF15 sunblock for 1 year following treatment.
- Protecting the skin from the elements and extreme temperatures.
- Avoiding the use of adhesive tape within the treatment field.
- One per cent hydrocortisone for itchy areas (Glean *et al.*, 2001). However other guidelines advise that this should not be a routine therapy and should 'only be prescribed following medical advice' (Best Practice Statement, 2007) and should not be used for more than 7 days.

For those head and neck patients who develop moist desquamation during treatment, management can be awkward, as it is a difficult area to apply dressings to (Glean *et al.*, 2001). Early effects of skin reactions can lead to a limitation in range of movement, poor limb positioning, poor posture and result in a decrease of functional ability.

The late effects include scaling, atrophy, fibrosis of soft tissue and the obliteration of superficial vessels and dermal lymphatics. Lymphoedema may occur as a result of damage to the soft tissue and lymphatic vessels. These effects can develop over a number of years (Isaacson, 1998).

Salivary function and xerostomia

Exposure to ionising radiation has an inflammatory and degenerative effect on salivary glands, causing fibrosis, acinar atrophy (salivary gland partial/total wasting) and cellular necrosis. This leads to a marked reduction in the production of saliva known as xerostomia. The symptoms will include:

- Dryness
- Burning sensation of the tongue
- Fissures at lips and sores
- Atrophy of dorsal surface of the tongue
- Difficulty wearing dentures
- Increased thirst
- Impaired speech and swallowing function
- An inability to neutralise acid, increasing susceptibility to mouth infection (Feber, 2000)

It has been shown that there is a reduction in salivary flow during the first 1–2 weeks of radiotherapy (Burlage *et al.*, 2001) and xerostomia 'becomes apparent' when doses exceed 10 Gy. Secretion progressively decreases with increased radiation dose and irreversible damage to the salivary glands occurs when doses exceed 54 Gy (Perkins *et al.*, 2007).

The parotid glands are thought to be more susceptible to the effects of radiation (Berk *et al.*, 2005) compared to submandibular, sublingual and other minor salivary glands. If there is recovery, it may take from 6 to 12 months but the amount of saliva produced may remain inadequate.

Management includes:

- Frequent sips of water
- Saline mouthwashes
- Mouthwashes designed to moisten the mouth
- Chewing sugar-free gum

Synthetic salvia solutions and substitutes have been of limited help in the majority of patients with dry mouth (Silverman, 2003).

Loss of taste

Taste buds are very sensitive to radiation and are included in the treatment field for most oral cancer patients. Therefore the majority of patients will develop a partial (hypogeusia) or, more usually, a complete (ageusia) loss of taste during treatment. Sometimes there may be an alteration to the taste buds, leading to a confused perception of taste known as dysgeusia.

Taste acuity is usually absent when 30 Gy of radiation has been delivered. Once radiotherapy is completed, the acuity of taste will recover rapidly at first and then progress more slowly. Most patients report some improvement within 20–60 days following treatment (Parsons, 1994).

Dysphagia

Dysphagia (impaired swallowing) is initially attributed either to disruption to the normal anatomy due to pressure of tumour, nerve involvement, soft-tissue tethering or tumour-induced pain. Dysphagia which persists following treatment is caused and influenced by the extent of surgery undertaken and/or the tumour and soft-tissue response to radiotherapy and chemotherapy (McCullough & Jaffe, 2006). The extent, type and location of surgical resection play a major role in determining both difficulties and outcomes (Pauloski *et al.*, 1998).

Following surgery, some degree of dysphagia may occur, such as:

- Total glossectomy – always have dysphagia.
- If less than 50% of the tongue is removed, followed by primary closure, most patients will regain nearly normal swallowing (Hirano, 1992).
- With intra-oral cancer involving bone, where the tumour is removed by a combination of glossectomy, mandibulectomy and radical neck dissection, a variety of swallowing difficulties can be experienced. Range and severity will depend on the amount of mandible and other surrounding structures that are removed.
- Tumours of salivary glands, tonsils and sinus may necessitate a resection of the hard and/or soft palate, affecting the oral stage of swallowing (Kronenberger & Meyer, 1994).

Radiation can have early and late side effects that impact on swallowing function. Those side effects already mentioned such as xerostomia, erythema and mucositis will all impact on the oral stage of the swallow. Later effects of radiation may include osteoradionecrosis (bone cell death thought to occur primarily because of vascular insufficiency), reduced capillary flow, dental caries, altered taste and trismus (Parsons, 1994). A reduction in blood supply to the muscles can result in fibrosis, causing a reduction in muscle size and replacement with collagen. This can severely impact on swallowing, sometimes not being evident until years after treatment are completed (Eisele *et al.*, 1991). Examples of dysphagia experienced include:

- Longer oral transit time.
- Pharyngeal residue (Pauloski *et al.*, 1998).
- Fixation of the hyolaryngeal complex.
- Reduced range of tongue movement.
- Reduced glottic closure and cricopharyngeal relaxation – all resulting in potential for aspiration (Lazarus, 1993).
- Reported incidents of cranial nerve palsies in patients undergoing radiotherapy as their primary mode of treatment. This can occur alone or in combination with cranial nerve palsy and may be uni- or bilateral. The most common cranial nerve involvement is CN XII (hypoglossal – provides motor innervation to intrinsic and some extrinsic muscles of the tongue) followed by CN X (vagus – supplies palatal muscles, pharyngeal constrictors and most of laryngeal muscles; taste and sensation to epiglottis). The mechanism by which damage occurs is 'not fully understood'

but is thought to be either directly (thought to be rare) or indirectly, where radiation damage to surrounding tissue may cause fibrosis, causing 'thickening of the neurilemma sheath, demyelinisation and fibrous replacement of some nerve fibrils resulting in entrapment' (Mok *et al.*, 2001).

Dysphagia has also been identified as a common debilitating and potentially life-threatening sequelae of chemoradiation. Nguyen *et al.* (2004) found that there was severe dysfunction of base of tongue, larynx and pharyngeal muscles, leading to poor bolus control, vallecular residue, poor epiglottic movement and, in severe cases, aspiration. For those patients who were neutropenic following chemotherapy and aspirating, there was increased risk of aspiration pneumonia, sepsis and respiratory failure.

Communication

Communication can be affected in a number of ways, as a result of the tumour and/or treatment. Often changes to the voice quality/phonation may be an initial onset symptom which can increase with medical treatment. Vocal cord immobility, tissue loss, fibrosis and 'lack of lubrication' all affect phonation (Boyle & Kraus, 1998). Any structural changes or impaired nerve functioning following surgery can influence speech quality/intelligibility in the following number of ways:

• Poor sound articulation due to impaired tongue movement
• Hypernasality due to impaired soft palate movement or resection of the hard palate
• Dysphonia (hoarse voice)
• Loss of voice due to laryngectomy, where the patient becomes reliant on surgical voice restoration or the use of an artificial larynx, e.g. Servox
• Reduced range of jaw movement
• Altered quality of speech due to dental clearance

Treatment of swallowing and communication difficulties

Ideally, the patient should be seen prior to surgery to record baseline functioning. Post-surgery a detailed swallowing and communication assessment is required. At this point or subsequently they may require regular input by a specialised speech and language therapist (SLT). This includes the use of strategies and postures to achieve a safe swallow, altered food consistencies and range of motion exercises to maintain/improve oral movement. Instrumental investigation of swallowing may also be required and the patient may attend for videofluoroscopy or a fiberoptic evaluation of swallowing (FEES) assessment.

It is suggested that prophylactic range of movement exercises during and after treatment is beneficial in preventing/minimising the effects of radiation (Gaziano, 2002). It is important to bear in mind that for those patients undergoing radiotherapy, the onset of the longer term side effects of radiation treatment might not be experienced until after treatment is complete. Therefore it is crucial that radiation dose, area being treated, number of fractions and anticipated difficulties are all considered when planning follow up for the individual, e.g. patients experiencing or at risk of developing trismus (reduced jaw opening). Those with post-surgical trismus may experience an increase in severity with radiotherapy. Others may experience radiation-induced trismus. Using devices such as the Therabite (which passively stretches the jaw muscles) (Hancock et al., 2003; Nicolaou, 2001) therapeutically and prophylactically has proved to be of benefit to both groups. While personal experience shows prophylactic use of Therabite is of benefit, many patients do not always appreciate the need for prophylactic use. For such patients support and encouragement are required as well as access to the SLT service to allow more intensive input if required. Further research is required to help refine practice.

Therapy to improve communication will depend on problems experienced and may include:

- Voice care advice and where appropriate therapy
- Range of oral exercises to increase/maintain movement
- Strategies to improve functional communication
- Use of communication aids if appropriate, e.g. amplifiers
- Education in the use and care of a voice prosthesis
- Learning how to use an artificial larynx, e.g. a Servox if SVR is not appropriate/has been unsuccessful

The emotional and psychological effects of impaired communication and/or swallowing, altered function and body image, e.g. presence of a stoma, should not be underestimated. Many patients will experience a complete change in social circumstances and find this very difficult to cope with. Continued management and support are essential to enable the individual to attain optimum function and a return as far as is possible to their previous level of social functioning (Sullivan, 1999).

Nutrition

At diagnosis many of these patients may have nutritional problems, often due to a high incidence of alcoholism. Other physical problems which may impinge on the nutritional status include poor oral hygiene, poorly fitting dentures, ulcerated mouth, oral swelling, presence of dysphagia and aspiration (Grant et al., 1989; Hunter, 1996).

The incidence of malnutrition at diagnosis can range from 40 to 58% (Connally, 2004; Grobbelaar et al., 2004). This risk increases with multi-modality treatments, e.g. surgery, radiotherapy and chemoradiation, with 75–80% of patients having significant weight loss (more than 10% of body weight) during treatment period (Hammerlid et al., 1998; Lopez et al., 1994). All three treatments will result in an increase of nutrient requirement and at the same time interfere with the patient's physical ability to eat (Williams & Meguid, 1989). Surgical resection of tumours of the head and neck region have the potential to severely restrict oral intake (Grobbelaar et al., 2004) due to anatomical disfigurement of the area. Malnutrition is harmful to the patient with cancer (Van Bokhorst-de van der Schuer *et al.*, 199) and is associated with increased morbidity and mortality (Bassett & Dobie, 1983). The malnourished patient has an increased risk of complications, including impaired wound healing, increased susceptibility to infection, decreased tolerance to effective cancer therapy, apathy, depression, fatigue, loss of will to recover and decreased survival (Goodwin & Byers, 1993; Grobbelaar *et al.*, 2004; Lees, 1999).

For many patients with a diagnosis of head and neck cancer oral nutrition will not provide adequate nutrition during treatment. This results from side effects of treatment such as dysphagia, mucositis, xerostomia and aguesia. When oral intake is not adequate, enteral feeding will be initiated. Enteral feeding can be delivered via a nasogastric (NG) tube or by a gastrostomy tube (percutaneous endoscopic gastrostomy – PEG). Gastrostomy tubes can be placed prior to treatment (prophylactically) or during treatment period. Nasogastric tubes are placed during treatment.

PEGs have been quoted as having advantages over NG tubes through enhanced mobility, improved quality of life and being able to use higher energy feeds (Bassett & Dobie, 1983; Beaver *et al.*, 1998). Prophylactic PEGs have been shown to decrease the incidence of weight loss and dehydration during treatment (Beaver *et al.*, 1998; Lee *et al.*, 1998), resulting in decreased treatment interruptions (Porter, 2003). Unplanned interruptions in radiotherapy treatment have a significant negative outcome for the patient by reducing disease-free period. The reduction in local control rate has been estimated to be approximately 0.7–1.4% for a 1-day gap rising to 14–20% for a 7-day gap (Huang *et al.*, 2003; James *et al.*, 2003; NICE, 2004). PEGs are not without complications; these include site infection, leakage around the gastrostomy site, local pain, gastric erosion, tube dysfunction, interperitoneal leakage (Bassett & Dobie, 1983; Deurloo *et al.*, 2001; Piquet *et al.*, 2002; Righi *et al.*, 1998) and metastasis of head and neck carcinoma to the percutaneous endoscopic gastrostomy site (Lee *et al.*, 1998; Pickhardt *et al.*, 2002).

NG feeding is considered for short-term feeding less than 30 days (Cannaby *et al.*, 2002). NG tubes are associated with patient discomfort, risk of aspiration, frequency of occlusion, nasopharyngeal ulceration and unintentional removal (Piquet *et al.*, 2002; Riera *et al.*, 2002). In a study comparing PEG feeding with NG feeding, significant dysphagia proved more persistent among the PEG patients than the NG patients at 3 months and at 6 months post-treatment. Patients NG fed are more likely to have their feeding tubes removed before patients who are PEG fed (Al-Othman *et al.*, 2003; Mekhail *et al.*, 2001).

Prior to surgery, chemotherapy and/or radiotherapy, the specialist oncology dietitian will undertake a comprehensive nutritional assessment. This assessment will be in conjunction with the specialist SLT who will give advice on safe food consistency.

The nutritional assessment will involve:

- Measurement of body weight, height and body mass index
- Recording of normal body weight
- Percentage of weight loss
- Assessment of the consistency and range of food and fluids
- Assessment of the nutritional value of the diet obtained from a diet history

- Evaluating the use of oral nutritional supplements and/or the use of enteral feeding
- Calculation of individual energy and protein requirements
- Interpretation of biochemical results

Advice on nutritional support may be initiated at the time of diagnosis or at any stage throughout the treatment or post-treatment. Depending entirely on the assessed nutritional status of the patient, nutritional support may range from:

- Food fortification
- Use of oral nutritional supplements
- Enteral feeding
- Combination of the above

Patients should be monitored throughout their treatment, on a weekly basis or more if required. Following the completion of treatment patients should continue to have access to a specialist oncology dietitian for ongoing advice and nutritional support. This will continue until symptoms of treatment have subsided and the patient's nutritional status has stabilized either with continued enteral feeding or on having returned to oral feeding.

Nausea and vomiting

Nausea and vomiting are common side effects of chemotherapy resulting in fatigue and low mood. It may also be caused by constipation due to medication, e.g. analgesia. Physical symptoms include severe dehydration, electrolyte imbalance and weight loss. Antiemetic medication may be required to alleviate symptoms.

Osteoradionecrosis

This is one of the more serious possible side effects of head and neck irradiation where the bone cells and blood supply can be irreversibly damaged. It is a progressive condition and can lead to severe pain or fracture and may necessitate jaw resection. The incidence of osteoradionecrosis will vary depending on the reporting institutions, aggressiveness of the radiotherapy and follow-up time. It is related to the dose of radiation delivered and to the volume of bone treated (Silverman, 2003).

Pain

Types of presenting pain in head and neck cancer may include oropharyngeal, facial, neck, shoulder or headache. The various treatments of head and neck cancer also have the potential to either reduce or increase pain. Extensive surgery, especially neck dissections, can lead to some degree of pain, which can be nociceptive, neuropathic or myofascial in nature (Feber, 2000). Nearly all patients who receive radiation therapy to the head and neck experience pain at some point during treatment (Carper *et al.*, 2004). Pain is often experienced in the throat, initially on swallowing and later more constantly. It can be caused by inflammation, oedema and ulceration of mucosa. This can impact on the patients' ability to swallow even saliva, and also decreases their ability to cough/clear any retained upper airway secretions, which can lead to the development of an upper respiratory tract infection (Chaplin & Morton, 1999).

Pain management for patients with head and neck cancer should follow established guidelines. Pain should be evaluated regularly and can be treated with pharmacological therapy and other modalities, i.e. transcutaneous electrical nerve stimulation (TENS) and the teaching of relaxation (Brooks, 1998) (refer to Chapter 13).

Cancer-related fatigue

Treatment for the cancer of head and neck can often be very aggressive in its nature and combined modalities are often recommended. Therefore, the possible cumulative effects of sequential treatments may increase the risk of occurrence of fatigue in such a population (Richardson, 1995) (refer to Chapter 12).

Lymphoedema

Drainage of lymph can be altered by the removal of lymph nodes or by damage to the tissues, and as such the lymphatic collectors. The medical management of head and neck cancer can, as has been discussed, cause both of these problems. This patient group is therefore at risk of developing localised lymphoedema (refer to Chapter 11).

Body image, disfigurement and dysfunction

The range of treatment modalities may cause disfigurement affecting a number of functions; e.g. with surgery the shoulder may (as previously discussed) become dysfunctional due to pain and reduced range movement (Scott *et al.*, 2007). This limits the patient's ability to carry out their activities of daily living independently, which can be distressing. Treatment in the form of pain control, stretching, muscle strengthening and posture correction and teaching compensatory techniques can enable the patient to regain his or her independence and as a result have a more positive mental attitude.

For many patients the physical signs of head and neck cancer cannot be concealed. The tumour itself could be visible and cause structural changes and disfigurement. As a consequence, patients can experience depression, social anxiety, reduced self-esteem, sexual difficulties and a generalised sense of reduced quality of life. Koster and Bergsma (1990) describe head and neck cancer as more emotionally traumatic than any other type of cancer.

For those patients experiencing an altered body image and negative reactions from others, Price (2000) suggests strategies designed to help the patient feel in control, not only of the body but also of social encounters with others. This should involve evaluating support networks available (identifying key people to work with) and developing information strategies (what the patient wants others to know). Measures designed to help the patient manage encounters should also be discussed, for example:

- Helping patients to appreciate the range of reactions that they may encounter
- Examining why others behave as they do and how this in turn makes them feel

Having assisted the patient to understand social reactions, different measures, e.g. challenging, dissipation and collusion, can be discussed as methods of managing these situations (Price, 2000).

A multidisciplinary approach to care provides an opportunity to address all the issues arising, where different professional disciplines can put their own perspective on the various problems (Machin & Shaw, 2001) in a timely manner.

Case study

This case study is based on a married 43-year-old female who has two teenage children and works full time. She was diagnosed with poorly differentiated nasopharyngeal cancer, graded at $T_3 N1 Mo$. Treatment consisted of two cycles of induction chemotherapy followed by concurrent chemoradiation two cycles and 70 Gy of radiotherapy.

On admission to the ward to begin her induction chemotherapy she was referred to the dietitian, speech and language therapist, physiotherapist and occupational therapist. At this stage she was not experiencing any difficulties in any area, but was seen by all disciplines, which carried out baseline assessments, discussed the anticipated side effects of treatment and explained potential input. Individual contact details were given and the patient agreed to be seen by all relevant disciplines as and when required. At this point she did not experience any difficulties with communication or swallowing, nutritional status was satisfactory and she had full range of movement in neck, jaw and shoulder. The first side effect experienced was fatigue post-chemo, which impacted on activities of daily living. As treatment progressed she experienced a number of anticipated treatment side effects and was seen regularly by all team members.

Dietetic intervention

This patient agreed to have a prophylactic PEG inserted prior to second cycle of induction chemotherapy. On completion of 18 Gy of radiotherapy, she began to experience pain on swallowing, hypogeusia and xerostomia and reported that her mouth felt 'sensitive'.

She was advised on:

- Increasing energy in her diet by adding additional snacks between meals and by using fortified foods.
- Avoiding foods that would irritate or heighten pain on swallowing and mucositis, such as highly spiced, salty and acidic foods.
- Keeping temperature of food to a level of tolerance, meaning for many patients' foods will only be tolerated at room temperature – extremes in temperature may increase levels of pain for patients.
- Eating moist foods that would be easier to swallow when experiencing xerostomia or to have a drink with foods to ease swallowing.
- Eating soft foods that do not require a lot of chewing will be better tolerated, such as scrambled eggs and minced foods.
- Despite having little incentive to eat due to pain, hypoguesia and xerostomia, this patient wished to continue with a soft, high-energy, moist diet supplemented with whole-protein-based nutritional supplements rather than commence PEG feeding.

Enteral feeding was commenced at 24 Gy of irradiation, as pain levels prevented adequate oral intake. Analgesia was increased to a morphine-based drug and the patient was made aware of increased risk of constipation. The feed used was a whole protein-fibre-containing feed. By 32 Gy of radiotherapy this patient was tolerating enteral feeding well via the PEG and receiving all of her nutritional requirements via the PEG.

As treatment progressed this patient was not keen to continue with 1500 mL of 1.5 Kcal/mL fibre feed as she felt 'too full'. The feed volume was decreased to 1000 mL and the energy deficit was corrected with the use of a fat emulsion via the PEG.

On completion of this treatment she remained as an inpatient to enable analgesia to be regulated and to observe skin reaction. Throughout this period she remained on 1000 mL of a 1.5 Kcal/mL fibrous feed and 30 mL three times per day of a fat emulsion. During her treatment period she experienced 9.5% of body weight loss. To increase energy intake she was encouraged to try a sip feed containing 1.5 Kcal/mL throughout the day.

On discharge this patient was reviewed by the specialist oncology liaison dietitian in the community. Four weeks post-completion of treatment little progress had been made with recovery. She remained sore to swallow and continued with PEG feed as previous. Five and a half weeks post-treatment, she had managed a bowl of soup but remained on her enteral feeding as previous. She continued to be monitored by the community dietitian.

Speech and language therapy intervention

Following her initial SLT appointment, potential communication and swallowing difficulties that may be experienced during/following treatment difficulties were discussed in detail. A programme of prophylactic oral exercises was given. By 18 Gy of radiotherapy she was experiencing difficulty at the oral stage of swallowing due to pain, poor taste and xerostomia. A soft, moist diet was suggested. This rapidly progressed to moist mashed diet and then to a puree diet. However, enteral nutrition was soon required.

The patient was encouraged to continue with her oral exercise programme throughout treatment, as tolerated. However, at the height of treatment toxicities and for a number of weeks after treatment completion, SLT input was limited, as pain levels would not permit active intervention. She agreed to attend for a review appointment approximately 7 weeks after treatment, by which point unfortunately a number of side effects were adversely affecting speech and swallowing:

- Severe trismus (only able to insert six wooden spatulas between upper and lower teeth)
- Reduced tongue movement
- Altered oral sensation
- Continued dry mouth and poor taste
- Oral intake limited to small amounts of fluid which she managed without difficulty

Initially, SLT aim was to increase jaw opening sufficiently to allow the use of a Therabite. This was achieved over the next 2 weeks, using tongue depressors and range of movement exercises. At that point jaw opening measured approximately 12 mm. The patient attended initially on a 2-weekly basis and then monthly.

Treatment included:

- Aiming to use the Therabite on a 7–7–7 routine as recommended by the manufacturers, i.e. 7 repetitions for 7 seconds, 7 times daily. The optimum achieved was 7–7–5. Jaw opening has so far improved by 11 mm.
- Tongue range of movement exercises.
- Exercises for bolus control.
- Exercises to improve oral residue.
- Planned trials of different food textures and tastes.
- Keeping a written record of foods taken over short periods. This was not only to help the SLT keep accurate information on textures being taken, but proved to be encouraging to the patient who was finding the progress slow and emotionally demanding.
- Videofluoroscopy, which confirmed problems experienced at the oral stage. No other difficulties at the pharyngeal stage of the swallow were identified.

The patient continues to attend SLT on a regular basis. Jaw opening is improving very slowly and she is gradually increasing the amounts and variety of food textures taken orally. Although effort is still required at the oral stage, there has been improvement, which is reflected functionally. PEG tube feeding has recently been reduced by the community dietitian and the lady has returned to work on a part-time basis.

Physiotherapy intervention

As a result of the combined modality treatment, the patient's main problems requiring physiotherapy intervention were:

- Severe skin and soft-tissue reaction of the neck area, limiting range of movement (occurring at approximately 16 Gy)
- Decreased jaw range of movement during course of radiotherapy
- The formation of copious amounts of sticky green secretions giving rise to infection

Exercises (active and active assisted with passive end of range stretch) were taught to maintain range of movement in all neck movements, i.e. flexion/extension/rotation and side flexion. The patient was also taught shoulder exercises, although as this area was not included directly in the treatment field, full movement was maintained.

As the patients jaw was in the field of treatment she experienced the onset of trismus. Active jaw exercises were practised and through liaison with the SLT, the aim was to introduce a Therabite. However, this was delayed due to severity of toxicities, as noted above.

As radiotherapy treatment progressed and skin reactions worsened, neck range of movement decreased and active exercises were carried out but only as tolerated. The patient was advised that once her skin began to heal post-radiotherapy, a more aggressive exercise programme would be recommenced.

The production of thick sticky secretions was problematic and the patient had great difficulty in clearing these. Part of the difficulty of expectorating secretions was also due to a painful throat. If these secretions were not cleared, they could cause the patient to develop upper respiratory tract infections. Physiotherapy treatment was carried out twice daily during or immediately post-nebuliser. Cheat physiotherapy, which included active cycle of breathing techniques and/or autogenic drainage, was used to initially transport and then aid expectoration of secretions with good results. Sputum samples were regularly sent to the laboratories to ensure infection was not present.

The patient and nursing staff were also advised of the importance of maintaining adequate humidification and this was provided by humidified oxygen and frequent saline nebulisers.

During the course of the treatment, the patient's mobility was also assessed and maintained by daily mobilisation, bed exercises and the practice of steps/stairs pre-discharge. A very simple exercise programme also helped to reduce the fatigue as a general level of physical fitness was gradually increased.

On discharge, a portable nebuliser was loaned to the patient until respiratory symptoms had eased. She was also referred to a local physiotherapy department to encourage her to achieve her full potential.

Occupational therapy intervention

The first side effect experienced was fatigue post-induction chemotherapy, which began impacting on her daily life. Occupational therapy assessment was carried out and she was advised on:

- Reconfiguring her daily routines
- Considering how much energy a task now required and adjusting her daily/weekly tasks accordingly
- Incorporating rest and relaxation techniques into that routine
- Strategies to aid delegation and simplification of tasks
- Use of daily living equipment to conserve energy, e.g. use of a shower stool

She found this advice on lifestyle management beneficial for carrying out her activities of daily living, and also by employing these coping strategies it aided in the alleviation of anxiety by helping her regain a sense of control, generally in her life and over her lifestyle choices.

A referral for continuity and follow-up care was made to her local community occupational therapy department. It was hoped that she would continue with the progress made whilst in hospital and incorporate the energy conservation and lifestyle management principles into her home and family life, with the long-term goal of returning to work.

As the treatment progressed, toxicities became more obvious (moist desquamation of the neck, the development of peripheral oedema), she felt very self-conscious and started to reduce her social contact with members of her family and friends, discouraging visitors. She reported missing her children, being frustrated at not being able to do things with them due to hospital admission and fatigue. Although she acknowledged that her mother was helping, by looking after her children, she felt frustrated by this. As a result, she withdrew more into her room and tended to spend much time resting on the bed. It was recognized by the health care team that while this was her method of dealing with her current situation, it might not be the most beneficial approach. Over a very short period she had to come to terms with a diagnosis of cancer and cope with an aggressive form of treatment, causing a number of distressing side effects. Her roles as wife, mother and worker had been significantly altered as she had been in hospital for 6 weeks. However such a reaction in withdrawing could be justified as 'we need to allow each individual patient their own style of reacting and recovery' (Owen et al., 2001). This behaviour was monitored as it was felt that should it become detrimental to her psychological state, a referral for psychological support would be offered.

She was encouraged to consider weekend leave, on a regular basis throughout the remainder of her treatment, in order for her to spend more quality time with her family in surroundings which were more relaxed and comfortable. She reported to enjoy these periods at home and it allowed to slowly readjust to home life and to plan her discharge.

Good psychosocial care of the patient and those that matter to them depends on effective multidisciplinary teamwork and aims to improve psychological and emotional well-being (Lloyd-Williams, 2003).

Key learning points

- The range and severity of side effects experienced by an individual will depend on tumour site and treatment(s) delivered.
- Due to the nature of the disease and types of treatment delivered, assessment and interventions from each professional may be initiated on diagnosis and span a period ranging from months to even years.
- The severity of side effects experienced will vary from individual to individual; hence, all interventions will be individually tailored to each patient's specific needs.
- All care delivered will be within a multi-professional setting to ensure complete holistic care.
- Difficulties that may be experienced can be as a direct effect of the treatment given, rather than the disease itself.

References

Agarwala, S. S. & Sbeital, I. (1999). Itraogenic swallowing disorders: chemotherapy. In: R. L. Carru & T. Murry (Eds.), *Comprehensive management of swallowing disorders* (pp. 125–129). San Diego, CA: Singular Publishing Group.

Al-Othman, M. O., Amdur, R. J., Morris, C. G., Hinerman, R. W. & Mendenhall, W. M. (2003). Does feeding tube placement predict for long-term swallowing disability after radiotherapy for head and neck cancer? *Head & Neck*, 25 (9), 741–747.

Bassett, M. R. & Dobie, R. A. (1983). Patterns of nutritional deficiency in head and neck cancer. *Otolaryngology – Head & Neck Surgery*, 91 (2), 119–125.

Beaver, M. E., Myers, J. N., Griffenberg, L. & Waugh, K. (1998). Percutaneous fluoroscopic gastrostomy tube placement in patients with head and neck cancer. *Archives of Otolaryngology – Head & Neck Surgery*, 124 (10), 1141–1144.

Berk, L. B., Shivnani, A. T. & Small. W. (2005). Pathophysiology and management of radiation induced xerostomia. *The Journal of Supportive Oncology*, 3 (3), 191–206.

Best Practice Statement (2004). *Skincare of patients receiving radiotherapy*. NHS Quality Improvement Scotland. Retrieved 25 September 2007 from www.nhshealthquality.org

Boyle, J. O. & Kraus, D. H. (1998). Functional rehabilitation. In: L. G. Close, D. L. Larson & J. P. Shah (Eds.), *Functional rehabilitation in essentials of head and neck oncology* (chapter 33, pp. 369–378). New York: Thieme Medical Publishers Inc.

Brooks, C. (1998). Radiation therapy – guidelines for physiotherapists. *Physiotherapy*, 84 (8), 387–394.

Burlage, F. R., Coppes, R. P., Meertens, H., Stokman, M. A. & Vissink, A. (2001). Parotid and submandibular/sublingual salivary flow during high dose radiotherapy. *Radiotherapy and Oncology*, 61, 271–274.

Cancerbackup (2005). Cancers of the head and neck information centre [online]. (Update 13 March 2006). Retrieved 22 August 2006 from http://www.cancerbackup.org.uk

Cannaby, A. M., Evans, L. & Freeman, A. (2002). Nursing care of patients with nasogastric feeding tubes. *British Journal of Nursing*, 11 (6), 366–372.

Carper, E., Fleishman, S. B. & Mc Guire, M. (2004). Chapter 8, Symptom management and supportive care for head and neck cancer patients. In: L. B. Harrison, R. B. Sessions & W. K. Hong (Eds.), *Head and neck cancer. A multidisciplinary approach* (2nd ed.). Philadelphia: Lippincott Williams & Wilkins.

Chaplin, J. M. & Morton, R. P. (1999). A prospective longitudinal study of pain in head and neck cancer patients. *Head and Neck*, 21 (6), 531–537.

Connally, C. (2004). Head and neck cancer: preventing malnutrition. *World of Irish Nursing*, 12 (8), 27–28.

Deurloo, E. E., Schultze Kool, L. J., Kroger, R., van Coevorden, F. & Balm, A. J. (2001). Percutaneous radiological gastrostomy in patients with head and neck cancer. *European Journal of Surgical Oncology*, 27 (1), 94–97.

Eisele, D. W., Koch, D. G. & Tarazi, A. E. (1991). Case report: aspiration from delayed radiation fibrosis of the neck. *Dysphagia*, 6 (2), 120–122.

Feber, T. (Ed.) (2000). *Head and neck oncology nursing*. London: Whurr Publishers Ltd.

Fee, W. E. (1998). Nasopharynx. In: L. E. Close (Ed.), *Essentials of head and neck oncology* (pp. 205–210). New York: Thieme Medical Publishers, Inc..

Gaziano, J. E. (2002). Evaluation and management of oropharyngeal dysphagia in head and neck cancer. *Cancer Control*, 9 (5), 205–210.

Glean, E., Edwards, S. & Faithful, S. L. (2001). Intervention for acute radiotherapy induced reactions in cancer patients: the development of a clinical guideline recommended for use by the College of Radiographers. *Journal of Radiotherapy in Practice*, 2, 75–84.

Goodwin, W. J., Jr. & Byers, P. M. (1993). Nutritional management of the head and neck cancer patient. *Medical Clinics of North America*, 77 (3), 597–610.

Grant, M., Rhiner, M. & Padilla, G. V. (1989). Nutritional management in the head and neck cancer patient.*Seminars in Oncology Nursing*, 5 (3), 195–204.

Grobbelaar, E. J., Owen, S., Torrance, A. D. & Wilson, J. A. (2004). Nutritional challenges in head and neck cancer. *Clinical Otolaryngology & Allied Sciences*, 29 (4), 307–313.

Hammerlid, E., Wirblad, B., Sandin, C., Mercke, C., Edstrom, S., Kaasa, S., Sullivan, M. & Westin, T. (1998). Malnutrition and food intake in relation to quality of life in head and neck cancer patients. *Head & Neck*, 20 (6), 540–548.

Hancock, P. J., Epstein, J. B. & Sadler, G. R. (2003). Oral and dental management related to radiation therapy for head and neck cancer. *Journal of Canadian Dental Association*, 69 (9), 585–590.

Haskins, N. (1998). Intensive nursing care of patients with a microvascular free flap after maxillofacial surgery. *Intensive Critical Care Nursing*, 14 (5), 225–230.

Hirano, M. (1992). Dysphagia following various degrees of surgical resection for oral cancer. *Annals of Otology, Rhinology and Laryngology*, 101 (21), 138–141.

Huang, J., Barbera, L., Brouwers, M., Browman, G. & Mackillop, W. J. (2003) Does delay in starting treatment affect the outcomes of radiotherapy? A systematic review. *Journal of Clinical Oncology*, 21 (3), 555–563.

Hunter, A. M. (1996). Nutrition management of patients with neoplastic disease of the head and neck treated with radiation therapy. *Nutrition in Clinical Practice*, 11 (4), 157–169.

Isaacson, S. R. (1998). Complications of radiation therapy. In: L. G. Close, D. L. Larson & J. P. Shah (Eds.), *Essentials of head and neck oncology* (p. 395). New York: Thieme Medical Publishers Inc.

James, N. D., Robertson, G., Squire, C. J., Forbes, H., Jones, K., Cottier, B. & RCR Clinical Oncology Audit, Subcommittee (2003). A national audit of radiotherapy in head and neck cancer. *Clinical Oncology, 15* (2), 41–46.

Koster, M. & Bergsma, J. (1990). Problems and coping behaviours of facial cancer patients. *Social Science Medicine, 30* (5), 569–578.

Kronenberger, M. B. & Meyer, A. D. (1994). Dysphagia following head and neck cancer surgery. *Dysphagia, 9* (4), 236–244.

Kuntz, A. & Weymuller, E. (1999). Impact of neck dissection on quality of life. *Laryngoscope, 109* (8), 1334–1338.

Lamont, E. B. & Vokes, E. E. (2001). Chemotherapy in the management of squamous cell carcinoma of the head and neck. *The Lancet Oncology, 2*, 261–269.

Lazarus, C. L. (1993). Effects of radiation therapy and voluntary manoeuvres on swallowing function in head and neck cancer patients. *Clinics in Communication Disorders, 3*, 11–20.

Lee, J. H., Machtay, M., Unger, L. D., Weinstein, G. S., Weber, R. S., Chalian, A. A. & Rosenthal, D. I. (1998). Prophylactic gastrostomy tubes in patients undergoing intensive irradiation for cancer of the head and neck. *Archives of Otolaryngology – Head & Neck Surgery, 124* (8), 871–875.

Lees, J. (1999). Incidence of weight loss in head and neck cancer patients on commencing radiotherapy treatment at a regional oncology centre. *European Journal of Cancer Care, 8* (3), 133–136.

Lloyd-Williams, M. (2003). *Psychosocial issues in palliative care.* Oxford: Oxford University Press.

Lopez, M. J., Robinson, P., Madden, T. & Highbarger, T. (1994). Nutritional support and prognosis in patients with head and neck cancer. *Journal of Surgical Oncology, 55* (1), 33–36.

Machin, J. & Shaw, C. (1998). A multi disciplinary approach to head and neck cancer. *European Journal of Cancer Care, 7* (2), 93–96.

McCullough, T. M. & Jaffe, J. (16 May 2006). GI motility [online]. *Part 1: head and neck disorders affecting swallowing.* Retrieved 16 October 2006 from http://www.nature.com

Mekhail, T. M., Adelstein, D. J., Rybicki, L. A., Larto, M. A., Saxton, J. P. & Lavertu, P. (2001). Enteral nutrition during the treatment of head and neck carcinoma: is a percutaneous endoscopic gastrostomy tube preferable to a nasogastric tube? *Cancer, 91* (9), 1785–1790.

Mok, P., Seshadri, R. S., Siow, J. K. & Lim, S. M. F. (2001). Swallowing problems in post irradiated NPC patients. *Singapore Medical Journal, 42* (7), 312–316.

National Institute for Clinical Excellence [NICE] (2004). *Improving outcomes in head and neck cancers.* London: National Institute for Clinical Excellence.

Nguyen, N. P., Moltz, C. C., Frank, C., Vos, P., Smith, H. J., Karlsson, U., Dutt, S., Midyett, F. A., Barloon, J. & Sallah, S. (2004). Dysphagia following chemoradiation for locally advanced head and neck cancer. *Annals of Oncology, 15* (3), 383–388.

NHS Direct Encyclopaedia: Mucositis (2004). Retrieved 29 January 2008 from http://wwwnhsdirect.nhs.uk. Updated 27 June 2007.

Nicolaou, N. (2001). Prevention and management of radiation toxicity. *Cancer management: a multidisciplinary approach* (5th ed.). Retrieved 25 September 2007 from www.cancernetwork.com/handbook/RadiationToxicity.htm

O'Rouke, M. E. (1987). Enhanced cutaneous effects in combined modality therapy. *Oncology Nursing Forum, 14* (6), 31–35.

Owen, C., Watkinson, J. C., Pracy, P. & Galholm, J. (2001). The psychosocial impact of head and neck cancer. *Clinical Otolaryngology*, *26* (5), 351–356.

Parsons, J. T. (1994). The effect of radiation on normal tissues of the head and neck. In: R. R. Million & N. J. Cassisi (Eds.), *Management of head and neck cancer: a multidisciplinary approach* (pp. 245–289). Philadelphia: J. B. Lippincott Company.

Pauloski, B. R., Rademaker, A. W., Logemann, J. A. & Colangelo, L. A. (1998). Speech and swallowing in irradiated and non irradiated post surgical oral cancer patients. *Otolaryngology Head and Neck Surgery*, *118* (5), 616–624.

Perkins, K., Hancock, K. C. & Ward, E. C. (2007). Speech and swallowing following laryngeal and hypolaryngeal cancer. Chapter 7 in: E. C. Ward & C. J. van As-Brooks (Eds.), *Head and neck cancer: treatment, rehabilitation and outcomes* (pp. 166–167). Oxfordshire: Plural Publishing Inc.

Pickhardt, P. J., Rohrmann, C. A. & Cossentino, M. J. (2002). Stomal metastases complicating percutaneous endoscopic gastrostomy: CT findings and the argument for radiologic tube placement. *American Journal of Radiology*, *179* (3), 737–739.

Piquet, M. A., Ozsahin, M., Larpin, I., Zouhair, A., Coti, P., Monney, M., Monnier, P., Mirimanoff, R. O. & Roulet, M. (2002). Early nutritional intervention in oropharyngeal cancer patients undergoing radiotherapy. *Supportive Care in Cancer*, *10* (6), 502–504.

Porter, G. (2003). *Nutritional considerations for Head and Neck Cancer Patients*. Grand Rounds Presentation. Texas: UTMB Department of Otolaryngology.

Price, B. (2000). Altered body image: managing social encounters. *International Journal of Palliative Nursing*, *6* (4), 179–185.

Pryor, J. A. & Prasad, S. A. (2002). *Physiotherapy for respiratory and cardiac problems: adults and paediatrics* (pp. 281–298). Edinburgh: Churchill Livingstone.

Richardson, A. (1995). Fatigue in cancer patients: a review of the literature. *European Journal of Cancer Care*, *4* (1), 20–32.

Riera, L., Sandiumenge, A., Calvo, C., Bordas, J. M., Alobid, I., Llach, J. & Bernal, M. (2002). Percutaneous endoscopic gastrostomy in head and neck cancer patients. *ORL; Journal of Oto-Rhino-Laryngology & Its Related Specialties*, *64* (1), 32–34.

Righi, P. D., Reddy, D. K., Weisberger, E. C., Johnson, Trerotola, S. O., Radpour, S., Johnson, P. E. & Stevens, C. E. (1998). Radiologic percutaneous gastrostomy: results in 56 patients with head and neck cancer. *Laryngoscope*, *108* (7), 1020–1024.

Robbins, T. (1998). Classification of neck dissection. *Otolaryngologic Clinics of North America*, *31* (4), 639–655.

Rose, P. & Yates, P. (2001). Quality of life experienced by patients receiving radiation treatment for cancers of the head and neck. *Cancer Nursing*, *24* (4), 255–263.

Sanderson, R. J. & Ironside, J. A. (2002). Squamous cell carcinomas of the head and neck. *British Medical Journal*, *325* (7368), 822–827.

Scott, B. Lowe, D. & Rogers, S. N. (2007). The impact of selective neck dissection on shoulder and cervical spine movements. *Physiotherapy*, *93*, 102–109.

See, A. Wright, S. & Denham, J. W. (1998). A pilot study of demofilm in acute radiation-induced desquamative skin reactions. *Clinical Oncology (Royal College of Radiologists)*, *10*, 182–185.

Silverman, S. (2003). *Oral cancer* (5th ed.). Ontario: B. C. Decker Inc.

Sullivan, P. A. (1999). Clinical dysphagia intervention in oncology in swallowing intervention in oncology. In: P. A. Sullivan & A. M. Guilford (Eds.), *Swallowing intervention in oncology*. London: Singular Publishing Group Inc.

Talmi, Y. P. (1999). Minimising complications in neck dissection. *The Journal of Laryngology and Otology*, *113* (2), 101–113.

Van Bokhorst-de van der Schuer, M. A. E., van Leeuwen, P. A. M., Kuik, D. J., Klop, W. M., Sauerwein, H. P., Snow, G. B. & Quak, J. J. (1999). The impact of nutritional status on the prognoses of patients with advanced head and neck cancer. *Cancer*, *86* (3), 519–527.

Watson, P. G. (1992). Cancer rehabilitation and overview. *Seminar Oncology Nursing*, *8* (3), 167–173.

Williams, E. F. & Meguid, M. M. (1989). Nutritional concepts and considerations in head and neck surgery. *Head & Neck*, *11* (5), 393–399.

Chapter 8

MULTI-PROFESSIONAL MANAGEMENT OF MUSCULOSKELETAL TUMOURS

Lena Richards, Merian Denning and Gemma Lindsell

Learning outcomes

After studying this chapter the reader should be able to:

- Discuss the presentation, importance of early diagnosis and prognosis of patients with primary bone tumours and soft-tissue sarcoma
- Discuss how bone metastases develop, the signs and symptoms and the various complications that might arise
- Implement a coordinated, seamless, evidence-based rehabilitation programme
- Recognise the importance of multi-professional team working in addressing the holistic rehabilitation needs of patients with musculoskeletal tumours

---

Introduction

Malignant tumours of the musculoskeletal system are lesions that may metastasise and are potentially lethal. These lesions may be primary in bone and derived from mesenchymal cells (osteosarcoma and chondrosarcoma) or from marrow elements (myeloma and lymphoma) (see Chapter 6), or they may be metastatic to bone (Levesque *et al.*, 1998).

Sarcomas are rare tumours; a general practitioner (GP) will on average see only one or two in their whole career. However, bone metastases are the most common malignant bone lesion and should always be considered in the differential diagnosis of malignant bone tumours, particularly in the older patient. In this chapter, the management of bone sarcomas, soft-tissue sarcomas (STSs) and metastatic bone disease will be described, paying particular attention to the role of the allied health professional (AHP) in the rehabilitation of this patient group.

Primary bone tumours

Bone sarcomas are rare tumours, with fewer than 500 people diagnosed each year in the UK. They are estimated to account for 0.2% of all malignancies. Symptoms vary with the most common being pain and swelling in the affected area. The most common histological types of malignant bone tumours are:

(a) Osteosarcoma – the most common primary malignant bone tumour, occurring predominantly in patients <20 years, 80% occurring in long bones
(b) Chondrosarcoma – incidence increases with age, 50% occurring in long bones, pelvis and ribs
(c) Ewing's sarcoma – incidence predominately occurs in the second decade of life, typically arising in the axial skeleton (pelvis, scapula and rib) or in the diaphysis of long bones
(d) Spindle cell sarcomas – three major types: fibrosarcoma, malignant fibrous histiocytoma and leiomyosarcoma, typically arising in an older population (National Institute of Clinical Excellence [NICE], 2006)

Epidemiology

Osteosarcoma and Ewing's sarcoma are described here, but the principles of rehabilitation will be similar for most bone sarcomas, regardless of the histological type.

Osteosarcoma

- Peak frequency is during the adolescent growth spurt, with 75% of cases occurring between the ages of 10 and 25 years.
- Ratio of males to females is 1.5:1.0.
- Males present most commonly at 15–17 years and girls slightly earlier at 13–15. This is thought to be linked to puberty and stimulation of osteoblasts (Parker Gibbs *et al.*, 2001).

Ewing's sarcoma

- It was first described by Dr James Ewing in 1918. It is the second most common bone cancer in children and adolescents, accounting for approximately 10% of all primary malignant bone tumours, 80% of tumours occurring in patients <20 years old (Arndt & Crist, 1999; Parker Gibbs *et al.*, 2001).
- Ratio of males to females is 1.5:1.0.

Clinical features

Diagnosis may be confused or delayed due to the variety of symptoms present on clinical presentation.

Pain is the most common presenting symptom:

- It occurs in 85% of patients with osteosarcoma and 96% of those with Ewing's sarcoma (Trueworthy & Templeton, 2002).
- It is non-mechanical; i.e. patients will often complain of deep ache, which worsens and persists and may be especially bad at night.
- It may be mistaken for musculoskeletal pain, as most common sites for musculoskeletal tumours are regions frequently involved in sports injuries, e.g. knee and hip.
- The most common misdiagnosis is tendonitis (Widhe & Widhe, 2000).
- Any bone or joint pain not responding to conservative therapy within a reasonable period of time, e.g. 3–4 weeks, should be investigated thoroughly.

Swelling is a feature of late presentation and indicates that the tumour has spread into the soft tissue.

Pathological fracture might be the initial presentation of disease.

Most common sites affected are as follows:

Osteosarcoma

- Metaphyses of long tubular bones, the area of most rapid growth.
- Distal femur, proximal tibia, proximal humerus and the proximal femur, with over 70% occurring around the knee joint.
- Occasionally the diaphysis, or shaft, of long bones and, more rarely, in flat bones.
- Twenty to twenty-five per cent of patients with both Ewing's sarcoma and osteosarcoma have metastatic disease at presentation, most commonly, in the lungs for osteosarcoma and bone and lungs for Ewing's (Arndt & Crist, 1999).

Ewing's sarcoma

- It occurs with almost equal frequency in flat bones (45% occur in pelvis, spine and chest wall) and diaphyses of tubular bones, the femoral diaphysis being the most common.
- It may occasionally arise in soft tissues only (Arndt & Crist, 1999).
- Systemic manifestations such as fever, weight loss and raised erythrocyte sedimentation rate (ESR) are common features. Alkaline phosphatase and lactate dehydrogenase (LDH) are seen in the blood tests of over one-third of patients and correlate reliably with the extent of disease and are usually associated with a poor prognosis.

Diagnosis and staging

Public awareness of sarcomas is low and many studies have shown that some patients wait a considerable time after the onset of symptoms before seeking medical advice (Goyal *et al.*, 2004; NICE, 2006). Radiological features include bone destruction, new bone formation, soft-tissue swelling and periosteal elevation (Grimer, 2005).

Following X-ray and magnetic resonance imaging (MRI), patients with a probable bone tumour should be referred to a bone tumour treatment centre for biopsy and staging. Other investigations include computed tomography (CT) scan of chest to exclude or confirm lung metastases and a bone scan to identify possible bone metastases elsewhere.

Prognosis

The single most predictive prognostic factor in bone sarcomas is the presence or absence of detectable metastatic disease at presentation (NICE, 2006; Parker Gibbs *et al.*, 2001). In the 1970s and 1980s, new chemotherapy agents and treatment protocols were developed and now long-term survival rates of patients with chemosensitive tumours have risen from 10–20% to 60–70%. Patients who have clear surgical margins and good response to chemotherapy (more than 90% tumour necrosis) following induction chemotherapy have a more favourable outcome (NICE, 2006). Patients who present with metastases have a much worse prognosis in the region of 20–30% 5-year survival.

Treatment

Treatment for bone sarcomas requires a combination of surgery, chemotherapy and, in certain cases, radiotherapy.

Chemotherapy

As haematogenous spread occurs early, adjuvant chemotherapy is a cornerstone of treatment, and given pre-operatively and post-operatively it contributes significantly to long-term survival. Chemotherapy for bone sarcomas is amongst the most toxic given for any solid tumour.

Radiotherapy

Radiotherapy is a key part of curative treatment for some patients with Ewing's sarcoma but it should be avoided in younger children, if possible, because of its adverse effect on growth and the increased incidence (10–20%) of a second cancer 20 or more years after treatment (Arndt & Crist, 1999; Parker Gibbs *et al.*, 2001). Radiotherapy is delivered by fractionation of the total dose over 4–6 weeks, with daily attendances for treatment.

Surgery

The aim of surgical management is to completely remove the primary tumour while preserving the limb and its function wherever possible. Surgical treatment is radical and sometimes disabling, even when limb-sparing surgery has been performed.

Amputation. The decision regarding amputation versus limb salvage surgery is not made until the response to chemotherapy is evident. It is important in the early stages to 'sow a seed' of possible amputation, especially if the response to chemotherapy is poor. Amputations are as radical as necessary; complete removal of the tumour offers the best outcome and chance of survival (Grimer, 2005). The advantages of an amputation include early mobilisation and independent and good functional outcome depending on the level of amputation (Grimer, 2005).

Osteosarcoma is relatively resistant to radiotherapy and complete surgical removal of the primary tumour and any metastases is essential for cure. For patients who present with lung metastases, or who develop recurrence following first-line treatment, lung metastasectomy can offer those with a limited number of pulmonary metastases a realistic chance of survival.

Limb salvage surgery. Reconstruction is recommended for patients who have a good expected outcome and where the function will be better than that with amputation (Grimer, 2005). Limb salvage options include:

- Resection of tumour without replacement
- Endoprosthetic replacement
- Rotationplasty
- Autografts or allografts

Resection of the tumour alone without reconstruction is possible only in some sites. The fibula, clavicle and rib are the most obvious expendable bones, but osteosarcoma is rare in these sites (Grimer, 2005).

Endoprosthetic replacements (EPR) are used in 75% of patients (Figures 8.1 and 8.2). It is most common in the knee region (proximal tibia and distal femur), and consists of a titanium alloy implant with a rotating hinged knee and a shaft segment according to the amount of bone resected. It can replace all or part of the humerus, radius, pelvis, femur or tibia. The success of the various implants depends on the site and on the amount of normal soft tissue that can be retained to provide function (Grimer, 2005).

Advantages of EPRs

- Provide immediate and stable fixation.
- Custom-made to fit the patient and EPR is extendable in young people who are still growing; limb length can be maintained non-invasively by lengthening the prosthesis every 6 months or more frequently depending on growth rate.
- Patients mobilise, as a rule, 48 hours post-operatively fully weight bearing (FWB) as able. The long-term function for patients having had limb salvage surgery, especially around the knee, is generally very good. Most achieve near-normal function and are able to do most things apart from contact sports and activities involving running, twisting, jumping and hopping.

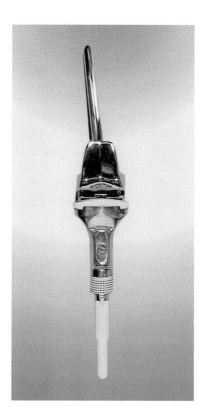

Figure 8.1 Proximal tibial EPR. [Reproduced with permission from Stanmore Implants Worldwide Ltd.]

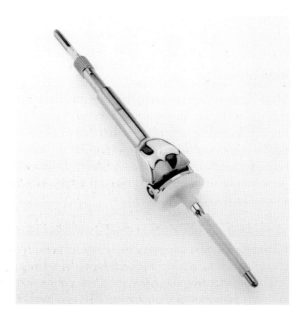

Figure 8.2 Extendable or growing distal femoral EPR. [Reproduced with permission from Stanmore Implants Worldwide Ltd.]

Disadvantages of EPRs

- Complications are common and include post-operative haematoma, infection, joint stiffness, delayed wound healing and nerve palsies, such as foot drop in tumours around the fibula (Grimer, 2005).
- Long-term risk of infection is significant (6–10% over a 10-year period) (Grimer, 2005). Signs of an infected prosthesis are pain, redness, sudden development of stiffness and an increase of temperature in the area. High-dose IV antibiotics may control the infection, but amputation may be required.
- Mechanical loosening of the prosthesis is rarer nowadays. The prosthesis will require revision at some stage, resulting in significant further hospitalisation and an increased risk of complications (Grimer, 2005).

Rotationplasty is resection of the distal femur and proximal tibia. The distal tibia is rotated 180° and attached to the proximal femur. The former ankle joint serves as a knee joint and creates a functional below-knee amputation. The main disadvantage is the appearance, which is cosmetically unappealing, and although it is functionally excellent, some patients have problems with body image.

An *autograft* uses the patient's own bone, e.g. fibula, to replace the removed tumour bone, and an *allograft* uses sterilised bone from a deceased donor. There is a high rate of complications associated with both these techniques, mainly non-union, infection and fracture. Another disadvantage is that the rehabilitation period is very long: patients are often non-weight bearing (NWB) for up to 6 months. However, with successful procedures, the advantage is that the reconstruction stabilises after 3–5 years and the patient would achieve almost full function and be able to lead a normal life.

Rehabilitation

Most patients require rehabilitation, involving intensive physiotherapy, occupational therapy (OT) and dietetics, to recover optimal physical, social and emotional functioning, including a return to school or work (NICE, 2006). Patients and their carers need a variety of support, information on managing symptoms and help with accessing social care and benefits. Many patients also have specific needs for lifelong provision of orthoses and prosthetic limbs. NICE (2006) recommends that patients should be allocated a key worker (specialist nurse or AHP) with specialist knowledge of bone tumours or STSs and their treatment and who can act as an advocate. The role of the specialist AHP as part of the multidisciplinary team (MDT) enables rehabilitation and supportive care to be provided in a timely and coordinated way, ideally in a setting local to the patient.

Many patients will require specialist equipment and environmental adaptations to aid their activities of daily living (ADLs) (Cooper, 2006) and dietetic advice particularly during chemotherapy.

Pre-operative management

Most patients undergo chemotherapy prior to their definitive surgery. This period is a useful time for the therapist to establish a relationship with the patient and to gain mutual trust. Ideally, adolescents and young adults should receive their treatment in specialist units where an expert health care professional can provide his or her patient with the very best chance of recovery (Whiteson, 2005).

Following diagnosis, the patient may need to mobilise partial weight bearing (PWB) or non-weight bearing (NWB) with elbow crutches, depending on the extent of bone destruction. If bone destruction is over 50%, there is a high risk of fracture, which would complicate the surgery as well as risk further spread of the tumour. Pain control is vital and opioids are often required in the early stages. The pain usually responds quickly to chemotherapy, with noticeable improvement even after the first cycle.

Early physiotherapy to encourage maintenance of range of movement and muscle strength should be commenced once good pain control has been achieved. A clear understanding of the implications of the forthcoming surgery and what is expected of the patient post-operatively is important. The physical and psychological aspects could be explored at this stage, such as body image issues, if the patient feels ready to do this.

Teenagers and young adults respond well to goal setting and are usually highly motivated to participate actively in their rehabilitation. It is vital that they take responsibility for this. For patients awaiting a planned amputation, a visit to their local disablement services centre (DSC) pre-operatively should be arranged. It will assist with the psychological preparation and adjustment. Pre-operative medication, e.g. anticonvulsants/antidepressants for neuropathic pain, may minimise phantom limb sensations post-operatively.

Early intervention by the OT assesses existing and potential functional independence, including home visits to address environmental problems. The OT analyses difficulties, advises on solutions and compensatory techniques and may suggest a range of equipment and adaptations (temporary or permanent) to facilitate independence. Early referral to and liaison with outside agencies and colleagues such as social service OTs in ordering equipment avoids unnecessary delays.

A gentle approach in the early stages is paramount, bearing in mind that patients are still likely to be in shock following diagnosis. Their normal routine will have been dramatically altered, e.g. education, work and social life. They will also just be coming to terms with the side effects of chemotherapy, such as hair loss, infertility, nausea and vomiting.

Post-operative management

Following amputation, physiotherapy treatment includes:

- Exercises to maintain muscle strength, range of movement of remaining joints, balance exercises and gait re-education, usually with elbow crutches.

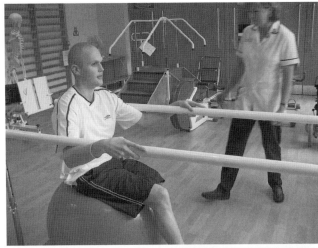

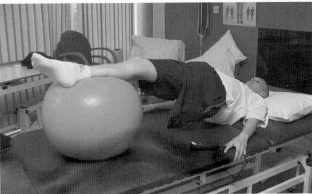

Figure 8.3 Rehabilitation 6-week post-hindquarter amputation.

- Stump and phantom limb pain/sensation respond well to gentle stump and scar massage and the use of transcutaneous electrical nerve stimulation (TENS).
- Use of a post-pneumatic amputation mobility (PPAM) aid is valuable in the early stages for patients having undergone above- and below-knee amputations.

Rehabilitation is functional and should ideally be carried out in a hospital gymnasium (Figures 8.3a and 8.3b). Early liaison with the patient's DSC for post-operative assessment for specialist prosthetic casting and fitting will ensure unnecessary delays. Prosthetic rehabilitation will be carried out by the specialist team at the DSC.

OT intervention depends on the level of amputation, particularly for patients undergoing hip disarticulation, hind and forequarter amputations. OT will be essential to facilitate discharge from hospital:

- A programme of functional activities is carried out to ensure that optimum functional independence is achieved in self-care and areas that have been identified as important to the patient.

- A second home visit, for example, would ensure that equipment previously ordered, e.g. stair rail, bathroom accessories and seating, are in place and suit the specific needs of the patient.
- A wheelchair and pressure-relieving cushion may be necessary, depending on the extent of the surgery, age and general health.
- For patients who have had limb salvage surgery, permanent adaptations are rarely necessary as the final function is expected to be good.

Rehabilitation following EPRs:

- Patients mobilise 48 h post-operatively FWB for prostheses around the knee. They are taught to 'clunk' or 'lock' prosthesis into extension which enables them to mobilise with weak quadriceps without the knee giving way.
- Protocols of rehabilitation vary depending on site of tumour and EPR. It is essential to liaise with the surgeon to ensure appropriate management.
- Post-operative physiotherapy to restore muscle strength, range of movement of joints affected, soft-tissue and scar massage and gait re-education, usually with elbow crutches or a stick.
- After 6 weeks, the emphasis of rehabilitation is functional, ideally carried out in a hospital gymnasium.

Whether limb salvage surgery offers a better psychological outcome than amputation has yet to be demonstrated because no long-term prospective or comparative studies have been completed (DiCaprio & Friedlaender, 2003). Functional outcome and patient satisfaction appear to be at least as good, and probably better, after skeletal reconstruction than after amputation. Outcomes should continue to improve as advances are made in surgical technique, implant design, autogenous bone allograft biology and post-operative management (DiCaprio & Friedlaender, 2003). For specific outcome measures (functional mobility assessment (FMA) and Toronto Extremity Salvage Score (TESS)), see the soft-tissue sarcoma section in this chapter.

Soft-tissue sarcomas

Connective tissue tumours not arising in bone are classified as soft-tissue sarcomas (STSs). They are a large and diverse group of tumours affecting any part of the body and this chapter describes those occurring in the limbs and limb girdles. STSs account for only 1% of all cancers (Kotilingam et al., 2006).

Epidemiology

Benign soft-tissue tumours outnumber malignant tumours by a factor of 100 (Clarke et al., 2005). As with many cancers, STSs increase in frequency with age (Rydholm, 1998). Although very rare in children, a recent pan-European study of incidence of childhood cancer showed a 1.8% rise in the incidence of STSs, especially among the 10–14 years age group (Kaatsch *et al.*, 2006).

Presenting features

These vary according to the anatomical site of the tumour. In the extremities:

- Patients will often present with a gradually enlarging painless lump, but sarcomas developing in the trunk or proximal thigh may grow unnoticed until patients present with symptoms of increased pressure on adjacent structures such as paraesthesia or oedema.
- Forty per cent of STSs occur in the lower limb and pelvis.
- Twenty per cent occur in the upper limb and shoulder girdle.
- Ten per cent occur in head and neck.
- Ten per cent occur in the trunk.
- Twenty per cent occur in the retroperitoneum/intraperitoneum (Clarke *et al.*, 2005).
- Tumours arising in organs will display symptoms relating to that organ; e.g. gastrointestinal stromal tumours present with non-specific GI symptoms including abdominal pain, nausea, vomiting and diarrhoea.
- While all patients with STS should be managed within the framework of a sarcoma MDT, some patients will require further specialist care; e.g. central nervous system sarcomas require the shared management of the sarcoma MDT and the neurosurgical MDT (NICE, 2006).

NICE (2005) recommends that a specialist opinion should be sought urgently if patients present with the following criteria (Table 8.1):

If there is any doubt regarding the need for referral, discussion with a local sarcoma specialist should be undertaken (NICE, 2006).

Classification

STSs are classified according to their cellular type. The World Health Organization (WHO)'s classification of tumours currently lists approximately 50 subtypes of STS (Fletcher *et al.*, 2002). The most frequent histological types are:

Table 8.1 Criteria for suspicion of an STS.

Refer urgently if a patient presents with a palpable lump that is:

- Greater than 5 cm in diameter
- Deep to fascia, fixed or immobile
- Painful
- Increasing in size
- Reoccurring following previous excision at the same site

Reproduced with permission from NICE (2005).

Table 8.2 Subtypes of rhabdomyosarcoma.

Subtype	Associated age distribution
Embryonal rhabdomyosarcoma	Children <6 years
Alveolar rhabdomyosarcoma	Children and adolescents
Pleomorphic rhabdomyosarcoma	Middle age

- Liposarcomas: Age 30–50 years, arising from deep-seated well-vascularised connective tissue, can appear anywhere, but are more commonly found in the extremities and trunk and less frequently in the head and neck.
- Leiomyosarcomas: These are found in smooth muscle but can occur anywhere in the body, e.g. uterus and GI tract.
- Fibrosarcoma: This sarcoma is more commonly found in the limbs and limb girdles being associated with tendons and ligaments.
- Dermatofibrosarcoma or desmoid tumours: They can occur anywhere in the body and are locally aggressive tumours that do not form distant metastases.
- Synovial sarcomas: They are more commonly located close to joints and they tend to occur in young adults.
- Pleomorphic sarcoma: Previously known as malignant fibrous histiocytoma, they are a histologically diverse group of tumours most commonly found in the limbs.
- Rhabdomyosarcoma: Arising in striated muscle, they can occur in the bladder, vagina, head and neck, limbs and trunk and, very rarely, in other parts of the body. There are three different subtypes (Table 8.2).
- Malignant peripheral nerve sheath tumours: These are sometimes called schwannomas or neurofibrosarcomas and can be associated with neurofibromatosis. They can occur anywhere in the body.

Aetiology

Very few aetiological factors have been identified. Many patients are perplexed that they have developed an STS perceiving themselves to be otherwise healthy, although many patients will describe how a recent trauma led them to discover their 'lump'. There are associations with certain rare medical conditions such as neurofibromatosis and human immunodeficiency virus. It is also known that prior radiotherapy can lead to development of STS later in life (Clarke *et al.*, 2005).

Clinical features

Most patients presenting with an STS will describe a gradually enlarging painless lump. They usually deny any systemic symptoms, although some patients presenting with large masses may have associated symptoms of compression on adjacent tissues, such as paraesthesia or oedema.

Table 8.3 TNM tumour staging.

Stage	Five-year survival (%)
I	86
II	72
III	52
IV	10–20

Clarke *et al.* (2005).

Diagnosis and staging

Patients presenting to their GP with a lump that fulfils the criteria set out by Table 8.1 should be referred to their local specialist sarcoma MDT without delay. A detailed history is taken, the mass is measured and its depth and proximity to other structures such as joints or major vessels are assessed. Baseline radiographic images are taken:

- Ultrasound for smaller lumps.
- MRI is preferred to CT scanning (Clarke *et al.*, 2005) for larger and deeper masses as the anatomical detail available enables both the surgeon and the oncologist to plan their treatment.
- Biopsy of the lump is carried out for definitive diagnosis, classified according to its histological type, e.g. liposarcoma, angiosarcoma, graded according to the degree of cell differentiation, the extent of necrosis and the mitotic count. Biopsy should be carried out by a specialist sarcoma surgeon as it is essential that the biopsy site is incorporated into the site of subsequent surgical excision.
- Baseline CT scan of the thorax is carried out, because the lungs are the most common site for metastatic disease (Kotilingam *et al.*, 2006).

The tumour is staged according to its tumour, node, metastasis (TNM) status, there being several subtypes dependent on size, anatomical location and depth (Table 8.3).

Surgery

The aim of curative surgery is to resect the tumour with optimal margins of disease-free tissue, maintaining maximal function with minimal morbidity (NCCN, 2006). Although STSs are known to expand spherically from their core compressing the external cells into a 'pseudocapsule' (Clarke *et al.*, 2005), some malignant cells may penetrate this and spread in a filament pattern along the tissue planes. The compartmental fascia is known to resist tumour spread, allowing the surgeon to completely resect the tumour together with adjacent soft tissues within that compartment.

Surgery, often supplemented by radiotherapy, is the treatment of choice and is often curative for localised STS (Clarke *et al.*, 2005). Some STSs are chemosensitive (Clarke *et al.*, 2005; Wolden *et al.*, 1999). Systemic use of chemotherapy is mainly reserved for metastatic disease where its role is chiefly palliative.

Preservation of function is paramount. This can be achieved by sparing some muscles within a compartment. For example knee extension, so vital for function, can be achieved by sparing one of the four quadriceps muscles within the anterior compartment of the thigh. Occasionally, major nerves or blood vessels are encased in the tumour. In a series of 15 patients requiring en-bloc sciatic nerve resection for surgical management of sarcoma, 14 returned to walking, 7 with a walking aid and 11 rated their overall function as good (Bickels *et al.*, 2002). Limb-sparing surgery has reduced the need to perform limb amputation, although, occasionally, this is required if local control cannot be obtained any other way. The estimated rate of amputation for STS is 5–10% (Clarke *et al.*, 2005). As these patients are frequently young, functional outcome is usually good (NICE, 2006).

Radiotherapy

Adjuvant radiotherapy is considered for all high-grade tumours and for all low- and intermediate-grade tumours where the margins are suboptimal (Clarke *et al.*, 2005). Occasionally, the treatment is administered as brachytherapy, involving the insertion of radioactive wires into the tumour bed (Clarke *et al.*, 2005). Radiotherapy is sometimes given pre-operatively particularly when the tumour lies in close proximity to radiosensitive normal structures.

Rehabilitation

Baseline levels of mobility and/or functional ability can be recorded using a sarcoma outcome tool, such as the functional mobility assessment (FMA) (Marchese *et al.*, 2006), Musculoskeletal Tumour Society (MSTS) score (Enneking, 1987) and Toronto Extremity Salvage Score (TESS) (Davis *et al.*, 1996). As resection of the sarcoma will involve en-bloc dissection, the physiotherapist will be able to give advice on the possible impact of the proposed surgery on future functional capability. Occasionally, an amputation may be considered. The specialist sarcoma therapist must provide a link with the rehabilitation team at the local DSC to ensure a seamless rehabilitation programme.

Post-operative rehabilitation

This will aim to regain maximal range of movement, muscle power and function. It should begin as soon as possible as the window of opportunity between surgery and radiotherapy is relatively short. Effective liaison between specialist therapists at the sarcoma centre and the patients' local therapist will ensure that appropriate and timely treatment is provided.

Functional outcome following surgery and radiotherapy has been shown to be linked to depth of tumour and its anatomical location (Gerrand *et al.*, 2004). Joint stiffness and lymphoedema are the two most common complications of radiotherapy. Joint stiffness is insidious in onset and can develop up to 2 years post-treatment (Davis *et al.*, 2005). Preservation of joint mobility through regular exercise commenced prior to radiotherapy can enhance the overall functional outcome, although very little clinical research has been done in this field. Advice on prevention strategies and early intervention can minimise the risk of developing lymphoedema (Box *et al.*, 2002) and is discussed in Chapter 11.

Physiotherapy and OT intervention, regardless of site, start with a clear understanding of the functional anatomy of the region and how surgical procedures, radiotherapy damage and postural and emotional factors are likely to compromise function. Scarring of the connective tissue, fascial and other soft-tissue structures is known to contribute to pain and stiffness. Connective-tissue mobilisation techniques, myofascial and fascial release techniques and stretching of tight structures become very useful additional treatment modalities in restoring movement and reducing pain.

Case study 1

Forty-six-year-old Mrs Z presented to her local accident and emergency with a lump in the back of her right calf. The medical team suspected a deep vein thrombosis and she was referred to the vascular surgery team. Following extensive scanning and vascular investigations over a period of 3 months, a low-grade liposarcoma, measuring 18 × 11 cm and 8 cm deep, was eventually resected (Figure 8.4). The surgical scar extended from the lower third of the posterior thigh to the lower margin of the popliteal fossa (Figures 8.5a and 8.5b).

Three months later Mrs Z was then referred to the specialist sarcoma clinic for radiotherapy.

When assessed by the physiotherapist in clinic, Mrs Z was clearly having considerable mobility problems. She had a fixed flexion deformity of 30° at the knee, decreased range of movement in the ankle and a very painful foot, which she could hardly put to the floor

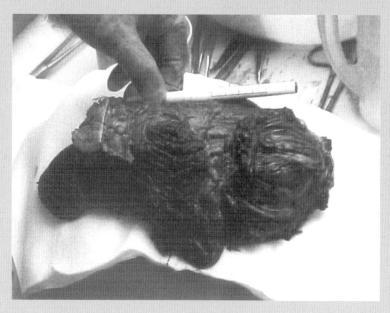

Figure 8.4 Radical dissection of a liposarcoma.

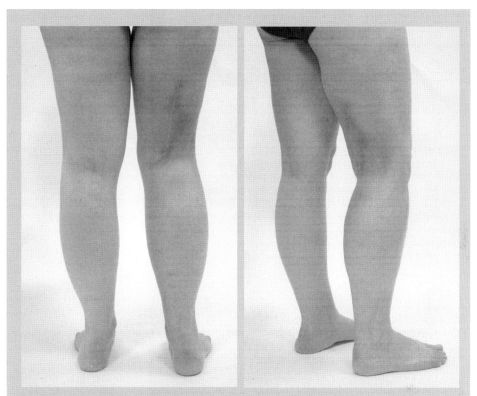

Figure 8.5 Surgical scar following radical dissection of a liposarcoma. Comorbidities post-surgery and radiotherapy include loss of knee extension and leg lymphoedema.

and was walking with elbow crutches. The foot was swollen, mottled, painful to touch and very stiff with a particularly painful first metatarsophalangeal (MTP) joint which she could not bear to touch. Her symptoms were consistent with early signs of complex regional pain syndrome (CRPS). The oncologist and physiotherapist decided that pain control was paramount. The specialist pain control team prescribed analgesia and TENS was applied to the common peroneal nerve and front of ankle.

On review a week later, Mrs Z reported a significant reduction in pain in her foot and a slight improvement in her mobility. The physiotherapist then commenced gentle connective-tissue mobilisation techniques. Foot, ankle and gentle knee extension exercises were taught and she was assessed by the OT whose intervention aimed at improving her ability to perform household tasks, in particular those activities requiring weight bearing, e.g. in the kitchen, bedroom and bathroom as well as self-care, childcare and energy con-servation.

Pain was slightly improved but, nevertheless, remained a significant problem. She was then referred to her local hospice physiotherapist for a 6-week course of hydrotherapy, after which her mobility greatly improved.

The increased demand on the circulatory system of the right foot and leg had caused the limb to become more swollen. Careful measurements were taken and a Class I or II compression stocking fitted to support the circulation.

At this point, Mrs Z was considered fit enough to tolerate a 6-week course of radiother-apy. Throughout her radiotherapy she continued her home exercise programme, adding stretching exercises to maintain the length of her hamstrings and calf muscles. The irradiated leg became sore towards the end of the treatment, which made her exercises difficult to perform, but as soon as the soreness subsided Mrs Z was encouraged to resume her previous regime. At the 6-week post-radiotherapy follow-up her knee remained slightly flexed (10° fixed flexion) but ankle movements were full. The foot continued to be very sensitive to touch, but the allodynia at the first MTP joint had resolved. She was walking without a walking aid, but her main complaint was swelling in the foot and lower leg. As a large volume of the leg had been irradiated and having had a vascular graft it was decided that Mrs Z would benefit from specialist management by the lymphoedema team, which is still ongoing.

Two years following the discovery of the lump in her leg, Mrs Z returned to her job as a learning support teacher. She remains well and is on continuing follow-up.

This case history highlights many facets of rehabilitation and the importance of teamwork but, above all, illustrates the crucial role of the multi-professional team (MPT) in managing patients with STS. Her pain and mobility problems may well have been avoided had Mrs Z been referred directly to the sarcoma MPT as per the NICE guidelines. Delays in diagnosis, treatment and specialist AHP input would not have occurred and loss of mobility, function and, possibly, the onset of CRPS symptoms may have been prevented.

Metastatic bone disease

Introduction

Sixty to eighty per cent of cancer patients will develop bone metastases at some point during the course of their disease (MacDonald & Hall, 2005). Metastatic bone cancer is most common in association with breast, prostate, lung, renal and thyroid tumours, in addition to sarcomas and multiple myeloma (Bower & Waxman, 2006). Metastatic disease to bone occurs much more commonly than primary bone tumours (Rubens, 2000a) and is the third most common form of metastasis after lung and liver (Brown & Healey, 2001). In most cases, multiple sites of bone metastasis are involved (Brown & Healey, 2001). Diagnosis is usually made via CT scan, MRI, X-ray and bone scan in addition to percutaneous needle aspiration of bone (Souhami & Tobias, 2003).

Clinical presentation

Pain is the most frequently reported symptom of metastatic bone disease. However, it has been estimated that up to 20% of women with breast cancer will present with a fracture or hypercalcaemia as the first sign of metastatic bone disease (McGarvey et al., 2006).

The most common bones to be affected by metastases are those of the axial skeleton, including the ribs, pelvis and the vertebral column, in addition to the proximal ends of the femur and humerus (McGarvey et al., 2006; Rubens, 2000a). It is thought that these areas are affected most frequently due to their highly vascularised nature (Rubens, 2000a). The bones of the appendicular skeleton are much less commonly affected, a fact which has been attributed to their lack of red marrow (O'Leary, 2001).

Although the process by which tumours metastasise to bone is not fully understood, it is generally considered that blood flow is the most likely mechanism of spread (Rubens, 2000a).

Cranial nerve syndromes can occur where bone metastases are situated at the base of the skull (Rubens, 2000a). These can cause facial pain, muscle weakness, sensory loss, hoarse voice and dysphagia (Portnow & Grossman, 2000). Metastases within the skull vault can cause increased pressure on the brain, leading to epilepsy or hemiparesis. Both of these complications are usually treated with local radiotherapy to the skull, in addition to steroids, such as dexamethasone (Hoskin & Makin, 2003).

Myelosuppression is a further complication, occurring when malignant cells invade the bone marrow. This can lead to decreased levels of white blood cells and also platelets, leaving patients at risk of developing infection and haemorrhage (Rubens, 2000a).

Pathology

Malignant cells detach from the primary tumour and travel, via the bloodstream, to bone (Lipton, 2004). Bone provides a rich supply of growth factors for malignant cells to reproduce. Once established within the bone, the metastatic cells generate growth factors that cause osteoclasts to begin destroying the bone; growth factors that stimulate bone formation are also released (Lipton, 2004). The process of bone metastases development is caused by a disruption in the normal bone remodelling process (Lipton, 2004), which involves a delicate balance between osteoclastic bone resorption and osteoblastic bone formation (MacDonald & Hall, 2005). The majority tend to be mainly lytic lesions (Bower & Waxman, 2006) and are usually seen in breast cancer and multiple myeloma (Maxwell *et al.*, 2001). Lytic lesions are characterised by areas of erosion of the bone structure, reducing bone density (McGarvey *et al.*, 2006; Reich, 2003). Most patients will present with multiple sites of metastatic spread to the bones (Rubens, 2000b).

Diagnosis

Many patients live with bony lesions for many years (Portnow & Grossman, 2000; Rubens, 2000a), which can present a challenge for the rehabilitation team, who are required to focus on optimising functional status and quality of life (Crevenna *et al.*, 2003) over the course of a progressing disease (Brown & Healey, 2001; Cooper, 2006). New developments in treatment, including the use of bisphosphonates, have increased life expectancies and are enabling patients to remain active for longer. The average survival time, following diagnosis with metastatic bone disease, is between approximately 6 months and 2.5 years (McGarvey *et al.*, 2006).

The main complications arising from the development of bone metastases are pain, reduced mobility and functional status, pathological fracture, hypercalcaemia, myelosuppression and nerve compression (Bower & Waxman, 2006). Lytic lesions are the most prone to pathological fracture (Rubens, 2000a).

Historically, patients that were considered to be at risk of pathological fracture were advised to remain on bed rest in order to avoid this from occurring. This had a significant impact on the ability of the patient to participate in rehabilitation (Bunting, 1995). However, it is now accepted that pathological fracture can be very difficult to predict (Bunting, 1995) and that the benefits of rehabilitation far outweigh the risks of fracture (Bunting & Shea, 2001). It is imperative that patients are encouraged to mobilise and maintain their functional abilities, in order to avoid deconditioning and deskilling (McDonnell & Shea, 1993). In addition, bed rest has been shown to have an exacerbatory effect on hypercalcaemia, can compromise respiratory function and present an increased risk of pressure sores and thromboembolic problems (Brown & Healey, 2001). Nevertheless, it is essential that the risk of fracture is considered when planning rehabilitation programmes (McGarvey *et al.*, 2006); falls prevention work plays an important role in this (Struthers *et al.*, 1998). Interventions to facilitate energy conservation (including the provision of assistive equipment including walking aids) are highly applicable to patients with metastatic disease to the bones (McDonnell & Shea, 1993).

Common sites

Fractures to the long bones and the vertebral bodies, causing damage to the spinal cord, are the most significant in terms of functional loss (Maxwell *et al.*, 2001). It is possible for bones that have been infiltrated by tumour to fracture after seemingly insignificant trauma, whilst others can fracture spontaneously; fracture can also occur in asymptomatic sites of metastasis (Hoskin & Makin, 2003). Hoskin and Makin (2003) state that bone lesions that are at high risk of pathological fracture can be identified using the following criteria:

- Lesions that have destroyed more than 50% of the bone cortex
- Painful sites that are greater than 2.5 cm in diameter
- Significant lytic destruction of a weight-bearing bone

Interventions

Lesions that fulfil the above criteria are considered for orthopaedic intervention, such as internal fixation (intermedullary nailing). The goal is to enable the patient to regain weight-bearing use of the affected limb and to reduce pain (MacDonald & Hall, 2005). Surgical stabilisation of the spine and long bones can be performed to prevent pathological fractures (Reich, 2003). Internal or external fixation may be used (Brown & Healey, 2001). Surgical decompression for spinal metastases may also be carried out (Brown & Healey, 2001). Surgical intervention for a fracture or potential fracture is usually followed by radiotherapy, in order to prevent local progression (Barton, 2005).

Metastatic spinal cord compression is an oncological emergency (Chapter 5). This condition occurs most commonly in association with breast, lung and prostate cancers (Brown & Healey, 2001). Prompt diagnosis of the condition and early subsequent intervention is necessary to prevent irreversible neurological damage (Reich, 2003).

Hypercalcaemia tends to be particularly prevalent in patients with multiple myeloma and breast cancer. Osteoclastic bone resorption causes calcium levels in the blood to rise, which is the method by which hypercalcaemia occurs, and thus it is more commonly associated with osteolytic lesions (Reich, 2003). Initial signs and symptoms of hypercalcaemia may be anorexia, nausea, constipation, confusion, thirst and polyuria (Cooper, 2006; Rubens, 2000a). As the condition progresses, symptoms may include vomiting, drowsiness, psychosis, coma, proximal muscle weakness, renal failure and cardiac arrest (Rubens, 2000a; Souhami & Tobias, 2003). Hypercalcaemia can also cause pain and is considered to be a poor prognostic indicator (de Kock, 2005).

Hormone therapies

Calcitonin is a hormone that has an inhibitory effect on osteoclastic activity and is used to reduce hypercalcaemia. It has a role in reducing the risk of pathological fractures occurring (MacDonald & Hall, 2005) and reduces pain both by increasing levels of natural opiates in the brain and by preventing the release of calcium into the bloodstream (Portnow & Grossman, 2000).

Hormone therapy is used to treat scattered, symptomatic bone metastases in cancers of the prostate and breast (Rubens, 2000b). Chemotherapy may also be used, with or without adjuvant radiotherapy (Hoskin & Makin, 2003).

Intravenous administration of bisphosphonates is widely used in the treatment of multiple sites of bone metastases. They work by inhibiting bone resorption and therefore assist in slowing the progression of bone metastasis, reducing pain and the risk of pathological fracture, and are often used prophylactically (MacDonald & Hall, 2005). Bisphosphonates have an important role in the treatment of hypercalcaemia, reducing the level of calcium in the bloodstream (Souhami & Tobias, 2003). A reduction in bone pain can be considered to be indicative that a patient has responded well to treatment (McGarvey et al., 2006).

Radiotherapy

Radiotherapy is often used as a highly effective method of management of pain from bone metastases (Souhami & Tobias, 2003), achieving some degree of pain relief in 80–90% of cases (Brown & Healey, 2001). The pain-relieving effects of radiotherapy can take between 2 and 3 weeks to appear (Miaskowski & Lee, 1999) and pain may be worsened for a brief time following treatment (MacDonald & Hall, 2005). Side effects of radiotherapy, including nausea and vomiting and fatigue, may affect patients' ability to participate in rehabilitation (Lowrie, 2006). Hemibody radiotherapy is often used in cases where there are diffuse sites of bone metastasis.

This is usually targeted at either the upper or lower body (above or below the umbilicus) and is commonly delivered in one dose (Hoskin, 2000).

Radioisotopes (such as strontium-89) are used for widespread bony metastases, although costly (MacDonald & Hall, 2005). The agents are injected and collect at sites of bone metastasis, administering a local dose of radiation (Barton, 2005). One of the benefits of this kind of therapy is that the incidence of toxicity is low as the isotope acts on the specific sites of metastasis, without affecting healthy cells (Houston, 2000).

Pain in metastatic bone disease

Usually, the first sign that a patient has developed bone metastasis is pain (Barton, 2005). Initially, this pain is commonly reported to be worse at night, or at rest. In the early stages of bone metastasis, pain may be relieved by activity (Brown & Healey, 2001). Over time, pain becomes unrelenting and may be present at rest (Barton, 2005); it is said to have a deep and dull quality to it (Maxwell *et al.*, 2001) with episodes of 'stabbing discomfort' (Rubens, 2000a). Pain that is exacerbated by movement is known as incident or mechanical pain and this usually accompanies metastases in the pelvis, femur or vertebrae (Rubens, 2000a).

Pain from bone metastases can be notoriously difficult to control and is known to shift from site to site in some cases (MacDonald & Hall, 2005). Bone pain tends to be nociceptive, but can also be neuropathic, where there is nerve involvement (Hoskin & Makin, 2003). Bone pain may also be accompanied by muscle spasm, so muscle relaxants can be prescribed for this (Hoskin & Makin, 2003). Pain can have a considerably detrimental impact on patients' functional status, which in turn can reduce quality of life (Kori *et al.*, 1997). It is thought that there is also a relationship between pain levels and fatigue (Miaskowski & Lee, 1999), which is discussed in Chapter 12.

Rehabilitation

A combination of pharmacological and non-pharmacological approaches to bone pain is recommended. Approaches using heat or ice have been found to be effective (MacDonald & Hall, 2005), as has the use of acupuncture (Filshie & Thompson, 2000). In addition, the use of pain diaries can be useful, as these can highlight patterns of pain occurrence and triggers, in addition to facilitating exploration and discussion of pain and its effects (Reich, 2003).

Modifications of the home environment and provision of equipment (e.g. mobility aid to reduce weight bearing) are also important interventions (MacDonald & Hall, 2005). The use of TENS may be helpful (Robb, 2002). The practice of relaxation has benefits in helping patients to cope with their pain (Skevington, 2000). For a more detailed discussion regarding pain management, please refer to Chapter 13.

Psychological interventions

Patients with bone metastases have been said to be a particularly vulnerable group with regard to development of depression and anxiety (Maxwell *et al.*, 2001). MacDonald and Hall (2005) describe the development of bone metastasis as a grave event for patients and, thus, the effect that such a diagnosis has on patients' psychological well-being must not be underestimated. Once cancer has metastasised to bone, it is generally accepted that the condition is palliative (Mundy & Guise, 2000) and this diagnosis can be the cause of great distress to patients (O'Leary, 2001). The increasing loss of function due to bone metastases can further exacerbate feelings of depression and anxiety (Reich, 2003).

It is therefore imperative that all members of the MDT are aware of the value of techniques to assist with ameliorating these symptoms as part of rehabilitation (Maxwell & Givant, 2001) and this is discussed in Chapter 15.

Case study 2

Susan was a 77-year-old woman, who presented to her GP with a right-sided breast lesion and left-sided hip pain. On referral to specialist oncology services, it was discovered via a bone scan that she had multiple bone metastases, involving her right iliac bone, sternum, several vertebrae and ribs. She was well aware at this stage that her condition was palliative. She was treated with letrozole (endocrine therapy) to inhibit growth of the primary tumour and clodronate (oral bisphosphonate therapy). Having shown a good response to systemic treatment, Susan was able to be treated with conservative wide local excision surgery for her breast tumour. At this stage, Susan was referred to the physiotherapist due to reduced mobility secondary to her bone pain and was discharged home, with Macmillan input to provide psychological support.

Eight months later, Susan was readmitted to the ward as she had developed an unsteady gait and symptoms of malignant hypercalcaemia (poor appetite, constipation and weight loss). An MRI scan was carried out, which excluded spinal cord compression. She was again treated with clodronate, but this was soon changed to hormone therapy, due to gastro-intestinal side effects. Susan was also seen by the physiotherapist with regard to her reduced mobility and given a daily exercise programme which included balance, strengthening and joint mobility exercises. Gait re-education with a walking stick enabled her to regain confidence and independence with her mobility and ADLs on the ward.

Following a 5-month stay at home, Susan was once again readmitted to the ward with symptoms of hypercalcaemia, generalised bone pain, particularly in her pelvis, and a further reduction in mobility. A bone scan taken at this time showed new lytic lesions to both shoulders and pelvis. A single fraction of hemibody radiotherapy was administered in order to achieve pain relief. During this admission, the physiotherapist reassessed Susan's mobility and provided her with a rollator frame, which gave her added support and enabled her to continue to mobilise. The exercise programme was resumed within Susan's capabilities and pain-free limits.

Susan was also assessed by the OT, who recommended provision of equipment in order to increase independence, facilitate fatigue management and reduce pain levels whilst attending to personal and domestic ADLs at home. The OT also recommended a package of care (to include daily assistance with personal care tasks), which was arranged by the hospital social worker.

During MDT meetings, Susan's mood was discussed and it was agreed that she was showing signs of depression. With her consent, Susan was referred to the hospital's psychological support team for counselling. She was subsequently commenced on antidepressant medication and discharged home soon after.

Within a month of discharge, Susan was readmitted with a 2-week history of acute confusion. Her mobility had deteriorated further and she was largely bed bound. She was treated with clodronate, calcitonin and was rehydrated. Her confusion lessened as her hypercalcaemia resolved. The physiotherapist and OT worked together to assess Susan's potential for mobility. With daily input, she was again able to mobilise with her rollator frame, but only a short distance, due to pain and fatigue. This was important to Susan, as it meant she was able to walk the few steps she needed to get to her bathroom and remained able to transfer into her chair.

Her consultant considered that Susan was no longer well enough for further chemotherapy and she was subsequently treated palliatively for pain and symptom control. As per her wishes to return home, Susan was discharged with an increased package of care. As a result of the teamwork and input from the AHPs and community services, it was possible for Susan to remain at home until the end stage of her illness. Susan's son moved in with her and was happy to attend to all domestic tasks. Due to her greatly reduced mobility, the hospital-community liaison nurse arranged provision of an electric profiling bed and pressure-relieving mattress, in order to prevent skin breakdown. The hospital OT referred Susan to the community palliative care OT, who provided an over-bed table and commode. Provision of a wheelchair plus pressure-relieving cushion was arranged via the local wheelchair service. A referral was made to the local hospice, and a few weeks later, Susan was admitted for end-of-life care.

Conclusion

Sarcomas are rare tumours. Their symptoms can vary, but the most common are pain and swelling in the affected area. STSs account for about 1% of all malignant tumours and can occur anywhere that connective tissue is present and the signs and symptoms vary greatly depending on the anatomic site. All patients with a probable bone sarcoma should be referred directly to a bone tumour treatment centre for diagnosis and the management and all patients with a confirmed diagnosis of STS should have their care supervised by a sarcoma MDT. A key worker should be allocated to each patient for all stages of his or her treatment and care.

Rehabilitation should be coordinated, promoting a seamless service, with the aim of achieving maximum function for all patients, from acute to advanced stages of disease.

Bone metastases occur most commonly in association with primary cancers of the breast, prostate, lung, kidney and thyroid. Key complications include pain, reduced mobility and functional status, pathological fracture, hypercalcaemia, bone marrow suppression and spinal cord compression. It is, therefore, vital that AHPs are involved at all stages of treatment. Rehabilitation of patients with bone metastases must be multi-professional and holistic in its approach. The role of the AHP is to provide timely and appropriate care at all stages of the cancer journey and liaison with other members of the MDT and colleagues in the community is essential.

Key learning points

- Discuss the presentation, importance of early diagnosis and prognosis of patients with primary bone tumours and soft-tissue sarcoma
- Discuss how bone metastases develop the signs and symptoms and the various complications that may arise
- Implement a coordinated, seamless, evidence-based rehabilitation programme
- Recognise the importance of multi-professional teamwork in addressing the holistic rehabilitation needs of patients with musculoskeletal tumours

References

Arndt, C. A. S. & Crist, W. M. (1999). Common musculoskeletal tumors of childhood and adolescence. *The New England Journal of Medicine, 341* (5), 342–352.

Barton, R. (2005). Managing complications of cancer. In: C. Faull, Y. Carter & L. Daniels (Eds.), *Handbook of palliative care* (2nd ed.). Oxford: Blackwell Publishing.

Bickels, J., Wittig, J. C., Kollender, Y., Keller-Graney, K., Malawer, M. M. & Meller, I. (June 2002). Sciatic nerve resection: is that truly an indication for amputation? *Clinical Orthopaedics and Related Research, 399*, 201–204.

Bower, M. & Waxman, J. (2006). *Oncology*. Massachusetts: Blackwell Publishing.

Box, R. C., Reul-Hirche, H. M., Bullock-Saxton, J. E. & Furnival, C. M. (2002). Physiotherapy after breast cancer surgery: results of a randomized controlled study to minimize lymphoedema. *Breast Cancer Research and Treatment, 75* (1), 51–64.

Brown, H. K. & Healey, J. H. (2001). Metastatic cancer to the bone. In: V. T. Devita, S. Hellman & S. A. Rosenberg (Eds.), *Cancer: principles and practice of oncology* (Vol. 2, 6th ed.). Philadelphia: Lippincott, Williams and Wilkins.

Bunting, R. W. (1995). Rehabilitation of cancer patients with skeletal metastases. *Clinical Orthopaedics and Related Research, 312*, 197–200.

Bunting, R. W. & Shea, B. (2001). Bone metastasis and rehabilitation, cancer rehabilitation in the new millennium. *Cancer, 92*(supplement), 969–1057.

Clarke, M. A., Fisher, C., Judson, I. & Thomas, M. N. (2005). Soft-tissue sarcomas in adults. *New England Journal of Medicine, 353*, 701–711.

Cooper, J. (2006). Occupational therapy approach in symptom control. Chapter 3 in: J. Cooper (Ed.), *Occupational therapy in oncology and palliative care* (2nd ed.). Chichester: Wiley.

Crevenna, R., Schmidinger, M., Keilani, M., Nuhr, M., Fiaika-Moser, V., Zettinig, G. & Quittan, M. (2003). Aerobic exercise for a patient suffering from metastatic bone disease. *Support Care Cancer, 11*, 120–122.

Davis, A. M., O'Sullivan, B. & Turcotte, R. (2005). Late radiation morbidity randomization to preoperative versus post-operative radiotherapy in extremity STS. *Radiotherapy and Oncology, 75*, 48–53.

Davis, A. M., Wright, J. G., Williams, J. I., Bombardier, C., mGriffin, A. & Bell, R. S. (1996). Development of a measure of physical function for patients with bone and soft tissue sarcoma. *Quality of Life Research, 5*, 508–516.

de Kock, I. (2005). Nausea and vomiting. In: N. Macdonald, D. Oneschuck, N. Hagen & D. Doyle (Eds.), *Palliative medicine: a case-based manual* (2nd ed.). Oxford: Oxford University Press.

DiCaprio, M. R. & Friedlaender, G. E. (2003). Malignant bone tumors: limb sparing versus amputation. *Journal of the American Academy of Orthopaedic Surgeons, 11* (1), 25–37.

Enneking, W. (1987). Modification of the system for functional evaluation in the surgical management of musculoskeletal tumors. In: *Limb salvage in musculoskeletal oncology* (pp. 626–639). New York: Churchill-Livingstone.

Filshie, J. & Thompson, J. W. (2000). Acupuncture and TENS. In: K. H. Simpson & K. Budd (Eds.), *Cancer pain management: a comprehensive approach*. Oxford: Oxford University Press.

Fletcher, C. D. M., Unni, K. K. & Mertens, F. (2002). World Health Organisation classification of tumours. In: *Pathology and genetics of tumours of soft tissue and bone*. Lyon, France: IARC Press

Gerrand, C. H., Wunder, J. S., Kandel, R. A., O'Sullivan, B., Catton, C. N., Bell, R. S., Griffin, A. M. & Davis, A. M. (2004). The influence of anatomic location on functional outcome in lower-extremity soft-tissue sarcoma. *Annals of Surgical Oncology, 11* (5), 476.

Goyal, S., Roscoe, J., Ryder, W. D. J., Gattamaneni, H. R. & Eden, T. O. B. (2004). Symptom interval in young people with bone cancer. *European Journal of Cancer, 40,* 2280–2286.

Grimer, R. J. (2005). Osteosarcoma and surgery. In: T. O. B. Eden, R. D. Barr, A. Bleyer & M. Whiteson (Eds.), *Cancer and the adolescent* (2nd ed., pp. 121–129). Oxford: Blackwell Publishing.

Hoskin, P. & Makin, W. (2003). *Oncology for palliative medicine* (2nd ed.). Oxford: Oxford University Press.

Hoskin, P. J. (2000). Bone metastases – radiotherapy. In: R. D. Rubens & G. R. Mundy (Eds.), *Cancer and the skeleton.* London: Martin Dunitz.

Houston, S. J. (2000). Clinical use of radioisotopes for bone metastases. In: R. D. Rubens & G. R. Mundy (Eds.), *Cancer and the skeleton.* London: Martin Dunitz.

Kaatsch, P., Steliarova-Foucher, E., Crocetti, E., Magnani, C., Spix, P. & Zambon, A. (2006). Time trends of cancer incidence in European children (1978–1997): report from the automated childhood cancer information system project. *European Journal of Cancer, 42,* 1961–1971.

Kori, S. H., Laperriere, J. A., Kowalski, M. B., Rodriguez, C. & Dinwoodie, W. (1997). Management of bone pain secondary to metastatic disease. *Cancer Control, 4* (2), 153–157.

Kotilingam, D., Lev, D. C., Lazar, A. & Pollock, R. E. (2006). Staging soft tissue sarcoma: evolution and change. *CA: A Cancer Journal for Clinicians, 56,* 282–291. Copyright American Cancer Society available from caonline.amcancersoc.org.

Levesque, J., Marx, R. G., Bell, R. S., Wunder, J. S., Kandel, R. & White, L. (1998). *A clinical guide to primary bone tumours.* Baltimore: Williams & Wilkins.

Lipton, A. (2004). Pathophysiology of bone metastases: how this knowledge may lead to therapeutic intervention. *Supportive Oncology, 2* (3), 205–213.

Lowrie, D. (2006). Occupational therapy and cancer-related fatigue. In: J. Cooper (Ed.), *Occupational therapy in oncology and palliative care* (2nd ed.). Chichester: Wiley.

Macdonald, S. & Hall, J. (2005). Bone pain. Chapter 4 in: N. Macdonald, D. Oneschuck, N. Hagen & D. Doyle (Eds.), *Palliative medicine: a case-based manual,* (2nd ed.). Oxford: Oxford University Press.

Marchese, V. G., Rai, S. N., Carlson, C. A., Hinds, P. S., Spearing, E. M. Zhang, L., Callaway, L., Neel, M. D., Bhaskar, N., Rao M. D. & Ginsberg, J. P. (15 June 2006). Assessing functional mobility in survivors of lower-extremity sarcoma: reliability and validity of new assessment tool. *Pediatric Blood & Cancer, 42* (2), 183–189.

Maxwell, R. N., Givant, E. & Kowalski, O. M. (2001). Exploring the management of bone metastasis according to the Roy adaptation model. *Oncology Nursing Forum, 28* (7), 1173–1181.

McDonnell, M. E. & Shea, B. D. (1993). The role of physical therapy in patients with metastatic disease to bone. *Journal of Back and Musculoskeletal Rehabilitation, 3* (2), 78–84.

McGarvey, C. L., Stout Gergich, N. L., Soballe, P. & Pfalzer, L. (2006). A case report: breast cancer metastasis and implications of bony metastasis on activity and ambulation. *Rehabilitation Oncology, 24* (1), 4–17.

Miaskowski, C. & Lee, K. (1999). Pain, fatigue and sleep disturbances in oncology outpatients receiving radiation therapy for bone metastasis: a pilot study. *Journal of Pain and Symptom Management, 17* (5), 320–332.

Mundy, G. R. & Guise, T. A. (2000). Pathophysiology of bone metastasis. Chapter 4 in: R. D. Rubens & G. R. Mundy (Eds.), *Cancer and the skeleton.* London: Martin Dunitz.

NCCN (2006). *Practice guideline in oncology* (v. 3). Washington, DC: National Comprehensive Cancer Network, Inc.

National Institute for Health and Clinical Excellence [NICE] (2005). Referral guidelines for suspected cancer. *NICE clinical guideline* (no. 27). Retrieved 22 November 2006 from www.nice.org.uk/CG027

National Institute for Health and Clinical Excellence [NICE] (2006). Improving outcomes for people with sarcoma: the manual. *NICE cancer service guidance*. London: National Institute for Health and Clinical Excellence. Retrieved 22 November 2006 from www.nice.org.uk

O'Leary, U. (2001). Bone metastasis: secondary illness, primary concern. *Nursing Times*, 97 (41), 32–34.

Parker Gibbs, C., Weber, K. & Scarborough, M. T. (2001). Malignant bone tumors. *The Journal of Bone & Joint Surgery*, 83 (11), 1728–1745.

Portnow, J. & Grossman, S. A. (2000). Pain – mechanisms, assessment and management. In: R. D. Rubens & G. R. Mundy (Eds.), *Cancer and the skeleton*. London: Martin Dunitz.

Reich, C. D. (2003). Advances in the treatment of bone metastases. *Clinical Journal of Oncology Nursing*, 7 (6), 641–646.

Robb, K. A. (2002). *Non-pharmacological interventions in the management in the management of chronic pain associated with breast cancer treatment*. Ph.D. Thesis. London: Kings College.

Rubens, R. D. (2000a). Bone metastases – incidence and complications. In: R. D. Rubens & G. R. Mundy (Eds.), *Cancer and the skeleton*. London: Martin Dunitz.

Rubens, R. D. (2000b). Bone metastases – general approaches to systemic treatment. In: R. D. Rubens & G. R. Mundy (Eds.), *Cancer and the skeleton*. London: Martin Dunitz.

Rydholm, A. (1998). Improving the management of soft tissue sarcoma. *British Medical Journal*, 317, 94–95.

Skevington, S. M. (2000). Psychological support. In: K. H. Simpson & K. Budd (Eds.), *Cancer pain management: a comprehensive approach*. Oxford: Oxford University Press.

Souhami, R. & Tobias, J. (2003). *Cancer and its management* (4th ed.). Massachusetts: Blackwell Science.

Struthers, C., Mayer, D. & Fisher, G. (1998). Nursing management of the patient with bone metastases. *Seminars in Oncology Nursing*, 14 (3), 199–209.

Trueworthy, R. C. & Templeton, K. J. (2002). Malignant bone tumors presenting as musculoskeletal pain. *Pediatric Annals*, 31 (6), 355–359.

Whiteson, M. (2005). A right, not a privilege. In: T. O. B. Eden, R. D. Barr, A. Bleyer & M. Whiteson (Eds.), *Cancer and the adolescent* (2nd ed., pp. 1–10). Oxford: Blackwell Publishing.

Widhe, B. & Widhe, T. (2000). Initial symptoms and clinical features in osteosarcoma and Ewing's sarcoma. *American Journal of Bone and Joint Surgery*, 82, 667–674.

Wolden, S. L., Anderson, J. R. & Crist, W. M. (1999). Indications for radiotherapy and chemotherapy after complete resection in rhabdomyosarcoma: a report from the intergroup rhabdomyosarcoma studies I to III. *Journal of Clinical Oncology*, 17 (11), 3468–3475.

Chapter 9

MULTI-PROFESSIONAL MANAGEMENT OF GASTROINTESTINAL TUMOURS

Tessa Aston, Sallyanne McKinney, Jennifer Miller and Heidi Williams

---

Learning outcomes

After studying this chapter the reader should be able to:

- Discuss the risk factors and incidence for upper and lower gastrointestinal (GI) tumours and guidelines for health promotion
- Describe the medical and surgical management of such tumours and the impact on patients' quality of life at key stages along the patient's pathway
- Discuss the importance of a holistic, collaborative and multidisciplinary approach to the management of each of the GI tumours from their diagnosis through to end-of-life or potential cure
- Implement an evidence-based approach to the therapeutic management of such tumours.

Introduction

Most people with upper gastrointestinal (GI) tumours survive only a few months after diagnosis. The overall 5-year survival for oesophageal cancer is around 10% and for gastric cancer it is around 15%. This is in contrast to lower GI cancers (Cancer Research UK, 2006).

The disease and its treatment can have a significant physical impact on the patient. Malnutrition is a common problem affecting up to 85% of patients with GI tumours during the course of their disease (Stratton *et al.*, 2003). Weight loss, deconditioning and fatigue can have functional and lifestyle changes. The psychological impacts of the disease include anxiety, reduced independence, loss of role in the family, coming to terms with change in body image, tube feeding, stoma bags and sexuality in addition to financial difficulties. As treatment options are increasing, patients are having more complex and challenging needs.

Table 9.1 Cancer incidence of upper GI cancers in the UK.

Cancer type	Number of registrations of cancer diagnosed in 2003 (approximate)
Oesophagus	7500
Stomach	9000
Pancreas	7100

Data from Cancer Research UK (2006).

This chapter discusses the multidisciplinary approach to managing the complex needs of patients with GI tumours whether this is active treatment with intent to cure, advanced disease or those requiring support at the end of life.

UPPER GI TUMOURS

Types, incidence and prevalence

Incidence is summarised in Table 9.1.

Oesophageal cancer is the ninth most common cancer in the United Kingdom (UK). It has a male-to-female ratio of 5:3 and is predominantly a disease of the older person (Cancer Research UK, 2006). Squamous cell cancer (generally affecting the mid-to-upper third of the oesophagus) accounts for a slightly lower rate of incidence in comparison to adenocarcinomas. The incidence of adenocarcinoma has increased dramatically in the last 20 years and accounts for approximately half of all remaining malignant oesophageal tumours (Cancer Research UK, 2006). It is thought to be associated with acid reflux and predominantly affects the lower third of the oesophagus (Cancer Research UK, 2006). Malignant GI stromal tumours occur rarely.

Stomach cancer accounts for 3% of all newly diagnosed cancers and is the seventh most common cancer in the UK (Cancer Research UK, 2006). Ninety per cent of stomach cancers are diagnosed in adults over the age of 55 years. Ninety-five per cent are adenocarcinomas, with the remaining 5% being either squamous-cell, lymphomas, sarcomas or neuroendocrine tumours (Cancer Research UK, 2006).

Pancreatic cancer is the eleventh most common cancer in the UK (Cancer Research UK, 2006). It has a high mortality rate with 5-year survival rates ranging from 0.4 to 4.0% (Quinn et al., 2001). This is partly because symptoms are non-specific, so the disease is almost always diagnosed at a late stage. It can occur in the head, the body or the tail of the pancreas. Around 70% of tumours are in the pancreatic head (Takhar et al., 2004). The majority are adenocarcinomas with early local spread to lymph nodes to the duodenum, obstructing bile duct and into the peritoneal cavity.

Table 9.2 Clinical presentation of upper GI cancers.

	Oesophageal cancer	Stomach cancer	Pancreatic cancer
Dysphagia	✓	In some cases	
Weight loss	✓	✓	✓
Pain	✓ (in throat/sternum)	✓ (in abdomen)	✓ (in abdomen)
Nausea/vomiting	✓	✓	✓
Acid reflux	✓	✓	
Early satiety		✓	
Altered bowel habit			✓
Obstructive jaundice			✓
Cachexia	✓	✓	✓

Data from Cancer Research UK (2006).

Risk factors

In identifying the following risk factors, allied health professionals (AHPs) can recognise the potential benefits of encouraging a healthy lifestyle in their patients, thereby hopefully reducing the incidence of upper GI cancers:

- Tobacco smoking
- Excessive alcohol intake
- Poor nutritional status
- Oesophageal disorders
- Obesity
- *Helicobacter pylori*
- Family history, e.g. familial adenomatous polyposis
- Pernicious anaemia/atrophic gastritis/partial gastrectomy
- Diabetes mellitus and chronic pancreatitis
      (Allum *et al.*, 2002; Cancer Research UK, 2006)

Clinical presentation

Upper GI cancers often present with late-stage disease. Indeed, 50–80% of patients with oesophageal cancer and 30–50% of patients with stomach cancer are deemed inoperable at diagnosis (Scottish Intercollegiate Guidelines Network [SIGN], 2006). Those undergoing surgery can only expect a 10–25% 5-year survival rate (Cancer Research UK, 2006).

The differences in symptoms at presentation for the cancer types are given in Table 9.2. In addition to the symptoms listed in Table 9.2, infiltration of the bowel causes duodenal obstruction, abdominal pain and ascites.

Diagnosis

Owing to the radical nature of surgery, accurate staging of an oesophageal or gastric tumour is extremely important and greatly influences treatment options. Diagnostic investigations may include:

- Oesophagogastroduodenoscopy (OGD)
- Biopsy
- Computer tomography (CT) scan of thorax and abdomen
- Endoscopic ultrasound (EUS)
- Laparoscopy prior to consideration of radical resection
- Barium swallow
- Magnetic resonance imaging (MRI)
- Positron emission tomography (PET)
      (Allum *et al.*, 2002; Gao *et al.*, 1994)

For pancreatic cancer, investigations include:

- Abdominal ultrasonography
- CT
- MRI scans
- Endoscopic retrograde cholangiopancreatography(ERCP)
      (British Society of Gastroenterology, 2005)

At diagnosis, all patients should have access to specialist nursing support (Allum *et al.*, 2002). Clinical nurse specialists have a pivotal role in coordinating all members of the multidisciplinary team (MDT) in order to provide a collaborative approach to cancer management. In addition, they have a major role in improving a patient's quality of life, offering support, advice and information to both patients and carers. The contributions of AHPs are highlighted in the Manual of Cancer Services (2004).

Multidisciplinary assessment and treatment of cancers of the oesophagus and stomach

Treatment is dependent on the cancer stage, the patient's age and general health/fitness. Oesophagectomy or radical gastric resection is only recommended for patients with T1, T2 and T3 tumours with minimal nodal involvement (SIGN, 2006). Surgery should only be undertaken in centres with a sufficiently large case volume and appropriate multidisciplinary support services (Allum *et al.*, 2002; Department of Health [DH], 2001). Unlike oesophageal resection, which is predominantly aiming for a curative outcome, surgery for gastric cancer can also be undertaken in an attempt to relieve symptoms (e.g. vomiting as a result of a pyloric obstruction).

Chemotherapy and radiotherapy

Chemotherapy may be given before and/or after gastrectomy in patients with T3 cancers and/or local nodal involvement (Cancer Research UK, 2006). Neoadjuvant (pre-operative) chemotherapy may be offered to oesophageal cancer patients prior to oesophagectomy. In some cases patients may have chemoradiotherapy pre- or post-operatively. Radical chemoradiotherapy may also be considered as definitive treatment in those patients with localised oesophageal tumours who are unsuitable for surgery (Allum *et al.*, 2002).

It should be noted that treatment methods are constantly changing and patients can receive combinations of treatment that can last for long periods. As a result, patients will require close monitoring by AHPs/MDT throughout and after treatment.

Decisions about treatment are made with consideration to predicted prognosis and the effect of any treatment intervention on quality of life. It is important that the MDT provides a holistic approach to patient care (Allum *et al.*, 2002).

The MDT must be aware of the need to look for and identify nutritional problems early on. By rectifying such problems patients may be better able to cope with the demands of the illness and the effects of any treatment given (Eberhardie, 2002).

Surgery

Due to the nature of surgery and similar pre- and post-operative symptoms, the roles of AHPs in both oesophageal and gastric cancer resection can, in the main, be grouped together.

Pre-operative preparation

All health professionals should encourage patients to stop smoking. However, any reduction in post-operative complications will only be seen in those that have stopped for at least 8 weeks (Barry *et al.*, 1989). Smoking cessation advice can be obtained via the patients' general practitioner (GP) or national organisations (National Institute of Clinical Excellence [NICE], 2006a).

Physiotherapist

The physiotherapist is an important member of the team when assessing a patient's fitness for surgery (Janke *et al.*, 2002). In addition to taking a full subjective history (Table 9.3) and physical examination (including auscultation and palpation), a

Table 9.3 Subjective respiratory risk factors – a checklist.

Risk factor	Subjective details
History of chest condition	For example chronic obstructive pulmonary disease, asthma, bronchitis
Smoking habits	Number of cigarettes, cigars, ounces of tobacco and for how long (N.B. This is often underestimated by patients.)
Presence of a cough	Persistent, productive, signs of infection; associated symptoms of breathlessness and wheeze
Functional status	Able to manage flight of stairs, distance walked on the flat, functional indicators, e.g. Duke Activity Status Index (Hlatky *et al.*, 1989)

Data from Janke *et al.* (2002).

physiotherapist may also carry out specific lung function tests, e.g. shuttle test (Singh *et al.*, 1992) and lung spirometry (Ferguson & Durkin, 2000). Patients are at increased risk of pulmonary complications when FEV1 (forced expiratory volume in 1 s) is reduced by 20% of the predicted value (Nagawa *et al.*, 1994).

Those patients undergoing upper abdominal/thoracic surgery are at an increased risk of respiratory complications due to the disruption of the abdominal and diaphragmatic muscles, which in turn causes large decreases in lung volumes (Janke *et al.*, 2002). Functional residual capacity may be reduced by up to 30%, 24 h postoperatively and remain low for several days afterwards (Pryor & Ammani Prasad, 2002). This fact coupled with an impaired mucociliary action (Houtmeyers *et al.*, 1999) may lead to small airway closure, a ventilation/perfusion mismatch and impaired gas exchange. Respiratory function will also be further affected in those patients with pre-existing lung disease, e.g. chronic obstructive pulmonary disease, bronchiectasis and asthma. Pre-operative optimisation of these patients is essential and the physiotherapist has a role to play in reducing sputum retention and maximising lung volumes in the pre-operative period (Pryor, 1999). However, in practice, preparation is often time limited due to the urgency with which these patients are brought for surgery.

It is important that all patients and carers have an opportunity to discuss details of the operation and recovery period in order to help reduce anxiety and appreciate their role in their own recovery. All information should be tailored to the individual and be appropriate to their level of understanding and openness to information.

Routine pre-operative physiotherapy should include instructions in prophylactic deep-breathing exercises, supported expectoration techniques, the importance of early mobilisation and the significance of adequate functional pain control. Some centres may also include the teaching of incentive spirometry with an opportunity to take the equipment home to practice.

Dietitian

The dietitian plays a key role in the nutritional management of upper GI cancers undergoing radical resection (Brooks-Bunn, 2000). An impaired nutritional status can affect response to treatment, the amount of treatment required and quality of life (Bruera & MacDonald, 1988). A patient with a poor nutritional status is less likely to be able to withstand the side effects of treatment (Thomas, 2007). In addition, the side effects of chemotherapy can further exacerbate an already poor nutritional status (Cancer Research UK, 2006). In some cases where patients are to have radical chemoradiotherapy, due to treatment toxicity, a percutaneous endoscopic gastrostomy tube (PEG) may need to be inserted prior to treatment being commenced in order to maintain nutritional status (Margolis *et al.*, 2003).

A detailed nutritional history will identify nutritional problems and can assist the dietitian in planning the post-operative management of these patients (see Table 9.4). Patients with a body mass index (BMI) below 18.5 kg/m² and/or unintentional weight loss of greater than 10% over the preceding 3-month period are associated with an increased risk of perioperative complications (Allum *et al.*, 2002; NICE, 2006b).

Table 9.4 Factors to obtain during nutritional assessment.

Current weight, height and BMI

Percentage of unintentional weight loss over a given time period

Current diet history, including eating pattern, food frequency and portion sizes

Unintentional changes to diet history over preceding 3–6 months, e.g. consistency of foods, portion sizes and problem foods

Likes and dislikes

Symptoms related to cancer site over given time period (refer to clinical presentation)

Data from Thomas (2007).

In addition, those patients with near total dysphagia may require oral nutritional supplements and/or artificial feeding prior to surgery, e.g. nasogastric or nasojejunal feeding (Thomas, 2007).

Speech and language therapist

Although speech and language therapy input is not routinely part of an upper GI cancer patient's pathway, intervention may be useful to aid differential diagnosis and/or to determine if aspiration whilst swallowing is evident. This may involve either a videofluoroscopy assessment or a clinical bedside assessment. Speech and language therapy advice can also be useful when considering various dietary modifications and textures pre- and post-operatively.

Post-operative management

In gastric surgery a large upper abdominal incision is performed. With an oesophagectomy, the surgical approach is dependent on the type of tumour and its location. The most widely practised approach is the two-stage operation with a midline abdominal incision and formation of a gastric tube and right thoracotomy to excise the tumour and form the anastomosis. During surgery, the anaesthetist instigates 'one lung ventilation' as the right lung is collapsed to allow access for the resection and two chest drains are inserted. Patients are routinely nursed in high-dependency units for intensive monitoring and support (Allum *et al.*, 2002).

Physiotherapist

Pulmonary complications (e.g. atelectasis, consolidation and pneumonia) occur in up to 50% of patients and the role of the physiotherapist is vital in these early stages (McCulloch *et al.*, 2003). Physiotherapy in the form of deep-breathing exercises, supported coughing and early mobilisation are commenced immediately post-operatively. Although used in many centres, the use of incentive spirometry remains controversial (Grosselink *et al.*, 2000). Adequate analgesia, normally provided by an epidural, is of the utmost importance in permitting effective physiotherapy and preventing respiratory complications (Watson & Allen, 1994).

Due to the high anastomosis associated with an oesophagectomy, physiotherapists must exercise caution in the use of the following adjuncts:

- Head-down postural drainage positions to avoid regurgitation of abdominal contents and risk of aspiration.
- Suctioning via an oropharyngeal/nasopharyngeal airway, to avoid inadvertently entering the oesophagus and compromising the anastomosis. A mini-tracheostomy may be required.
- Positive pressure techniques (i.e. intermittent positive pressure breathing (IPPB), positive expiratory pressure mask (PEP) or continuous positive airway pressure (CPAP)) should be used only with caution (American Association for Respiratory Care [AARC], 2003). This is due to the risks associated with positive pressure and possible disruption to the anastomosis, particularly in high oesophageal surgery. In practice, these treatment modalities may be used post-operatively, although pressures should ideally be kept as low as possible and following discussion with the surgeon/anaesthetist involved (Pryor & Ammani Prasad, 2002).

Patients are normally nursed in bed the day after surgery and circulatory exercises should be instigated as soon as possible. Although patients have many drips and drains (e.g. central line, epidural, urinary catheter, chest drains and wound drains), the physiotherapist should play a key role in early mobilisation (Figure 9.1).

Within several days the patient should be aiming towards independent walking and, if possible, have access to a static cycle or other appropriate forms of cardiovascular exercise. In addition to chest clearance and mobilisation, upper limb exercises should also be encouraged (Reeve et al., 2007). The presence of the two chest drains is documented to be particularly painful (Fox et al., 1999) and this in turn may lead to a reduction in shoulder movement on the affected side. Some patients will continue to suffer with pain and a reduced range of movement once the drains have been removed and may require additional outpatient physiotherapy on discharge.

At all times the physiotherapist, collaborating with the occupational therapist, encourages patient's independence and self-management.

Dietitian

Post-pyloric feeding (either through a nasojejunal or surgical jejunostomy tube) can be used during the early post-operative period until the anastomosis has healed and the patient is able to take adequate diet and fluids orally (Reichle et al., 1995; Wakefield et al., 1995). The use of feeds enriched with arginine, omega-3 fatty acids and nucleotides pre- and post-operatively remains controversial (Braga et al., 2002; Daly et al., 1995). More recent studies have supported the use of such substrates in enteral feeds for major cancer surgery of the abdomen (Arends et al., 2006; Weimann et al., 2006). The patient recommences oral intake usually 7–10 days following surgery. If the patient is receiving jejunal feeding, the volume should be reduced as the patients' oral intake gradually increases.

Reported symptoms following surgery are shown in Table 9.5.

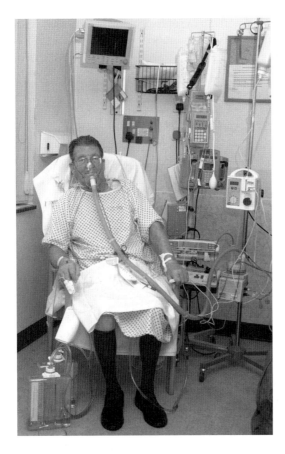

Figure 9.1 Patient sitting out of bed 2 days following an oesophagectomy.

Table 9.5 Potential nutritional problems following oesophagogastric surgery.

Poor appetite and lack of interest in eating

Early satiety, bloating and/or discomfort after eating

Fear of eating, particularly if problems pre-operatively

Weight loss and difficulty maintaining or regaining weight

Bland taste to foods/taste changes during early post-operative stage

Nausea, vomiting and delayed gastric emptying

Diarrhoea – related to increased intestinal motility and/or rapid emptying of gastric remnant

Constipation – during early post-operative stage, particularly if poor food/fluid intake and lack of mobility

'Dumping' – can occur immediately after eating or 2–3 h later. Can cause symptoms of sweating, dizziness, feeling faint and/or a rapid pulse

Acid reflux, indigestion and/or increased belching – primarily following oesophagectomy

Food 'sticking' particularly during early post-operative recovery – some patients may require dilatation if anastomosis too 'tight'

Data from Thomas (2007).

Regular dietetic advice and supervision during the early weeks and months following surgery are essential in order to reassure patients about their progress and help control the potential problems highlighted in Table 9.5. Oral nutritional supplements may need to be used if nutritional needs cannot be met by diet alone (Thomas, 2007). Written information regarding dietary advice and common post-operative symptoms should be provided to the patient and carer prior to their discharge home. The Oesophageal Patients Association produces a useful post-operative information booklet (see Support Organisations).

Dietary advice following surgery can be summarised as follows:

- Ensure food is chewed well and eaten slowly.
- Advice on protein and energy-dense foods and fluids and food fortification.
- Take fluids after eating a meal/snack rather than with food.
- Try to take small, frequent meals and snacks during the day even if not hungry.
- Avoid eating too late at night.
- If problems occur with some foods initially, leave them for a couple of weeks and then try them again.
- Limit intake of 'bulky' high-fibre foods as they will exacerbate the feelings of early satiety and bloating.
- Reassure patients that they can try any food and fluid and that this can be a normal texture.
- Oesophagectomy patients may be given a proton pump inhibitor , in order to help control acid reflux post-operatively. They should avoid lying flat in bed (by using well-propped pillows) and sit upright during and immediately after eating.
- Gastrectomy patients require vitamin B12 injections, usually every 3 months, due to the loss of intrinsic factor (needed for the absorption of vitamin B12).
  (Thomas, 2007, p. 437)

Occupational therapist

The occupational therapist can address a number of issues with the patient at this stage, particularly if anxiety is exhibited due to previous experiences. Through exploration of anxiety and identification of how it impacts on the patient's participation in meal preparation and eating, the occupational therapist can work with the patient in goal setting and implementation of anxiety management techniques. Such techniques commonly include breathing exercises, guided visualisation and challenging negative thought patterns. Additionally, the occupational therapist is ideally placed to provide advice on meal and drink preparation including the use of equipment to minimise energy expenditure and optimise independence within this activity.

The physiotherapist and occupational therapist will work collaboratively to provide specific discharge advice (Cheville, 2001). Advice on activities of daily living, work and hobbies should ideally be covered in written format and patients can be directed to appropriate support services in the community, including the Oesophageal Patients' Association (see Support Organisations).

Palliative treatment

Depending on symptoms, staging and the general health/fitness of the patient, options may include one or more of the following (Allum *et al.*, 2002; Cancer Research UK, 2006):

- Chemotherapy
- Radiotherapy (not used as frequently in gastric cancers but can be used to control pain and/or bleeding)
- Stent insertion (generally used to treat dysphagia in oesophageal cancer or pyloric outlet obstruction in gastric cancers)
- Brachytherapy (oesophageal cancers)
- Argon beam treatment

Physiotherapist

Some patients with advanced oesophageal cancer may develop tracheo- or bronchooesophageal fistulas. These patients are at extremely high risk of aspiration and consequently pulmonary complications, exacerbated by associated decreases in white cell counts. Chest clearance can be problematic as breathing exercises and coughing are often ineffective. Patients may require drug therapy (i.e. antimuscarinics) to help dry out oral secretions and improve patient comfort.

Patients can have significant muscle weakness and mobility issues particularly if their nutritional status is poor. Working within the MDT, the physiotherapist works with the occupational therapist to prepare the patient and family for safe discharge into the community, ensuring appropriate equipment and adequate support is in place (Cheville, 2001).

Dietitian

Patients having palliative chemotherapy often find the side effects of treatment have an impact on their already-poor oral intake. Assessment and advice by a dietitian can be of benefit during treatment and may include advice on food fortification, nutritional supplementation and, if appropriate, artificial nutritional support (Thomas, 2007).

Side effects from radiotherapy may initially cause dysphagia to worsen before it improves, particularly towards the end of the treatment period and a few weeks after completion. Patients may find that foods of a smooth, soft consistency are better tolerated during this time. Advice should be given on appropriate foods to choose and avoid. Many of these patients are likely to have lost weight and may already be malnourished. It is important that such patients are monitored by the MDT and the dietitian providing nutritional support in order to prevent further deterioration (Thomas, 2007).

As a result of the limited evidence around dietary advice for managing patients with oesophageal stents, the Oncology Group of the British Dietetic Association produced a professional consensus statement (Oncology Group of the British Dietetic Association, 2003). This gives information to support good practice rather than providing an evidence base. Thomas (2007) also gives general guidelines, but it should be noted that dietetic advice should be tailored to meet the patient's individual needs and tolerance to such foods.

Occupational therapist

The role of the occupational therapist in palliative care is varied, depending on the patient's functional and psychological needs; the primary aim is to facilitate patients in achieving optimum control within their lives (Penfold, 1996). As patients experience significant problems associated with nutritional status, engagement in usual routines including leisure activities can be affected. Treatment and hospital appointments can be all consuming and the occupational therapist can assist the patient to consider ways of reincorporating pleasurable activities of his or her choice into daily routines. In addition, increased activity levels can positively influence appetite. Such activities may include kitchen tasks, e.g. being involved in aspects of food preparation that are manageable, planning menus and writing shopping lists. Continued engagement and maintaining a useful role can be important for people.

Following collaboration with the patient and family, returning home, either for short periods of time or for terminal care, requires preparation within the MDT to ensure that all necessary equipment, care and adequate community support are in place. Occupational therapists play an integral part in safe discharge planning (Cheville, 2001), and this may include a home visit to identify equipment and minor adaptation needs, educating carers on the use of such equipment and providing psychological support throughout the transition.

Multidisciplinary assessment and treatment of pancreatic cancer

More than 80% of pancreatic cancers are unresectable at diagnosis. Consequently, prognosis is very poor with only 3–5% of patients alive after 5 years (Ellis & Cunningham, 1994). Patients with liver or peritoneal metastases and distant lymph node metastases are unlikely to be considered for resection (Alexakis *et al.*, 2004). The Kausch–Whipple procedure and the pylorus-preserving procedure are the most common approaches for cancer of the head of pancreas. The majority of patients develop disease recurrence within 1–2 years after resection (Amikura *et al.*, 1995; Karpoff *et al.*, 2001). Adjuvant chemotherapy is now standard post-operative treatment in the UK.

Treatment is mainly with palliative interventions in order to relieve symptoms and should have the ultimate aim of enhancing quality of life. These include biliary bypass or stenting to relieve obstructive jaundice and duodenal obstruction, pain relief, pancreatic enzyme supplementation and diabetes management (British Society of Gastroenterology, 2005).

Palliative radiotherapy is used as an option to manage pain and delay the need for analgesics. Gemcitabine chemotherapy is offered as a treatment option for well-motivated patients with good performance status and hence is gaining psychological benefit (British Society of Gastroenterology, 2005).

Referral to AHPs depends on the MDT but tends to be at the palliative stages of intervention when symptoms present rather than routine referral as in the case of oesophageal and gastric cancers.

Physiotherapist

As with most major surgery, physiotherapy is involved in the initial stages, ensuring effective chest clearance and early mobilisation. Patients will also require detailed information on reducing fatigue, improving general activity levels to promote conditioning and returning to exercise/hobbies/work as appropriate following discharge, which can be done in collaboration with the occupational therapist.

Dietitian

Since cancer cachexia has such an important part in the mortality and morbidity of pancreatic cancer patients, there has been much interest in alternative nutritional interventions to improve nutritional status. Several studies have been carried out evaluating the effectiveness of an omega-3 fatty acid, eicosapentaenoic acid (EPA) that is thought to attenuate the altered metabolic processes, which lead to cancer cachexia (Barber et al., 1999; Wigmore et al., 2000). Results have been mixed and it has been difficult to interpret these results and apply them to clinical practice due to the small numbers in the studies. Fearon et al. (2006) reported no statistically significant improvements in survival or weight in patients taking EPA supplement capsules. Arends et al. (2006) suggest that EPA is unlikely to prolong survival in advanced cancer. A systematic review of EPA for the treatment of cancer cachexia concluded that it was not possible to recommend the use of EPA in clinical practice (Dewey et al., 2007).

Assessment by the dietitian should take into account treatment options and patient-reported symptoms. In addition to obtaining the information as shown in Table 9.4 the following additional information should be obtained:

- Evidence of malabsorption/abdominal symptoms such as steatorrhoea, altered stool pattern and abdominal pain.
- Assessment of blood glucose control if patient has diabetes mellitus.
- Dietetic interventions should focus on nutrition support through dietary counselling, pancreatic enzyme replacement therapy (PERT) adjustment and oral nutritional supplementation. Guidelines for the management of PERT can be found in Thomas (2007, pp. 444–445).

As the disease advances patients can experience vomiting with solids as the tumour invades the duodenum. Stenting is attempted to give temporary relief and the dietitian can offer guidance and reassurance regarding diet at this stage.

Occupational therapist

Weight loss due to anorexia or cachexia may potentially result in the individual developing an altered body image, which can cause anxiety and stress to both the patient and his or her family (Bruera, 1997). Weight loss also impacts on functional tasks such as getting in and out of the bath due to reduced energy levels for completing the transfer and also discomfort while sitting in the bath.

Taking this into account, the occupational therapist will assess for equipment such as bathing equipment and padded toilet seats and make the appropriate referrals to external agencies for provision. Patients will also be advised to change their position regularly to distribute the pressure more evenly.

Fatigue is also a significant symptom and the occupational therapist is an appropriate member of the MDT to address such anxieties and adaptive strategies (Shearsmith-Farthing, 2001) (see Chapter 12).

Case study 1: Oesophagogastric junction tumour

Background

Mr P (76 years old) initially presented with a 3-month history of increasing dysphagia to solids. He reported episodes of nausea, vomiting and some weight loss. His weight at diagnosis was 67 kg, height 1.8 m and BMI 20.7 kg/m^2. He was referred to his GP under the '2-week rule' (DH, 2000) and underwent an OGD. A stricture was discovered at the oesophagogastric (OG) junction and subsequent biopsies revealed a poorly differentiated adenocarcinoma of the cardia and OG junction. Following a CT scan Mr P was staged as T3 N0.

His past medical history was unremarkable and in spite of his advanced age, the centre MDT decided to pre-assess him with a view to transabdominal resection.

Mr P lived alone, although plans were made for him to stay with his son for a period of convalescence if he went on to have surgery.

Pre-operative assessment

In addition to medical and nursing clerking (including physical examination, chest X-ray, ECG and arterial blood gases), Mr P underwent a full dietetic and physiotherapy assessment.

Physiotherapist

Assessment was carried out, including pulmonary function testing (PFT). He had no history of chest pathology and had stopped smoking many years before. He reported a good exercise tolerance (easily climbing three flights of stairs) and PFTs exceeded values for a man of his height and age. Following the combined anaesthetic and physiotherapy assessment, it was felt that Mr P was fit for resection via an abdominal approach as planned.

Mr P was taught the active cycle of breathing technique, supported coughing, the use of an incentive spirometer and was given general advice on mobilisation post-operatively. This was reinforced with a patient leaflet.

Dietitian

Assessment revealed that Mr P had lost 10.6% of his body weight over the preceding 4-month period ('normal' weight 75 kg) due to increasing problems with dysphagia and pain on eating. A diet history showed that Mr P was reliant on a smooth, blended diet but was managing to consume three to four small meals daily.

He reported a reduction in appetite and portion sizes over 3–4 months and was recently experiencing some regurgitation (mainly frothy and 'acid-like' rather than food) over the last few weeks. He had previously enjoyed a good variety of foods, although preferred 'traditional English dishes' rather than pasta, rice and spicy foods. Mr P reported that he consumed approximately six units of alcohol weekly.

Post-operative interventions

Physiotherapist

Mr P underwent a transabdominal oesophagogastrectomy via an upper midline incision as planned. He was transferred to the high-dependency unit for post-operative management, where his initial stage of recovery was unremarkable.

He cooperated well with physiotherapy, independently clearing his own chest with active cycle of breathing technique (ACBT) and mobilised out of bed with assistance of two people on the second day.

In the following days, Mr P progressed slowly, walking increasing distances on the ward under direct physiotherapy supervision. However, the prolonged presence of the jejunostomy tube did hamper his independence as he remained reliant on staff to assist with the feed dripstand when walking. It also necessitated an extended hospital stay and the physiotherapist maintained contact, encouraging independence in activities of living in collaboration with the occupational therapist (washing, dressing and social interactions) and prevention of disuse atrophy, fatigue, general weakness and feelings of isolation.

Dietitian

Mr P commenced jejunostomy feeds on day 1 post-operatively. He tolerated feeding well and achieved final rate/volume by day 5. His bowels initially opened by day 6 and remained slightly loose until oral intake had resumed. A Gastromiro swallow on day 7 identified a small anastomotic leak; hence, Mr P remained nil by mouth and on full jejunal feeding until day 20 post-operatively.

Once the integrity of the anastomosis had been confirmed, the dietitian instructed on gradual reduction of jejunal feeding to overnight and reintroduction of 'solid' food. Mr P remained on the ward for a further 10 days after resumption of oral intake due to his reluctance to eat and drink. His pre-operative nutritional problems had contributed to his anxieties, in addition to the delay in resuming oral intake following surgery. Further dietary advice was discussed with Mr P and his son prior to his discharge home and written information provided. Although Mr P was not discharged home on jejunal feeding, the jejunostomy tube remained in situ on discharge and Mr P was independent with tube care and flushing the tube daily at home.

Mr P was reviewed 2 weeks after discharge in therapy clinic with the nurse specialist and physiotherapist. He was continuing to consume a very smooth, soft diet (mainly cereals, soups and puddings) and felt anxious to try more 'solid' food for fear of food 'sticking' and affecting the anastomosis. The dietitian provided further reassurance and encouragement and gave advice on particular foods to reintroduce over the next few weeks. After a further 4 weeks, Mr P was starting to regain his confidence and had tried 'main meals' with extra sauces/gravy and sandwiches with soft fillings. Another 4 weeks later he was managing foods of a 'normal' consistency and was starting to enjoy food, with a gradual increase in portion sizes and variety of foods consumed. His jejunostomy tube was removed at this clinic appointment without any problems.

Occupational therapist

Mr P experienced a great deal of anxiety related to his nutritional problems and, on admission, became very low in mood and withdrawn. He was referred to occupational therapy for relaxation sessions whilst on the ward which focused on identifying his anxieties, challenging the negative thoughts he was having and practising relaxation techniques such as guided visualization where the occupational therapist guided him to use his imagination to help him picture himself in a pleasant and safe environment.

It was imperative to commence discharge planning at an early stage due to the functional deterioration that Mr P experienced as a result of the surgery and his reduced performance status. Although Mr P would be staying with his son on discharge, his son was at work during the day and so while he recuperated, Mr P required a visit from a carer each morning to assist him with personal care activities (washing and dressing). An access visit was completed by the occupational therapist and a referral made to the community occupational therapists for provision of a second stair rail and equipment to assist with showering which were delivered prior to discharge.

Following discharge, the occupational therapist saw Mr P for four further relaxation sessions as an outpatient and encouraged Mr P and his family to make further contact if any other issues arose at home.

Key learning points

- To understand the importance of the MDT to help decide on suitability of surgical intervention and consideration of patient's quality of life pre- and post-treatment
- To be able to initiate rehabilitation interventions immediately post-operatively to aid recovery
- To be aware of complications that may delay intervention strategies and the need to review planned interventions
- To appreciate the importance of providing support and reassurance to patients throughout their treatment to help aid their recovery and improve quality of life

---

LOWER GI TUMOURS

Types, incidence and prevalence

In 2004, there were 36 100 people diagnosed with colorectal cancer (Cancer Research UK, 2006). The occurrence of colorectal cancer is strongly related to age, with nearly 85% of cases arising in people who are 60 years or older (Cancer Research UK, 2006). They are the second most common cause of cancer death after lung cancer (Office National Statistics, 2004).

Most tumours are adenocarcinomas that evolve from polyps, which may be present for several years before malignancy develops (NICE, 2004). Small bowel tumours are not common and are often benign. There are four main types of small bowel cancer. These are adenocarcinoma, carcinoid, sarcoma and lymphoma. Adenocarcinoma is more common in patients with familial adenomatous polyposis, Peutz–Jeghers syndrome and Crohn's disease. Coeliac disease increases the risk of small bowel lymphoma.

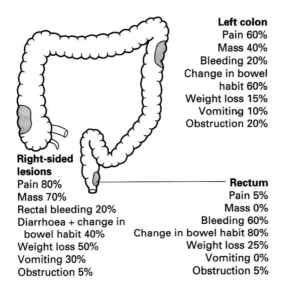

Left colon
Pain 60%
Mass 40%
Bleeding 20%
Change in bowel
habit 60%
Weight loss 15%
Vomiting 10%
Obstruction 20%

Right-sided lesions
Pain 80%
Mass 70%
Rectal bleeding 20%
Diarrhoea + change in
bowel habit 40%
Weight loss 50%
Vomiting 30%
Obstruction 5%

Rectum
Pain 5%
Mass 0%
Bleeding 60%
Change in bowel habit 80%
Weight loss 25%
Vomiting 0%
Obstruction 5%

Figure 9.2 *Symptoms of colorectal cancer according to site.* [Taken from Souhami & Tobias, 2005.]

Risk factors

It has been suggested that about two-thirds of cases of colorectal cancer may be preventable by changes in diet and lifestyle (Doll & Peto, 1981).

- Nutritional status (DH, 1998; Norat *et al.*, 2005)
- Obesity (Bergstrom *et al.*, 2001)
- Alcohol intake (Cho *et al.*, 2004)
- Aspirin and resistant starch (Cancer Research UK, 2006; Logan *et al.*, 1993)
- Family history (Cancer Research UK, 2006)

The NHS Bowel Screening Programme was launched in England in 2006. It offers screening every 2 years for people between 60 and 69 years. It is hoped that it will facilitate earlier intervention that is cost effective and result in better outcomes and decreased mortality from the disease. Scotland has a similar programme commencing in 2007 (NHS Quality Improvement Scotland, 2006).

Clinical presentation

Bowel tumour symptoms vary with the site of the tumour and may be absent in early disease. Patients with small bowel tumours commonly present with no abnormal physical signs. The symptoms of colorectal cancer are illustrated in Figure 9.2. Some patients may also present with ascites.

Diagnosis

NICE (2004) recommends that colonoscopy is available for diagnosis of colorectal cancers. Virtual colonoscopy is also being used increasingly. CT or MRI scans are used to stage the tumour and plan treatment.

The Duke's system is often used for staging, but the TMN classification is also used to give more detail (Cancer Research UK, 2006). Five-year survival rates range from 83% for Duke's stage A to 3% for Duke's stage D colorectal cancer.

Multidisciplinary assessment and treatment

Surgery is the most important method of treatment for approximately 80% of tumours of the small and large bowel (NICE, 2004). Surgery is performed even as palliation of symptoms particularly if patients suffer intestinal obstruction or perforation. In such cases patients may benefit from a defunctioning colostomy before attempting to remove the tumour. Where the tumour cannot be removed a colostomy can offer improved quality of life. In other cases of intestinal obstruction, stenting is carried out preventing the need for resection or stoma formation. Chemotherapy is offered following surgery for Duke's stage C if patients are well enough to tolerate it. It is also considered for recurrent and metastatic large bowel cancers, Duke's stage D (Cancer Research UK, 2006).

Pre-operative radiotherapy is used increasingly commonly in patients with operable rectal cancer. Post-operative adjuvant radiotherapy is associated with an increased risk of long-term toxicity. Pre-operative radiotherapy is used in preference. It can also be useful for inoperable or recurrent cancers (NICE, 2004; SIGN, 2003).

Patients with metastases to the liver or lung who have had resection of the primary tumour may undergo further resection. In the case of liver resection pre-operative chemotherapy is sometimes offered.

Whether the intention is to cure or for palliation, treatment side effects can impact on patient's recovery as well as quality of life. Patients can struggle to cope with a stoma whether this is physical management problems and/or the psychological impact of its appearance. NICE (2004) recommends that nursing and dietetic support should be provided following surgery. The Manual of Cancer Services (2004) recommends that the extended team for the colorectal MDT includes a dietitian. The MDT may choose additional extended members including occupational therapist. However, in spite of these recommendations, in practice, dietetic support for these patients is sometimes overlooked until the patient presents with nutritional problems such as weight loss, reduced appetite and malabsorption. This is in contrast to the approach to managing nutrition in patients with upper GI cancers.

Surgical patients

Physiotherapist

Post-operative physiotherapy should include chest clearance and early mobilisation, although patients do tend to have a lower incidence of pulmonary complications compared with those undergoing upper abdominal surgery (Arozullah et al., 2000). The emphasis should be on independent exercises and encouraging a gradual return to normal function. The use of individualized exercise prescription should also be utilised in the multi-professional management of cancer-related fatigue.

Table 9.6 Commonly reported food-related problems for ileostomy/colostomy patients.

Symptoms	Foods commonly associated
Increased stool frequency	Fruit, fruit juice, vegetables, fried food, spicy food, alcohol
Flatulence/bloating	Pulses, onions, garlic, brassica vegetables, salad, vegetables, fizzy drinks, lager, beer
Stool odour	Onions, garlic, brassica vegetables, pulses, fish, eggs
Poorly digested foods/risk of blockage	Mushrooms, sweetcorn, skin of fruit or vegetables, peas, nuts, seeds, coconut, fibrous vegetables, Chinese food

Data from Thomas (2007).

Dietitian

Pre-existing malnutrition is shown to be a major clinical problem in surgical patients and nutritional screening should commence on admission to hospital (NICE, 2006b).

There is growing evidence to support further dietary manipulation immediately prior to surgery. Noblett *et al.* (2006) compared patients who were overnight fasted. Study results showed significant reduction in post-operative length of hospital stay and a trend towards earlier return of bowel function in those patients who received oral carbohydrate.

Patients can have nutritional difficulties following surgery especially if they have had a history of poor food intake. Patients with ileostomies can experience large stomal losses immediately post-operatively, requiring extra fluids and sodium. This can last for 6–8 weeks. Patients can have concerns about stoma leakage and odour and restrict their diets to try to reduce stoma function. Certain foods can cause problems with wind and altered stomal output (see Table 9.6). Some patients may avoid eating out or socialising because of these symptoms.

All patients should have a dietetic assessment immediately alongside the colorectal nurse specialist to include reassurance as the patient adjusts to living with the stoma. Early post-operative nutrition is acknowledged as an important part of the patient's recovery. Silk and Gow (2001) report no evidence to suggest that bowel rest and a period of starvation are beneficial for wound healing and anastomotic integrity. They also highlight that post-operative infections can be reduced and hospital stay shortened by starting early post-operative enteral nutrition.

The key points for consideration in the dietetic assessment of bowel cancer patients post-operatively are summarised as follows:

- Stomal fluid losses/diarrhoea and their replacement
- Additional salt requirements (especially for ileostomies)
- Odour, flatulence, poorly digested foods and blockage
- Appetite that may be suppressed by symptoms such as pain
- Pronounced weight loss requiring additional nutritional support (oral, enteral or parenteral)
- Range of foods for a varied and well-balanced diet

- Individual tolerance
- Follow-up, to encourage good nutritional status and avoidance of unnecessary food restrictions

Dietary advice for patients with colostomies and ileostomies is based on anecdotal reports from patients rather than evidence. Commonly reported associations are shown in Table 9.6 and summarised by Thomas (2007). Green and Mullan (2001) provide further guidance on management of stoma patients.

Patients who have radiotherapy pre- or post-operatively, such as for anal cancer, can have altered bowel habit, e.g. diarrhoea. This can exacerbate the patient's symptoms of fatigue from treatment and increase anxiety (see Chapter 12). It is important that these patients are assessed by a dietitian to help reduce such symptoms, working closely with the MDT, including the occupational therapist.

Occupational therapist

Taking into account physical, psychological and social functioning the occupational therapist will work with the patient and other members of the MDT to develop a rehabilitation programme. This will encompass personal care, home care and activities of the patients' choice.

There may be functional issues to address that may include:

- Access and mobility to the toilet
  - Provision of adjustable height commodes
  - Aids to help transfer on and off the toilet
- Long-handled equipment such as shoehorns and sponges to minimise bending and twisting particularly if the patient is experiencing abdominal pain
- Pressure-relieving cushions
  - To optimise comfort
  - Minimise the risk of developing or exacerbating existing pressure sores
- Clothing
  - Requiring minimum effort to get on
  - Comfortable particularly with patients with stomas

Identification of such equipment may be carried out by the occupational therapist or nurse, and this equipment can then be sourced from community services via the district nurse.

As previously mentioned, the patient may experience extreme fatigue as a result of disease or treatment side effects, which may present as exhaustion, a lack of energy, disturbed sleep patterns and cognitive deficits (Wagner & Cella, 2004). This, understandably, can have implications for the individual's performance within his or her valued activities of daily living.

The occupational therapist may initiate the use of a fatigue diary to identify which activities are being affected by the patient's current level of function. Typical interventions that the occupational therapist may use include education on the symptoms of fatigue, the implementation of energy conservation techniques, the use of goal setting, advice on achieving restorative sleep, relaxation and provision of equipment (Shearsmith-Farthing, 2001).

Advanced colorectal cancer

A specialist palliative care team coordinates palliative interventions which aim to alleviate symptoms or delay their onset (SIGN, 2003). The patient can experience distressing symptoms, including change in stomal function, reduced appetite and fatigue in addition to the psychological impact of the disease.

Physiotherapist

Some patients may develop abdominal ascites, which can hamper mobility. In addition, due to poor nutritional status, patients with low albumin may have associated lower limb swelling which may interfere with walking. Physiotherapists should take a lead role in assessing mobility and advising on appropriate exercises and walking aids. Following chemotherapy in particular, patients are at an increased risk of developing a deep vein thrombosis. All health professionals should be vigilant in identifying warning signs (including lower limb swelling and a red, hot painful calf) and alert medical staff as necessary.

Fatigue can be a real problem for patients (see Chapter 12). Recent evidence suggests that cancer-induced fatigue does not improve with rest and gentle mobilisation may be advisable in end-stage disease (Tompkins-Stricker *et al.*, 2004).

Dietitian

A review of the patient's nutritional status and advice on nutrition support should be offered by a dietitian to help give relief of symptoms (SIGN, 2003). The dietitian should also provide advice and guidance for family and carers as food can often be a source of conflict.

Bowel obstruction

Bowel obstruction is a common complication of advanced disease.

Symptoms may include:

- Feeling bloated and full
- Pain
- Feeling sick and/or vomiting
- Constipation

Treatment options for bowel obstruction

Patients may have surgery to reduce tumour bulk and relieve intestinal obstruction or have stenting. In some cases surgery may result in the formation of a colostomy (Cancer Research UK, 2006). Where surgery is not appropriate the aim is on relief of symptoms.

Pain, nausea and vomiting can be controlled using analgesics, antiemetics and antisecretory drugs by a syringe driver with relaxation methods used as a non-pharmacological adjunct (Carty, 1997). This can then help the patient to reintroduce fluids and a reduced fibre diet without the need for intravenous fluids or a draining nasogastric tube (SIGN, 2003).

Dietetic management includes:

- Aiming to maintain nutritional status whilst the obstruction is treated or palliated.
- Advising on gradual reintroduction of high-fibre foods to tolerance. If the patient experiences abdominal bloating or discomfort after eating, the fibre intake should be reduced.
- Patients following any dietary restrictions should be monitored and reviewed by a dietitian whilst taking account of change in symptoms.
- Parenteral nutrition is sometimes indicated if it is uncertain whether the condition will resolve particularly if the patient is going to have surgery.

Currently there is no evidence to support the role of a reduced fibre diet in patients who experience constipation and griping abdominal pain without vomiting (Thomas, 2007).

The MDT including the dietitian should consider the patients' performance status, ethical considerations and medical outcomes when deciding on treatment of such patients (Philip & Depczynski, 1997).

Case study 2: Duke's C colorectal carcinoma

Background

Mrs F was 35 years old when she presented to her GP with faecal urgency and a change in bowel habit. Antibiotics were prescribed as the cause was thought to be bacterial. She then returned 3 months later with a history of recurrent abdominal pain, fatigue, weight loss and nausea. Colonoscopy followed by CT scan revealed Duke's C colorectal carcinoma, indicating evidence of spread to the lymph nodes in the tissue around the colon.

She was divorced and living with her partner and 6-year-old daughter.

Mrs F was given the diagnosis with the colorectal nurse specialist present who then provided counselling. It was explained to Mrs F that she would be discussed at MDT to decide on treatment options with a view to surgery and stoma formation. Information was provided about bowel cancer and other information and support services for her and her family.

Pre-operative assessment

Mrs F was discussed at the colorectal MDT. Diagnostic, staging and pathological information was used to help the team decide on the treatment plan. It was agreed that Mrs F would be pre-assessed with a view to carrying out a sigmoid colectomy and formation of a temporary colostomy, aiming to rejoin the bowel at a later date.

Mrs F was then seen by the colorectal nurse specialist who gave further support and counselling regarding the operation and managing a stoma. The nurse specialist explained that there was a possibility that the stoma may need to be permanent despite pre-operative investigations and that this would not be confirmed until the time of the surgery. Mrs

F's assessment included screening for nutritional state, assessment of performance status, comorbidity and psychological state.

The nurse specialist again saw Mrs F at hospital admission to offer further advice and support. Mrs F also underwent further nutritional screening on admission using the hospital's nutrition screening tool.

Post-operative interventions

Mrs F underwent a sigmoid colectomy and colostomy as planned. The colorectal nurse specialist immediately began education on management of the stoma.

Physiotherapist

The physiotherapist carried out a baseline assessment during her recovery period. The purpose was to demonstrate circulatory and breathing exercises to minimise the risk of blood clots and chest infections. The physiotherapist gave Mrs F an exercise programme to begin during her hospital stay and to continue with post-discharge to aid her recovery.

Dietitian

Dietetic assessment was provided immediately post-surgery and intervention to enhance post-operative recovery through oral nutritional support and specific stoma dietary advice (Thomas, 2007, pp. 500–502). Written dietary information including contact details was provided to Mrs F prior to her discharge.

Mrs F raised concern about her change in body image due to the stoma and her concerns about the impact this would have on her relationship with her partner and their sex life. With Mrs F's consent the dietitian discussed this issue with the colorectal nurse specialist who gave her information on support organisations and referred her, along with her partner, for specialist counselling (see Support Organisations).

Adjuvant chemotherapy

Prior to discharge the consultant explained to Mrs F that she was going to be referred to the oncologist with a view to commencing chemotherapy within the following 4–6 weeks.

Dietitian

During the 6-month period of chemotherapy, the colorectal nurse specialist, supported by the dietitian, provided ongoing support with stoma care. This proved invaluable particularly with the side effects she experienced, including diarrhoea and nausea.

Mrs F's partner became concerned that she was beginning to isolate herself and contacted the nurse specialist. On discussion with Mrs F it became apparent that she was concerned about how other people would react to the stoma and was having panic attacks and difficulty sleeping.

Occupational therapist

Referral was made to the occupational therapist, who helped Mrs F to learn how to recognise the symptoms of anxiety and develop strategies for managing them, including breathing exercises and regular relaxation interventions.

Mrs F had hoped to return to work but the side effects of the chemotherapy (fatigue, nausea and diarrhoea) meant that this was not possible. To help manage her financial situation she obtained financial support through advice from the benefits advisor at the Macmillan Information Centre at the hospital.

Palliative care

Mrs F was readmitted to hospital only after her third course of chemotherapy with worsening intestinal distension attributable to ascites, abdominal pain, reduced appetite and reduced mobility. Further investigations revealed multiple liver metastases and significant disease progression. Diuretic therapy was initiated for daily monitoring of electrolytes and body weight. Unfortunately, this gave limited response, so a paracentesis (cannula inserted into the peritoneal cavity to remove fluid) was performed and IV crystalloid given to replace protein lost from fluid drained.

Dietitian

Dietetic intervention focused on encouraging Mrs F to have frequent small meals and snacks through the day choosing high-protein and high-energy foods. Her partner also brought in some of her favourite sweets that were not available in the hospital.

Discharge plans were discussed with Mrs F and her partner and she was introduced to the specialist palliative care team for advice on symptom control and psychological support for her, her partner and daughter. She was referred to social services and home support was approved for a carer to visit in the morning to assist in washing and dressing.

Physiotherapist and occupational therapist

She was also reassessed by the physiotherapist to ensure that she was mobilising safely. Once at home she was seen by the occupational therapist who gave advice on energy conservation techniques to minimise tiredness, such as avoiding unnecessary exertion by ascending and descending the stairs too many times during the day. A range of equipment was also provided to assist in daily activities, such as getting in and out of the shower safely and independently.

Mrs F began to experience a perceived loss of her maternal role as she was unable to do the things she used to with her daughter due to frequent hospital visits and her extreme fatigue. The occupational therapist worked with her to prioritise which activities during the week she valued the most and identify which tasks she could delegate to others. Mrs F was also encouraged to put together a memory box for her daughter.

The dietitian and occupational therapist continued to monitor and support Mrs F regarding nutritional anxieties and functional abilities, liaising closely with the specialist palliative care team, district nurses and GP through to end-of-life care.

Key learning points

- To understand the importance of the MDT to help decide on suitable treatment plan with consideration to patients' quality of life post-treatment, particularly the impact a stoma can have on a young woman
- To understand the importance of initiating rehabilitation interventions immediately post-operatively to aid recovery
- To be aware of treatment side effects that may impact on patient's recovery and be able to review rehabilitation strategies to meet the needs of the patient
- To appreciate the importance of providing support and reassurance to patients and their carers, whether cure or palliation, throughout their treatment to enhance their quality of life

References

Alexakis, N., Halloran, C., Raraty, M., Ghaneh, P. & Neoptolemos, J. P. (2004). Current standards of surgery for pancreatic cancer. *British Journal of Surgery*, *91* (11), 1410–1427.

Allum, W. H., Griffin, S. M., Watson, A. & Colin-Jones, D. (2002). Association of Upper Gastrointestinal Surgeons of Great Britain and Ireland, the British Society of Gastroenterology and the British Association of Surgical Oncology. Guidelines for the management of oesophageal and gastric cancer. *Gut*, *50* (Suppl V), v1–v23.

American Association for Respiratory Care [AARC] (2003). Clinical practice guideline. Intermittent positive pressure breathing. *Respiratory Care*, *48* (5), 540–546.

Amikura, K., Kobari, M. & Matsuno, S. (1995). The time of occurrence of liver metastasis in carcinoma of the pancreas. *International Journal of Pancreatology*, *17* (2), 139–146.

Arends, J., Bodoky, G., Bozzetti, F., Fearon, K., Muscaritoli, M., Selga, G., van Bokhorst-de Van Der Schueren, M. A. E., von Meyenfeldt, M., Zürcher, G., Fietkau, R., Aulbert, E., Frick, B., Holm, M., Kneba, M., Mestrom, H. J. & Zander, A. (2006). ESPEN guidelines on enteral nutrition: non-surgical oncology. *Clinical Nutrition*, *25*, 245–259.

Arozullah, A. M., Daley, J., Henderson, W. G. & Khuri, S. F. (2000). Multifactorial risk index for predicting post-operative respiratory failure in men after major noncardiac surgery. *Annals of Surgery*, *232*, (2), 243–253.

Barber, M. D., Ross, J. A., Voss, A. C., Tisdale, M. J. & Fearon, K. C. H. (1999). The effect of an oral nutritional supplement enriched with fish oil on weight-loss in patients with pancreatic cancer. *British Journal of Cancer*, *81* (1), 80–86.

Barry, J., Mead, K., Nabel, E. G., Rocco, M. B., Campbell, S., Fenton, T., Mudge, G. H. & Slewyn, A. P. (1989). Effect of smoking on the activity of ischaemic heart disease. *JAMA*, *261* (3), 398–402.

Bergstrom, A., Pisani, P., Tenet, V., Wolk, A. & Adami, H. O. (2001). Overweight as an avoidable cause of cancer in Europe. *International Journal of Cancer*, *91*, 421–430.

Braga, M., Gianotti, L., Nespoli, L., Radaelli, G. & Di Carlo, V. (2002). Nutritional approach in malnourished surgical patients: a prospective randomised study. *Archives of Surgery*, *137*, 174–180.

Brooks-Bunn, J. (2000). Oesophageal cancer: an overview. *Medsurg Nursing*, *9* (5), 248–254.

Bruera, E. (1997). ABC of palliative care: anorexia, cachexia, and nutrition. *BMJ*, *315*, 1219–1222.

Bruera, E. & MacDonald, R. N. (1988). Nutrition in cancer patients: an update and review of our experience. *Journal of Pain Symptom Management*, *3*, 133–140.

Cancer Research UK (2006). Information Resource Centre [online]. Retrieved November 2006 from http://info.cancerresearchuk.org/

Carty, J. L. (1997). Relaxation to reduce nausea, vomiting, and anxiety chemotherapy in Japanese patients. *Cancer Nursing*, *20*, 342–349.

Cheville, A. (2001). Rehabilitation of patients with advanced cancer. *Cancer*, *92* (4), 1039–1048.

Cho, E., Smith-Warner, S. A., Ritz, J., Van Den Brandt, P. A., Colditz, G. A., Folsom, A. R., Freudenheim, J. L., Giovannucci, E., Goldbohm, R. A., Graham, S., Holmberg, L., Kim, D. H., Malila, N., Miller, A. B., Pietinen, P., Rohan, T. E., Sellers, T. A., Speizer, F. E., Willett, W. C., Wolk, A. & Hunter, D. J. (2004). Alcohol intake and colorectal cancer: a pooled analysis of 8 cohort studies. *Annals of Internal Medicine*, *140* (8), 603–613.

Daly, J. M., Weintraub, F. N., Shou, J., Rosato, E. F. & Lucia, M. (1995). Enteral nutrition during multimodality therapy in upper gastrointestinal cancers. *Annals of Surgery*, *221* (4), 327–338.

Department of Health [DH] (2000). Referral guidelines for suspected cancer [online]. Retrieved November 2006 from http://www.dh.gov.uk/prod_consum_dh/groups/dh_digitalassets/@dh/@en/documents/digitalasset/dh_4014421.pdf

Department of Health [DH] (2001). Guidance on commissioning cancer services. Improving outcomes in upper gastrointestinal cancers. *The Manual* [online]. Retrieved March 2007 from http://www.dh.gov.uk/prod_consum_dh/groups/dh_digitalassets/@dh/@en/documents/digitalasset/dh_4063792.pdf

Dewey, A., Baughan, C., Dean, T., Higgins, B. & Johnson, I. (2007). Eicosapentaenoic acid (EPA, an omega-3 fatty acid from fish oils) for the treatment of cancer cachexia. *Cochrane Database of Systematic Reviews*, Issue 1.

Doll, R. & Peto, R. (1981).The causes of cancer: quantitative estimates of avoidable risks of cancer in the United States today. *Journal of the National Cancer Institute*, 66 (6), 1191–1308.

Eberhardie, C. (2002). Nutritional support in palliative care. *Nursing Standard*, 17 (2), 47–52.

Ellis, P. & Cunningham, D. (1994). Current issues in cancer: management of carcinomas of the upper gastrointestinal tract. *BMJ*, *308*, 834–838.

Fearon, K. C., Barber, M. D., Moses, A. G., Ahmedzai, S. H., Taylor, G. S., Tisdale, M. J. & Murray, G. D. (2006). Double-blind, placebo-controlled, randomized study of eicosapentaenoic acid diester in patients with cancer cachexia. *Journal of Clinical Oncology*, 24 (21), 3401–3407.

Ferguson, M. K. & Durkin, A. E. (2000). Pre-operative prediction of the risk of pulmonary complications after oesophagectomy for cancer. *Journal of Thoracic and Cardiovascular Surgery*, *123* (4), 661–669.

Fox, V., Gould, D., Davies, N. & Owens, S. (1999). Patients' experience of having an underwater seal chest drain: a replication study. *Journal of Clinical Nursing*, 8, 684–692.

Gao, Y. T., McLaughlin, J. K. & Blot, W. (1994). Risk factors for oesophageal cancer in Shanghai, China. Part II: Role of diet and nutrients. *International Journal of Cancer*, *58*, 197–202.

Green, J. & Mullan, A. (2001). Gynaecological and urological cancers and intestinal failure. In: C. Shaw (Ed.), *Current thinking: nutrition and cancer* (p. 27). Basel, Switzerland: Novartis Consumer Health.

Grosselink, R., Schrever, K., Cops, P., Witvrouwen, H., De Leyn, P., Troosters, T., Lerut, A., Deneffe, G. & Decrammer, M. (2000). Incentive spirometry does not enhance recovery after thoracic surgery. *Critical Care Medicine*, 28 (3), 679–683.

Hlatky, M. A., Boineau, R. E., Higginbotham, M. B., Lee, K. L., Mark, D. B., Califf, R. M., Cobb, F. R. & Pryor, D. B. (1989). A brief self-administered questionnaire to determine functional capacity (The Duke Activity Status Index). *Journal of American College Cardiology*, *64*, 651–654.

Houtmeyers, E., Gosselink, R., Gayan-Ramirez, G. & Decramer, M (1999). Regulation of mucociliary clearance in health and disease. *European Respiratory Journal*, *13*, 1177–1188.

Janke, E., Chalk V. & Kinley, H. (2002). *Pre-operative assessment. Setting a standard through learning*. Southampton: University of Southampton.

Karpoff, H. M., Klimstra, D. S., Brennan, M. F. & Conlon, K. C. (2001). Results of total pancreatectomy for adenocarcinoma of the pancreas. *Archives of Surgery*, *136* (1), 44–48.

Logan, R. F., Little, J., Hawtin, P. G. & Hardcastle, J. D. (1993). Effect of aspirin and non-steroidal anti-inflammatory drugs on colorectal adenomas: case-control study of subjects participating in the Nottingham faecal occult blood screening programme. *BMJ*, *307*, 285–289.

Manual of Cancer Services (2004). [Online]. London: Department of Health. Retrieved November 2006 from http://www.dh.gov.uk/PolicyAndGuidance/HealthAndSocialCare-Topics/Cancer/CancerArticle/fs/en?CONTENT_ID=4135595&chk=CSpbzI

Margolis, M., Alexander, P., Trachiotis, G. D., Gharagozloo, F. & Lipman, T. (2003). Percutaneous endoscopic gastrostomy before multimodality therapy in patients with esophageal cancer. *Annals of Thoracic Surgery*, 76, 1694–1698.

McCulloch, P., Ward, J. & Tekkis, P. P. (2003). Mortality and morbidity in gastro-oesophageal surgery: initial results of ASCOT multicentre prospective cohort centre. *BMJ*, 327 (7425), 1192–1196.

Nagawa, H., Kobori, O. & Mutto, T. (1994). Prediction of pulmonary complications after transthoracic oesophagectomy. *British Journal of Surgery*, 81, 860–862.

National Institute of Clinical Excellence [NICE] (2004). *Guidance on cancer services improving outcomes in colorectal cancer* [online]. Manual update. Retrieved November 2006 from http://www.nice.org.uk/page.aspx?o=CSGCCguidance

National Institute of Clinical Excellence [NICE] (2006a). *Public health intervention guidance. Brief interventions and referral for smoking cessation in primary care and other settings* [online]. Retrieved November 2006 from http://www.nice.org.uk/guidance/PHI1

National Institute of Clinical Excellence [NICE] (2006b). *Nutrition support in adults: oral supplements, enteral and parenteral feeding* [online]. Retrieved March 2007 from http://guidance.nice.org.uk/CG32/guidance/pdf/English

NHS Bowel Cancer Screening Programme (2006). [Online]. Retrieved November 2006 from http://www.cancerscreening.nhs.uk/bowel/index.html

NHS Quality Improvement Scotland (2006). Draft clinical standards. Bowel screening programme [online]. Retrieved March 2007 from http://www.nhshealthquality.org/nhsqis/3161.html

Noblett, S. E., Watson, D. S., Huong, H., Davidson, B., Hainsworth, P. J. & Horgan, A. F. (2006). Pre-operative oral carbohydrate loading in colorectal surgery: a randomized controlled trial. *Colorectal Disease*, 8 (7), 563–569.

Norat, T., Bingham, S., Ferrari, P., Slimani, N., Jenab, M., Mazuir, M., Overvad, K., Olsen, A., Tjonneland, A., Clavel, F., Boutron-Ruault, M. C., Kesse, E., Boeing, H., Bergmann, M. M., Nieters, A., Linseisen, J., Trichopoulou, A., Trichopoulos, D., Tountas, Y., Berrino, F., Palli, D., Panico, S., Tumino. R., Vineis, P., Bueno-de-Mesquita, H. B., Peeters, P. H., Engeset, D., Lund, E., Skeie, G., Ardanaz, E., Gonzalez, C., Navarro, C., Quiros, J. R., Sanchez, M. J., Berglund, G., Mattisson, I., Hallmans, G., Palmqvist, R., Day, N. E., Khaw, K. T., Key, T. J., San Joaquin, M., Hemon, B., Saracci, R., Kaaks, R. & Riboli, E. (2005). Meat, fish and colorectal cancer risk: the European prospective investigation into cancer and nutrition. *Journal of the National Cancer Institute*, 97 (12), 906–916.

Office for National Statistics (2004). *Mortality statistics: cause*. Series DH 2, No. 31.

Oncology Group of the British Dietetic Association (2003). *Professional consensus statement: dietetic advice post oesophageal stent placement* [online]. Retrieved March 2007 from http://members.bda.uk.com/professional_guidance_docs.html

Pancreatic Section of the British Society of Gastroenterology, Pancreatic Society of Great Britain and Ireland, Association of Upper Gastrointestinal Surgeons of Great Britain and Ireland, Royal College of Pathologists, Special Interest Group for Gastrointestinal Radiology (2005). Guidelines for the management of patients with pancreatic cancer periampullary and ampullary carcinomas. *Gut*, 54 (Suppl V), v11–v16.

Penfold, S. (1996). The role of the occupational therapist in oncology. *Cancer Treat Review*, 22, 75–81.

Philip, J. & Depczynski, B. (1997). The role of total parenteral nutrition for patients with irreversible bowel obstruction secondary to gynaecological malignancy. *Journal of Pain and Symptom Management*, 13 (2), 104–111.

Pryor, J. A. (1999). Physiotherapy for airway clearance in adults. *European Respiratory Journal*, 14, 1418–1424.

Pryor, J. A. & Ammani Prasad, S. (2002). *Physiotherapy for respiratory and cardiac problems. Adults and paediatrics* (3rd ed.). London: Churchill Livingstone.

Quinn, M. J., Babb, P. J., Brock, A., Kirby, E. A. & Jones, J. (2001). *Cancer trends in England and Wales, 1950–1999. Studies on medical and population subjects no. 66*. London: The Stationery Office.

Reeve, J., Denehy, L. & Stiller, K. (2007). The physiotherapy management of patients undergoing thoracic surgery: a survey of current practice in Australia and New Zealand. *Physiotherapy Research International, 12* (2), 59–71.

Reichle, R. L., Venbrux, A. C., Heitmiller, R. F. & Osterman, F. A. (1995). Percutaneous jejunostomy replacement in patients who have undergone esophagectomy. *Journal of Vascular and Interventional Radiology, 6* (6), 939–942.

Scottish Intercollegiate Guidelines Network [SIGN] (2003). *Management of colorectal cancer: a national clinical guideline*. SIGN publication 67. Edinburgh: Scottish Intercollegiate Guidelines Network. Retrieved 25 November 2006 from http://www.sign.ac.uk/guidelines/published/index.html

Scottish Intercollegiate Guidelines Network [SIGN] (2006). *Management of oesophageal and gastric cancer. A national clinical guideline*. SIGN publication 87. Edinburgh: Scottish Intercollegiate Guidelines Network. Retrieved November 2006 from http://www.sign.ac.uk/guidelines/published/index.html

Shearsmith-Farthing, K. (2001). The management of altered body image: a role for Occupational therapy. *The British Journal of Occupational Therapy, 64* (8), 387–392.

Silk, D. B. A. & Gow, N. M. (2001). Post-operative starvation after gastrointestinal surgery. Early feeding is beneficial. *BMJ, 323* (7316), 761–762.

Singh, S. J., Morgan, M. D., Scott, S., Walters, D. & Hardman, A. E. (1992). Development of a shuttle walking test of disability in patients with chronic airways obstruction. *Thorax, 47*, 1019–1024.

Souhami, R. & Tobias, J. (2005). *Cancer and its management* (5th ed., p. 275). Oxford: Blackwell Publishing.

Stratton, R. J., Green, C. J. & Elia, M. (2003). *Disease-related malnutrition: an evidence-based approach to treatment*. Wallingford: CABI Publishing.

Takhar, A. S., Palaniappan, P., Dhingsa, R. & Lobo, D. N. (2004). Systemic treatment of pancreatic cancer. *European Journal of Gastroenterology & Hepatology, 16*, 265–274.

Thomas, B. (2007). *The manual of dietetic practice* (4th ed., pp. 430–433, 769–779). Oxford: Blackwell Science Ltd.

Tompkins-Stricker, C., Drake, D., Hoyer, K. & Mock, V. (2004). Evidence-based practice for fatigue management in adults with cancer: exercise as an intervention. *Oncology Nursing Forum, 31* (5), 963–976.

Wagner, L. I. & Cella, D. (2004). Fatigue and cancer: causes, prevalence and treatment approaches. *British Journal of Cancer, 91*, 822–828.

Wakefield, S. E., Mansell, N. J., Baigrie, R. J. & Dowling, B. L. (1995). Use of a feeding jejunostomy after oesophagogastric surgery. *British Journal of Surgery, 82*, 811–813.

Watson, A. & Allen, P. R. (1994). Influence of thoracic epidural analgesia on outcome after resection for oesophageal cancer. *Surgery, 115*, 429–432.

Weimann, A., Braga, M., Harsanyi, L., Laviano, A., Ljungqvist, O., Soeters, P., Jauch, K. W., Kemen, M., Hiesmayr, J. M., Horbach, T., Kuse, E. R. & Vestweber, K. H. (2006). ESPEN guidelines on enteral nutrition: surgery including organ transplantation. *Clinical Nutrition, 25* (2), 224–244.

Wigmore, S. J., Barber, M. D., Ross, J. A., Tisdale, M. J. & Fearon, K. C. (2000). Effect of oral eicosapentaenoic acid on weight loss in patients with pancreatic cancer. *Nutrition Cancer, 36* (2), 177–184.

Further Reading

National Institute of Clinical Excellence (2004). *Guidance on cancer services. Improving supportive and palliative care for adults with cancer. The manual* [online]. Retrieved November 2006 from http://www.nice.org.uk/pdf/csgspmanual.pdf

NHS Cancer Services Collaborative 'Improvement Partnership'. Retrieved November 2006 from http://www.cancerimprovement.nhs.uk/patinfopath/

Valentini, L., Schutz, T., Allison, S., Howard, P., Pichard, C. & Lochs, H. (2006). ESPEN guidelines on enteral nutrition. *Clinical Nutrition, 25* (2), 177–360.

Chapter 10

MULTI-PROFESSIONAL MANAGEMENT OF GENITOURINARY TUMOURS: GYNAECOLOGICAL AND PROSTATE

Dr Doreen McClurg, Pippa McCabe and Karen Chambers

Learning outcomes

Having read this chapter the reader should be able to:

- Discuss prostate cancer and the most common types of gynaecological cancers and their treatments
- Describe and implement an evidence-based holistic, collaborative and multidisciplinary team approach to the therapeutic management of these cancers
- Describe and critically discuss the associated complications which are relevant to allied health professionals

---

Introduction

Over the past decade the treatment of gynaecological and prostate cancers has become increasingly complex with more radical surgery, adjuvant chemotherapy and radiotherapy. The needs of the patient and their carers are therefore much more complex necessitating a multi-professional approach to ensure that quality of life is maximised. Comorbid conditions such as incontinence, sexual dysfunction, lymphoedema, altered body image, generalised debility and pain are often associated with these cancers. After the initial trauma of undergoing life-saving treatment, these issues come to the fore and require appropriate sensitivity and treatment. Palliative care may be required for adequate pain relief and other symptom management. This often involves input from the voluntary and health care sectors with specialist palliative training. Further contribution from the multidisciplinary team (MDT) is required

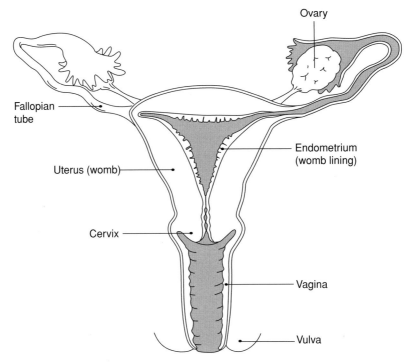

Figure 10.1 The female pelvis.

to devise practical and humane ways of delivering care, attenuating and decelerating the assaults cancers can deliver on functional autonomy. This chapter examines the specialist areas of gynaecological and prostate cancers.

GYNAECOLOGICAL CANCERS

For a better understanding of these conditions an explanation of the most common cancer investigations and treatments must first be considered.

Common gynaecological procedures

Bilateral salpingoophorectomy
This is the removal of both ovaries and fallopian tubes and, if indicated, is usually performed at the time of hysterectomy (Figure 10.1).

Colposcopy
This is performed at an outpatient clinic when abnormalities have been detected on a cervical smear. The colposcope is a microscope which magnifies the cervix. Biopsies

may be taken. A cone biopsy may also be performed, which removes a cone-shaped piece of cervix either by laser or by using a wire loop.

Cystoscopy
Cystoscopy is an examination under anaesthetic using a thin 'telescope' which is inserted into a fluid-filled bladder and used to examine the bladder lining. The procedure may also be conducted under local anaesthetic using a flexible cystoscope.

Debulking
Debulking is used for ovarian tumours and may include removal of ovaries, uterus, cervix and omentum.

Dilatation and curettage
Under anaesthesia, the cervix is dilated and the contents or a sample of the inner lining of the uterus are removed by suction.

Hysteroscopy
This is a thin flexible tube with a light at the end and is used to look inside the uterus and take a biopsy.

Inguinal node dissection
In this procedure, lymph nodes near the vulva are removed usually following a vulvectomy (unilateral or bilateral). Drain(s) may be in situ for a few days.

Laparoscopy
The laparoscope is a narrow telescope which allows the surgeon to view the organs inside the pelvis. Laparoscopic staging, pelvic lymphadenectomy, vaginal hysterectomy or total hysterectomy is an alternative to laparotomy. Blood loss and hospital stay are usually reduced; however, complications such as bladder or bowel perforation are higher for malignant disease (Hatch, 2005).

Laparotomy
A laparatomy is an incision in the abdomen which allows the surgeon to inspect the contents. A transverse suprapubic incision may be employed (Pfannenstiel). A vertical incision is preferred in ovarian malignancy or where access to the upper abdomen is required.

Large-loop excision of the transition zone
Large-loop excision of the transition zone (LLETZ) outpatient treatment for cervical dysplasia (pre-malignant lesions) aims to totally remove the abnormal cells from the cervix. A wire loop with an electric current (diathermy) is used to shave off these cells.

Omentectomy
This involves removal of the fatty tissue overlying the bowel.

Pelvic exenteration

It is indicated in recurrent cancer of the cervix after radiation therapy and is tailored to remove the tumour and only those organs that are involved (Hatch & Berek, 2005). Anterior pelvic exenteration includes removal of the bladder, uterus and varying amounts of the vagina, depending on the extent of the disease. Total pelvic exenteration removes the uterus, vagina and portions of the rectosigmoid colon with colonic re-anastamosis.

Pelvic node dissection

In cases of suspected malignancy, pelvic and para-aortic nodes may be excised.

Radiotherapy (external/brachytherapy)

Radiotherapy for gynaecological cancer may be used pre- or post-operatively, as an alternative to surgery or as palliative treatment. External beam radiotherapy uses an X-ray beam directed at the malignant area. Internal radiotherapy (brachytherapy) involves insertion of an X-ray-emitting applicator into the uterus or vagina. The device is usually inserted under general anaesthetic and may remain in place for up to 24 h. A Selectron machine can be used to insert the radioactive material into the applicator. Microselectron may be used for internal radiotherapy and delivers the radiotherapy more rapidly.

Radical total abdominal hysterectomy

This involves the removal of the uterus, fallopian tubes, ovaries and upper one-third of the vagina usually via a midline incision (Figure 10.2).

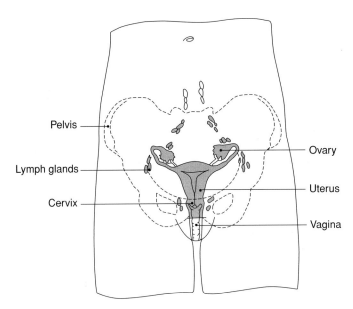

Figure 10.2 Total abdominal hysterectomy. The shaded areas show the organs that are removed.

Radical trachelectomy

Performed for fertility preservation in patients with early stage cervical cancer with no metastases to regional lymph nodes and involves removal of the uterine cervix plus the adjacent parametria while conserving the uterine body and the ovaries (Grant, 2006).

Sentinel lymph node biopsy

The technique is used to locate the primary lymph node(s) that drain lymph from the area in which the cancer developed. These are assessed for any cancer spread. Currently, this is a novel approach and not recognised as standard treatment, but can help to reduce the side effects of inguinal node dissection, such as lymphoedema.

Subtotal abdominal hysterectomy

The uterus is removed through an incision in the abdominal wall; cervix and ovaries are conserved.

Total abdominal hysterectomy

This involves the removal of the uterus, body and cervix, usually through a transverse suprapubic incision in the abdominal wall.

Vulvectomy

There are several stages of vulvectomy, which include laser surgery for pre-invasive abnormal cells, simple vulvectomy when the entire vulva is removed and radical vulvectomy (partial or complete). The latter incorporates the vulva, deep tissues and the clitoris. Occasionally, skin grafting is required.

Types of gynaecological cancers

There are eight major gynaecological cancers, seven of which are usually treated with intra-abdominal surgery, and vulval cancer, by removal of the affected area. Each cancer is an individual disease and must be considered independently.

Uterine sarcoma

The uterus is a hollow pear-shaped organ in the pelvis. Uterine sarcoma forms in the uterine muscles or in the tissues that support the uterus (the stroma). This is a very rare cancer accounting for 1% of all gynaecological cancer; previous radiotherapy to the pelvis is a risk factor. Symptoms include bleeding that is not part of the menstrual cycle or after menopause, a mass in the vagina, pain or 'fullness' in the abdomen and frequent urination (Hacker, 2005a).

Surgery is the most common treatment, usually involving total abdominal hysterectomy (TAH), bilateral salpingoophorectomy (BSO) and lymphadenectomy. This may be followed by chemotherapy and radiotherapy depending on the stage of the disease.

The prognosis is primarily dependent on the extent of disease at the time of diagnosis. The 5-year survival for patients with Stage I disease (confined to the corpus) is approximately 50%, versus 0–20% for the remaining stages (El Husseiny *et al.*, 2002).

Endometrial cancer

The uterus is divided into two parts: the body and the cervix. The walls of the uterus are composed of muscle called myometrium. The endometrium is the membrane that lines the body of the uterus. This cancer is associated with the hereditary non-polyposis colon cancer and occurs in 40% of female gene carriers. It typically affects post-menopausal, nulliparous, obese women, with tendency to diabetes and cardiovascular disease. There is increasing evidence linking endometrial cancer with prolonged tamoxifen use (Fisher *et al.*, 1994; Saadat *et al.*, 2007). Post-menopausal bleeding is the classic presenting symptom. Pre-menopausal women may experience heavy and/or irregular periods which can be associated with vaginal discharge. General symptoms can include anorexia, weight loss and malaise.

Primary treatment is a TAH and BSO, which may be performed laparoscopically. Radiotherapy is mainly given as an adjunct to surgery where disease is advanced and margins are small. It may be internal, external beam or in combination. Chemotherapy is not commonly used.

The majority of patients present with Stage I endometrial cancer, which has cure rates of 85%. For advanced stages, prognosis rates fall:

Stage II – 65% 5-year survival
Stage III – 35% 5-year survival (Pessini *et al.*, 2007)

Cervical cancer

The cervix forms the lower part of the uterus and lies partly in the upper vagina and partly in the retroperitoneal space, behind the bladder and in front of the rectum. Cervical cancer accounts for around 20% of female cancers and is predominantly a disease of women between 40 and 50 years. The incidence of diagnosis in younger age groups, and commonly in lower socioeconomic groups, is however increasing (Campion, 2005). Risk factors include intercourse commenced before the age of 20 and multiple sexual partners; however, the most important risk factor is exposure and infection of the cervix with the human papilloma virus (HPV), which has also shown a synergistic effect with smoking (Gunnell *et al.*, 2006). Cervical cytology (smear test) is still the most accurate diagnostic method for assessing those at most risk (Irico *et al.*, 2006). The recent development of an HPV vaccination provides an opportunity to profoundly affect cervical cancer incidence (Roden & Wu, 2006). This cancer is frequently asymptomatic in early stages. Later stage symptoms include vaginal bleeding (particularly after intercourse) and vaginal discharge.

Definitive treatment for invasive cervical cancer involves surgery, chemoradiation or a combination of these approaches. Radical hysterectomy and pelvic lymphadenectomy are most commonly used for tumours less than 4 cm, which do not exceed a clinical Stage IIA (IIA = cancer extends beyond the cervix into the upper vagina but does not involve the parametrium). More advanced cancer (20%) will require post-operative external beam and/or intracavity irradiation; National Institute for Health and Clinical Excellence (NICE) (2006) states that current evidence would support the use of high-dose brachytherapy (intra-cavity) as a curative treatment (following surgery) in suitable patients, which delivers the maximum radiotherapy dose to the cervix and surrounding tissue (parametrium). Concurrent (cisplatin-based) chemotherapy is the current standard intervention for cervical cancer (Eifel, 2006). Keskar *et al.* (2006) have reported on the use of a novel insertable device which enables the delivery of sustained drug levels at the site of action, thereby reducing systemic side effects.

Prognosis depends on the disease staging:

Stage II–IIA – 80% 5-year survival
Stage III – 20–30% 5-year survival
Stage IV – less than 5% 5-year survival (Lukaszuk *et al.*, 2007)

Fallopian cancer

The fallopian tubes are a pair of thin ducts that transport ova from the ovaries to the uterus. The incidence of fallopian cancer is rare (1% of all gynaecological cancer) and peaks in women aged 60–64 (Benoit & Hannigan, 2006). It can be difficult to diagnose and there may be some association with chronic infection and/or inflammation of the fallopian tubes (e.g. due to untreated sexually transmitted diseases) and in those with the *BRCA1* or *BRCA2* gene mutation. The most common symptoms include vaginal bleeding, vaginal discharge and pelvic pain. It is usually diagnosed by the pathology and therefore rarely considered pre-operatively.

Treatment will usually entail TAH, BSO, omentectomy and lymphadenectomy and can be responsive to multi-agent chemotherapy.

The prognosis depends on the stage at diagnosis and the treatments provided. At 5 years, Stage I and II survival rates range from 60 to 90%. These rates decline in Stages III and IV to a 25% 5-year survival rate (Clayton *et al.*, 2005; Singhal *et al.*, 2006).

Gestational trophoblastic cancer

This is a rare cancer of unknown cause in which malignant cells grow in the tissues that are formed following conception. Gestational trophoblastic (GTT) tumours start inside the uterus and can be divided into two types: hydatidiform mole and choriocarcinoma. If a patient has a hydatidiform mole (also called a molar pregnancy), the sperm and egg cells join without the development of a baby. Instead, the tissue resembles grape-like cysts. Hydatidiform mole does not spread outside of the uterus to other parts of the body.

The management of molar pregnancies is relatively simple; problems arise when they are neglected as choriocarcinoma is very aggressive, metastases widely and can bleed profusely. A dilatation and curettage (D&C) is used for molar pregnancies, a hysterectomy sometimes followed by chemotherapy and/or radiotherapy for choriocarcinomas. Most GTTs are extremely chemosensitive.

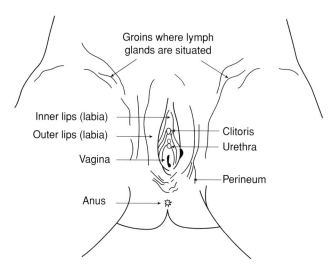

Figure 10.3 The vulva.

Vaginal cancer

The vagina is the canal leading from the cervix to the outside of the body. Vaginal cancer is relatively rare, accounting for about 2% of gynaecological malignancies. Typically, squamous carcinoma is found between 60 and 80 years of age, and adenocarcinoma in young women under 30 years old. There are often few early symptoms; however, bleeding and discharge or pain on intercourse may be present. A lump may be evident or it may occasionally be detected during a smear test. Vaginal cancer is thought to be associated with the HPV, exposure to DES (a 1950s miscarriage prevention drug) and the use of vaginal pessaries for prolapse support (Hacker, 2005b).

Treatment consists of a radical total abdominal hysterectomy (RTAH) possibly followed by radiotherapy to the pelvis. The type of radiation depends on the stage of the cancer and may be combined with chemotherapy.

Survival depends on the size of the tumour, whether it has spread to other areas, age and general health. The 5-year survival rate is 61%, and 54% at 10 years (Hacker, 2005b).

Vulva cancer (Figure 10.3)

The vulva is the fatty fold surrounding the clitoris, urethra and vagina. Vulvar cancer is primarily a disease of elderly women but has also been observed in pre-menopausal women. It is often preceded by condyloma or squamous dysplasia and is mostly squamous cell in type (Canavan & Cohen, 2002; Hopkins & Nemunaitis-Keller, 2001). Prevailing evidence favours HPV as a causative factor, particularly in younger patients (Canavan & Cohen, 2002). The labia majora accounts for approximately 50% of disease and the labia minora 15–20%. The clitoris and Bartholin's glands are less frequently involved (Canavan & Cohen, 2002; Hopkins & Nemunaitis-Keller, 2001; Macnab *et al.*, 1986). The presenting symptoms include local irritation, pain or burning sensations, a lump or change in the skin, bleeding and an unusual odour (Canavan & Cohen, 2002).

Treatment can vary from local excision to radical vulvectomy with bilateral inguinal and femoral node dissection (Canavan & Cohen, 2002; Hopkins & Nemunaitis-Keller, 2001). There is a trend towards vulvar conservation and individualised management of patients with early vulvar cancer because of the psychosexual consequences and significant morbidity associated with standard radical vulvectomy. External beam radiation is used to treat involved groin nodes or for palliation of symptoms in advanced disease (American Cancer Society, 2007). Chemotherapy and radiotherapy may be used for large-lesion pre-operative shrinkage where radical excision would involve disruption of the urethra, anal sphincter or anus (Hacker, 2005c).

Survival is very dependent on the pathologic status of the inguinal nodes. The overall 5-year survival rate is 90% for patients without and 50% for those with nodal involvement (Canavan & Cohen, 2002; Hopkins & Nemunaitis-Keller, 2001).

Ovarian cancer

The ovaries are a pair of oval-shaped organs lateral to the uterus. Ovarian cancer ranks as the leading cause of death in gynaecological cancers. Risk factors include increasing age, a genetic link accounting for approximately 10% of disease (Lynch *et al.*, 1993), low or nulliparity and a history of breast cancer (American Cancer Society, 2007). The symptoms are vague, such as abdominal discomfort, pelvic pain and enlargement of the abdomen due to tumour, ascites, urinary or bowel disturbances. Symptom absence in early stage disease explains the high mortality rate (Berek, 2005; Berek & Hacker, 2005).

All patients with operable disease will undergo staging laparotomy (mid-line incision) with RTAH and omentectomy, with careful examination/biopsy of the surrounding tissues and organs. This cancer is moderately sensitive to chemotherapy which can be given pre- or post-operatively. It may also be used as a second-line treatment for tumour recurrence. For those who fail chemotherapy, hormonal therapy is a viable treatment option. The role of radical radiotherapy in this area remains uncertain.

Prognosis depends on the stage of the disease:

Stage I – 80% 10-year survival
Stage II+III – 35–50% year survival
Stage IV – a few months (American Cancer Society, 2007; Omura *et al.*, 1991)

The multi-professional management of gynaecological cancers

The multi-professional management of gynaecological cancers can be divided into three stages:

1. Perisurgical
   - Pre-operative management
   - Post-operative management (including complications relating to surgery)

2. Perichemotherapy/radiotherapy/surgical (combinations)
   - Short-term side effects
   - Long-term complications relating to all treatment
3. Palliative management

Perisurgical

Pre-operative management. Surgery is often complex and a pre-operative assessment is recommended (Cook, 2004; Devine, 1992). This should include:

- Assessment of risk factors, such as obesity, cigarette smoking, debilitative state, previous or planned radiotherapy/chemotherapy, diabetes, chest, heart or circulatory conditions.
- Patient education regarding knowledge and skills for the post-operative and recovery periods. Some centres have their own specific literature or use booklets such as BACUP. These are an invaluable resource for patient information. Time spent talking to the patient can also be of great benefit.

Post-operative management (patient returned to ward). The course of the post-operative period depends on the extent of the surgery, pre-existing perimorbid conditions and the development of complications.

Following extensive surgery, the patient may have in situ:

- Epidural or patient-controlled analgesia (PCAS)
- Intravenous drip
- Nasogastric tube
- Intra-abdominal drains
- Saline drip
- Antiembolitic stockings or Flowtron
- Intra-vaginal pack
- Stoma
- Indwelling urinary catheter
- Supplementary oxygen (nasal specs/face mask) as prescribed by the anaesthetist
- Central line, intravenous line, arterial line (Sharpe, 1998)

AHP intervention should include:

1. Respiratory care
   Upper abdominal surgery is known to cause severe and prolonged alterations in pulmonary mechanics. Opiates and sedatives can also affect the natural 'sigh' mechanism (Richardson & Sabanathan, 1997). Respiratory physiotherapy is essential to prevent the development of atelectasis and chest infections. Active cycle of breathing techniques with supported huff/cough should be taught, and incentive spirometry provided for those at most risk. Thought must be given to the position of the wound when teaching supported breathing as this can vary greatly from the abdomen to the pelvic and vulval areas. Active treatment should be

undertaken when pain relief is most effective and independent work encouraged. For patients who develop respiratory complications, oxygen therapy, humidification and nebulisers may be necessary. Positive pressure devices, such as CPAP, can aid lung expansion (Cook, 2004).

2. Initial bed activity exercises
   When an epidural is in situ, the presence of equal, bilateral lower limb sensation and general mobility must be assessed. Simple active ankle and knee exercises should be encouraged; gentle pelvic rocking/knee rolling may help relieve flatulence (Cook, 2004).

3. Initial transfers
   Patients should be taught how to move in bed, e.g. from lying to sitting via side lying to minimise intra-abdominal pressure, moving up the bed by bending their knees and using their thigh muscles, digging in with their heels, pushing up with their hands and straightening their knees so that the hips lift up off the bed and back towards the pillow (Cook, 2004). The occupational therapist (OT) may need to assess regarding any assistive equipment and techniques; e.g. a bed lever may be supplied to aid general bed mobility.

4. Positioning
   Supported resting positions such as half lying with a pillow under their thighs and side lying with pillows between the knees and under the lower abdomen may be beneficial.

5. Posture
   Good posture in standing and supported positions in sitting, using appropriately placed pillows or lumbar rolls, may also help to reduce backache in the postoperative period. Patients may benefit from a recliner chair or specialist pressure relief; a graded sitting tolerance programme should be instigated for the most severely debilitated (Reed & Sanderson, 1992).

6. Mobility
   Early ambulation should be encouraged. On day 1, the patient should be assessed regarding ability to transfer out to a chair, including the potential use of a hoist. Standing should be encouraged and the need for a walking aid assessed. By day 2 most patients should be able to walk, with the assistance of two, for a short distance and progressed to independent mobilisation as able (Cook, 2004). Less extensive or laparoscopic surgery would require similar MDT input, although progress is usually quicker.

Complications:
Tumour-related complications can include:

- Renal failure due to bilateral ureteric obstruction
- Acute haemorrhage from tumour occasionally resulting in hypoglycaemic shock

- Fistulae between vagina and bladder or rectum
- Pyometra (pus in the uterine cavity) due to obstruction of cervical canal by tumour (Hatch & Berek, 2005)

Immediate post-operative complications can include:
Bleeding (internal), deep venous thrombosis, respiratory problems, paralytic ileus, urinary tract and wound infection (Cook, 2004; Sharpe, 1998). Lower limb, lower abdominal or groin lymphoedema may also develop in those who have had pelvic or groin node dissection (see Chapter 11). Bladder and bowel dysfunction are common in the immediate post-operative period; suprapubic or urethral catheterisation and laxatives are therefore desirable in the first week. In a study undertaken by Behtash *et al.* (2005) comparing the symptoms post-radical and post-simple hysterectomy in the 2 weeks after surgery, it was demonstrated that those who had undergone an RTAH were more prone to bladder complications. It is therefore essential to monitor the patient's ability to void after removal of the catheter, and the OT and physiotherapist may need to assess function regarding access to and transfers on/off the toilet, rearranging clothing and cleaning of the perianal area and hands (Reed & Sanderson, 1992) alongside adequate control of bladder and bowel.

MDT management in the convalescent/post-acute phase

(a) Counselling/information provision
    This may be an anxious time for patients as they await pathology results. Gynaecological cancers have profound psychosocial implications in addition to the obvious physical manifestations. Women are confronted with cancer and its related treatments, which may impact adversely on body image, sexuality and relationships, including the possibility of imposed infertility and/or menopause. Altered body image is an important factor and becomes problematic when it affects the *individual's* quality of life (Shearsmith-Farthing, 2001). Although there is a lack of evidence-based interventions for addressing altered body image, there is anecdotal evidence for the use of such interventions as the adaptation through occupation model (Reed & Sanderson, 1992), which incorporates the physical, psychological and social well-being of individuals in a holistic manner.

    It is important that appropriate, timely and confidential information is provided. Literature and websites sponsored by cancer charities are useful; some details are supplied at the end of the chapter. Eighty per cent of centres now offer aromatherapy for the relief of stress and anxiety (Kohn, 2003).

    Menopausal symptoms may begin quite quickly after BSO; advice on the control of symptoms should be provided by the consultant surgeon/oncologist; HRT can be contraindicated in some cancers (Biglia *et al.*, 2006).

(b) Rehabilitation (including pelvic floor retraining)
    Pelvic tilting, knee rolling, abdominal bracing and knee bends may be taught as exercises for the lower abdominal muscles and lower back. Expert opinion also suggests that pelvic floor muscle training (PFMT) after gynaecological surgery

may mitigate problems such as urinary incontinence both in the short and long term (Cook, 2004). Many physiotherapists delay instruction until the catheter is removed, although there is no evidence of harmful effects resulting from undertaking pelvic floor exercises whilst a urinary catheter is in situ (Haslam & Pomfret, 2002).

Ideally, these exercises should have been taught pre-operatively; however, in both scenarios a vaginal assessment is unlikely to be possible. Therefore, the use of diagrams and models to verbally describe the anatomy and function of these muscles is essential as many women find it difficult to achieve correct pelvic floor contraction on verbal instruction alone (Bø et al., 1988; Bump et al., 1991). A combination of fast, slow and anticipatory pelvic floor muscle contraction should be taught to prevent leakage and control urgency. Patients may present with bladder problems ranging from hesitancy and poor flow, to incontinence, frequency and urgency, which may or may not have been present before surgery and/or related to the underlying malignancy. Individualised advice is required as this can be difficult to manage. Cranberry juice may be recommended to help prevent urinary tract infections, although this is contraindicated for patients on warfarin (Aston et al., 2006; Jepson et al., 2004).

(c) Constipation management
Some patients may also develop constipation; therefore, education regarding correct diet and defaecation position and technique should be taught. This includes sitting with the knees apart and higher than the hip joints; this may require the feet to be on a support. The trunk should be flexed forward at the hips supported on the forearms and with the neutral spinal curves maintained. A bracing technique should be adopted, which means to make the waist wide and let the abdominals bulge anteriorly (Chiarelli & Markwell, 1992; Markwell & Sapsford, 1995). Straining should be avoided. The use of a pad to support the perineal area may be useful.

(d) Diet
Dietary advice can be helpful, including information on supplementary feeding for those with depressed appetite and for those with stomas.

(e) Ascites
Ascites (the presence of fluid in the abdomen) may sometimes be present before surgery or in the later stages of the disease. This makes deep breathing and expansion of the bases of the lung difficult; patients should be encouraged to breathe as deeply as possible and provided with oxygen therapy if appropriate. Ascites can also affect functional activities because range of movement can be restricted and tolerance reduced. Some relief may be gained from paracentesis (Krishnan et al., 2001).

(f) ADL
Following assessment and advice, the provision of ADL equipment can promote independence in personal care, toileting, bathing, transfers, seating and pressure

relief. Written and verbal advice on a graded return to domestic, social and work activities is also essential.

(g) Discharge preparation

Before discharge, patients with stairs at home should have a supervised trial. If required ADL reports should be completed and adequate home care provision organised by liaison between the hospital and community or social services. District nursing services to assist with the management of continence/wound/stoma and input from the community MDT to assess, facilitate and encourage mobility and independent activities are often required. For some, nursing home or respite care is needed, and input from voluntary sectors, such as hospice, Marie Curie and Macmillan, can also be essential for palliative support.

Perichemotherapy/radiation therapy
Short-term side effects

(a) Bladder

Acute radiation injury results primarily from damage to rapidly dividing cells such as the bladder mucosa. This usually occurs during treatment and for a short while afterwards with symptoms of dysuria, cystitis, frequency and urgency (Denton *et al.*, 2002a). Patients are often advised to drink plenty of water and occasionally cranberry juice (Raz *et al.*, 2004).

(b) Bowel

After intracavity irradiation, a minor degree of rectal irritation (tenesmus: a feeling of wanting to empty the bowel), rectal bleeding and slight diarrhoea can be expected. During external beam radiotherapy diarrhoea is often a problem and advice would usually include a low-fibre diet, an antidiarrhoeal agent and avoidance of eating fruit and vegetables (Gibstone & Keefe, 2006). Post-treatment chronic proctitis (inflammation of the anus and/or the lining of the rectum) can occur with symptoms of tenesmus, urgency, diarrhoea or constipation, sphincter dysfunction and mucoid/bloody discharge or frank bleeding per rectum (Denton *et al.*, 2002b). In the small bowel obstruction is the commonest complication.

(c) Vaginal symptoms

Atrophic vaginitis may occur as a result of radiation and/or lack of oestrogen. Vaginal shortening, stenosis and atrophy may continue after treatment has ceased. Personal hygiene is important; vaginal lubricants, dilators and local oestrogen may be recommended (Denton & Maher, 2003).

(d) Anxiety

Psychological distress often accompanies external and internal radiation treatment. Research has shown that the provision of simplified-repetitious information helps patients cope with the emotional distress (Long, 2001). Relaxation techniques may be taught for use during brachytherapy (or at any time) and referral for complementary therapies can be beneficial (Decker *et al.*, 1992).

(e) Anorexia

Anorexia can be a feature of the disease or a side effect of many drugs. Several commonly used drugs can also cause a dry mouth, which alters sensation and food palatability. Nutritional support may be required and guidelines adhered to (Heber, 2005).

(f) Cancer-related fatigue

Cancer-related fatigue (CRF) can be a profound symptom and is discussed in depth in Chapter 12.

(g) Skin

Reactions are most likely to occur in treatment of the vulva where the perineum is relatively intolerant to radiotherapy due to natural moisture and friction. Painful desquamation (the skin sheds its outer layers, becomes thin and may start to weep) is inevitable (Symonds & Foweraker, 2006) and provides a challenge for hygiene requirements, seating and mobility. If submersion in water is recommended for wound healing, it is important to have ready access to a toilet/bath and also assessment regarding pressure-relieving devices (Bolderston et al., 2006).

(h) Osteoporosis

Radiation can cause depletion of bone marrow elements which can be transient or permanent. The risk of fracture depends on the bone irradiated, volume of bone in the high-dose region, bone density and coexistent steroid use. Assessment for falls prevention advice, mobility aids, pain relief (e.g. transcutaneous electrical nerve stimulation (TENS)) and positional information are necessary to facilitate independence (Reed & Sanderson, 1992).

Long-term implications of treatment (surgical and chemo/radiotherapy)

There are five main long-term problems which affect quality of life:

(a) Bladder dysfunction

Long-term bladder dysfunction may occur as a result of surgery and/or radiation treatment and has been reported to be the most distressing late complication. Although there are conflicting reports (Koelbl, 2006), clinically significant long-term bladder dysfunction can occur in 76% of patients who have undergone a radical hysterectomy and neoadjuvant chemotherapy (Benedetti-Panici et al., 2004). In this study, three main disturbances were found: detrusor overactivity (21%), mixed urinary incontinence (24%) and de novo (not present before treatment) stress incontinence (21%). There is also evidence that a significant proportion of patients report severe urinary incontinence symptoms that are not detected by gynaecologic oncologists during routine consultations (Priore et al., 2005). Benedetti-Panici et al. (2004) have suggested that the introduction of a specific and validated quality-of-life questionnaire would improve the detection and assess the severity of urinary symptoms. Bacterial infection of the urinary tract is also considered a major factor in the development of urinary symptoms post-radiotherapy. This can delay healing and worsen symptoms.

Treatment of long-term bladder dysfunction can include:
1. Anticholinergic drugs to decrease muscle tone of bladder/prostate
2. Bladder-retraining techniques
3. Pelvic floor exercises
4. Acupuncture
5. Behavioural interventions
6. Adaptation of clothing
7. Condition-specific urinals/continence products
8. Adaptation of toileting facilities
9. Lifestyle management (Sharpe, 1998)

No high-quality studies were found to report on the effects of these treatments and bladder dysfunction within this population. However, Naik *et al.* (2001) reported that non-fistulous urinary incontinence following radical pelvic surgery is a common long-term problem. These authors state that physiotherapy in the form of pelvic floor exercises should be offered to those with incontinence before proceeding to surgery with a reported improvement cure rate of 87%.

Several studies have indicated that PFMT following radical prostatectomy may reduce incontinence (see later). To date no quality data regarding the benefits of PFMT following radical gynaecological surgery has been found; however, it would seem reasonable to suggest that appropriate advice and PFMT, with or without biofeedback, may improve pelvic floor muscles which have maintained some nerve supply and can therefore be re-educated and strengthened. It is often several months after treatment completion that side effects, such as incontinence, affect quality of life. Further research is necessary to establish the extent of bladder and bowel dysfunction and the effect of these treatment modalities for short- and long-term quality of life. At present the use of intravaginal electrical stimulation following gynaecological cancer should be considered only after consultation with the surgeon/oncologist.

Intrauteric or intraurethral stenosis may also occur, and should be suspected, if voiding patterns change. Patients should be referred for treatment and exclusion of disease progression. The development of a urethral/vaginal fistula should be suspected if a sudden severe increase in leakage is reported.

(b) Sexual dysfunction
Retrospective studies of post-treatment outcomes report diminished sexual functioning in up to 78% of patients following radical hysterectomy, 44–79% of patients after radiotherapy and 35–46% of patients after combined treatment (Jensen *et al.*, 2003). Surgery and/or radiotherapy may reduce the vaginal length and shape, alter the outward appearance of the vulva area and cause tightening or fibrosis of scar tissue. Loss of ovarian function also leads to reduced vaginal lubrication. These physical changes can lead to dyspareunia (painful intercourse), telangiectasia (superficial blood vessels), post-coital bleeding and loss of sensation (Grumann *et al.*, 2001).

Many patients also report emotional changes that affect their sexuality and sexual functioning (Sundquist & Yee, 2003) and feel shame and unease when talking of their sexual problems. It has been shown that 80% want to be informed of strategies for alleviating pain during intercourse or the schedule for resumption of sexual activity after treatment (Neises, 2002; Wright *et al.*, 2002). Health professionals are in an ideal position to listen to these fears and liaise with other members of the MDT. Provision of written advice, e.g. 'Sexuality and Cancer' (Cancer BACUP, 2006), and information on self-help groups and websites can also be helpful. (Some appropriate contacts can be found at the end of the chapter.) Therapeutic interventions include infection control, use of vaginal dilators, lubricant and HRT when indicated (Fraunholz *et al.*, 1998; Robinson *et al.*, 1999). Sexual counselling has been shown to be of benefit to patients (Robinson *et al.*, 1999); a recent study recommends that sexual rehabilitation interventions should consider not just the anatomical and physiological effects, but also partner relationships, perceived physical appearance and women's attitudes towards themselves as sexual beings (Donovan *et al.*, 2006).

(c) Lymphoedema (see Chapter 11)

Lymphoedema is a late complication of pelvic lymphadenectomy and is under-reported in the medical literature. In a study of 233 patients having pelvic lymphadenectomy, 20% developed lymphoedema. The addition of pelvic radiation post-operatively further increases this risk (Hacker, 2005d).

(d) Pain (see Chapter 13)

Patients with gynaecological malignancies may experience chronic pain from a variety of causes which can be associated with sleep disturbance, impaired concentration appetite and functional ability.

(e) CRF (see Chapter 12)

This can be a persistent and/or late complication.

Palliative management

Functional impairment is common in advanced cancer patients and, according to Cheville (2001), has the capacity to engender significant psychosocial morbidity. The goal of palliative care is to achieve the best possible quality of life for patients and their carers. As an integral part of the team, rehabilitation professionals aim to improve function and symptom management whilst maintaining a balance between optimal function and comfort. Therapies such as relaxation techniques, TENS, massage, heat and cold, positioning, assistive devices for mobility, environmental modification and simple equipment provision can have a significant impact on pain control, overall function and preserve ADL independence (Reed & Sanderson, 1992). Exercise can counteract the effects of inactivity and improve psychological status. Energy conservation and work simplification techniques can help relieve fatigue. A balance is required between increasing rest to alleviate asthenia and preventing deconditioning (Watanabe & Bruera, 1996).

PROSTATE CANCER

The incidence of prostate cancer has increased markedly over the past 20 years and it is now the most common cancer in men (20%) and the second leading cause of cancer-related death (Lee & Patel, 2002). It is not clear if this increase in incidence is due to actual increased disease or improved diagnostic techniques (e.g. prostate-specific antigen (PSA) test) (Hameed, 2006; Harris & Lohr, 2002). Most prostate cancers are primary adenocarcinomas originating within the cortex of the gland with a firm, single- or multi-focal nodule. As the tumour volume increases it causes enlargement of the prostate, which may give rise to the symptoms of bladder outlet obstruction. There is no definitive cause, but genetic, racial, viral and dietary factors have been suggested; more recently, obesity has been linked to a more aggressive form of prostate cancer (Giovannucci & Michaud, 2007; Mazar & Waxman, 2002).

Increasingly, treatment can be a 'watch-and-wait' process. Patient choice regarding treatment is increasing and may include brachytherapy, chemotherapy and/or radical prostatectomy. Traditionally, men with clinically localised prostate cancer and a life expectancy of 10 years or more have been offered potentially curative treatment with either radiotherapy or radical prostatectomy. The latter involves the removal of the entire prostate gland, attached seminal vesicles and some nearby tissue either by the open retropubic or perineal approach or, more recently, laparoscopically (McLeod, 2004). Nerve-sparing techniques have been developed which help to preserve potency and continence. A 2005 review reported that early functional outcomes of laparoscopic surgery were comparable to the results obtained with open radical retropubic prostatectomy (Trabulsi & Guillonneau, 2005).

Radiotherapy, either by external beam or by brachytherapy, is an alternative radical approach widely used for the treatment of prostate cancer. Candidates tend to be not suitable for, or do not want, surgery. Disease-specific survival appears to be similar when compared to surgical management (McLeod, 2004). For those with positive surgical margins (i.e. evidence that all the cancer has not been removed), adjuvant radiotherapy is routinely considered; for those in whom the PSA becomes detectable post-surgery, salvage radiotherapy is also considered. Prolongation of disease-free survival is demonstrated in both scenarios (Kadmon, 2002).

Newer treatments include various forms of conformal radiotherapy to reduce the incidence of positive surgical margins and adjuvant hormonal therapy, which aims to control undetected cancer cells as well as to target any cancer in tissues outside the surgical margins or radiation fields. However, the latter is associated with loss of libido, impotence, fatigue and hot flushes, with long-term osteoporosis and anaemia implications (McLeod, 2004).

Prostate cancer may grow slowly in the elderly patient who may die 'with', rather than 'of', the disease. Over 90% of patients whose tumours are confined to the prostate have a 5-year disease-free survival; patients with positive surgical margins have a 28–49% incidence of biochemical failure within 5 years of surgery. Most patients whose cancer recurs within 2 years of surgery and whose PSA rises rapidly develop clinical metastases, with or without local recurrences (Lee & Patel, 2002).

Post-operative complications

Immediate post-operative complications include respiratory problems, bleeding wound, wound infection and urinary tract infection, with similar MDT input as described for gynaecological cancers.

Long-term implications of treatments

Pre-operative counselling and provision of booklets, e.g. 'Living and Loving after Prostate Surgery', which discuss potential problems, are important. Similarly, there should be links with specialist urology nurses and the MDT. NICE (2002) states that 'all patients with urological cancers should be managed by multidisciplinary urological cancer teams' and 'patients should receive individual support and guidance from members of the MDT team, and should be provided with well produced information leaflets'.

Problems include bladder dysfunction (incontinence or retention), erectile dysfunction, urethral stricture, faecal problems following radiotherapy, pain and potential spinal cord compression due to metastatic disease, primarily in the bones (see Chapters 5 and 13), fatigue (see Chapter 12) and psychological and psychosexual issues associated with these symptoms (NICE, 2002).

Bladder dysfunction

Incontinence affects the quality of life in men following radical prostatectomy and can be one of the main factors in returning to work. In a study by Donnellan *et al.* (1997), urinary incontinence was reported to be the most distressing post-operative problem. Improvement can be demonstrated for at least 1 year after surgery with conservative treatments, but for those with residual severe problems there are a number of surgical options. Before the advent of nerve-sparing surgery, incontinence was reported to be 87% at 6 months following radical prostatectomy. At 12 months the incidence varies between 2 and 87%, with significant leakage in 0.3–12.5% (Floratos *et al.*, 2002; Fontaine *et al.*, 2004). Patients may present with stress incontinence, urge incontinence or a mixture of both. Post-micturition dribble may also be present.

Treatment modalities include PFMT, biofeedback, urge suppression techniques and lifestyle changes. Anticholinergic medication may also be used to treat severe urge incontinence. A review of the literature (level II evidence) reported that PFMT is effective for an early return to continence after radical prostatectomy (Dorey, 2006). Ideally, PFMT should be taught before surgery (Porru *et al.*, 2001; Sueppel *et al.*, 2001) and commenced as soon as possible post-operatively, including when the catheter is still in situ (depending on the surgeon). There is debate as to whether intra-anal electrical stimulation should be used to try and improve muscle function in patients who have had cancer. According to Dorey (2006) it is contraindicated as we do not know if electrical stimulation will cause a proliferation of abnormal cells; however, it has been used in quite a few studies apparently without adverse effects (Wille *et al.*, 2003). Also, Watson (2007), an expert in the field of electrotherapy, states that it is contraindicated when the disease is being actively treated, but if it is being monitored but not 'treated' as such, then a clinical judgement has to be made (www.electrotherapy.org). The patient must also be provided with information regarding suitable clothing and containment devices, and if necessary an ADL assessment, such as accessing toileting facilities.

Erectile dysfunction

Erectile dysfunction is common in patients following radical prostatectomy. This can be due to nerve damage at the time of surgery or post-operative swelling leading to nerve compression and may take up to 1 year to resolve. According to Dorey (2006), PFMT may help to improve healing and erectile dysfunction. However, there have been no high-quality studies to support this following radical prostatectomy. Oral medication may be prescribed to help with erectile dysfunction. A referral may be made to an erectile dysfunction clinic if long-term problems exist. Further options, such as the use of topical therapies and vacuum devices, can be discussed and help provided with psychological issues.

Urethral stricture

This can occur after the catheter is removed; the patient reports hesitancy and poor flow. It is due to the formation of scar tissue at the anastomosis between the bladder and the urethra. Treatment usually consists of stretching the urethra or, occasionally, resection under anaesthetic.

Summary

A multidisciplinary approach to facilitate problem solving, whether for functional, psychological or physical difficulties, for patients (and their families) with gynaecological or prostate cancer, is essential. The holistic integration of disparate disciplines ensures that the unique challenges of individual cases may be met at all stages of the disease process.

Case study 1: Patient A – cervical cancer

Judith, a 48-year-old female, underwent a colposcopy and LLETZ procedure following an abnormal cervical smear. Two years later, following intermittent vaginal bleeding, a further biopsy revealed an intracervical lesion. Stage IB cervical carcinoma was diagnosed with possible lymphatic involvement and early parametrial extension. Surgery and/or chemoradiation with a 20–50% possibility of post-surgery chemoradiation were proposed. After discussing the options with Judith, a radical hysterectomy was performed.

Post-operatively, Judith self-administered pain relief and had a saline drip, urinary catheter, drains and antiembolitic stockings. Post-operative physiotherapy was commenced; however, she developed right lower lobe pneumonia and required treatment with antibiotics, nebulisers and intensive chest physiotherapy.

Independent mobilisation was achieved at day 4 and stair practice at day 7. Verbal and written advice was provided regarding a graded return to personal and domestic activities, pelvic floor exercises and lymphoedema prevention. The patient had excellent home support and did not require the input of social services or ADL aids.

Unfortunately, on removal of the urethral catheter at day 5, and again at day 8, Judith was unable to void and it had to be replaced. As a result, she went home with catheter in situ and was readmitted 10 days later for catheter removal, but continued to have a urine residual of 150–200 mL. Judith's sister was taught intermittent catheterisation, initially three times a day, gradually reducing as voiding improved.

Five cycles of chemotherapy were followed by brachytherapy. During this period several side effects such as an excoriated vagina with atrophic vaginitis, cystitis, chest infection, severe constipation, bowel spasms, CRF and poor bladder control were reported. MDT input included management of anxiety, CRF and vaginal discomfort. Relaxation techniques were discussed and a relaxation tape provided.

Judith remained independent throughout this period; however, fatigue was a problem. A graded exercise programme was prescribed by the physiotherapist and energy conservation principles were discussed by the OT, including the use of a perching stool, shower chair and bath board. A pressure cushion was provided and tea tree baths recommended.

Post-cancer treatment, Judith was referred to physiotherapy with bladder dysfunction. A 3-day, 24-h bladder diary showed an input of 2300 mL, mainly of tea and coffee and output of 1500 mL. This also recorded frequent leakage, including stress incontinence, urge incontinence and passive incontinence. At night Judith had to go to the toilet at least three times (nocturia) and had to change the pad each time (nocturnal enuresis). A post-void scan revealed a residual of less than 30 mL. Examination demonstrated poor strength and endurance of the PFMs. Based on this assessment, a training programme was commenced. As proprioception and sensation were reduced, intravaginal EMG biofeedback was used to enhance feedback.

Advice was provided regarding caffeine reduction, optimum fluid intake and the importance of continuing PFMT. Several weekly treatment sessions were undertaken and progress noted, including a reduction of stress incontinence and urgency. Bi-weekly sessions followed. Over several months stress incontinence further decreased, nocturia was reduced to once a night and urgency was controlled.

During this time, lymphoedema developed in the right lower leg and Judith was referred to the lymphoedema therapist. She also began to complain of a painful right hip. A bone density scan/MRI reported osteoporosis in the thoracolumbar spine and pelvis. Fosamax was commenced and a stick provided.

Although Judith's general health was quite good, several comorbid conditions affected her quality of life: bladder dysfunction, lymphoedema, increasing mobility problems and fatigue. Her weight also increased and this confounded her mobility, fatigue and depression. Physiotherapy and OT continued and the advice of a dietitian sought. At times Judith was depressed but did not want to take medication. She also reported that, although happily married, intercourse had not been attempted since surgery. This was due to a lack of desire, fatigue and fear (physical due to pain and psychological due to feeling less attractive). The use of an intravaginal device for EMG biofeedback opened discussion regarding the use of vaginal dilators and lubrication as a means of preparing for intercourse.

Case study 2: Patient B – prostate cancer

Bill, a 53-year-old lorry driver, attended his GP for routine blood tests, which revealed a raised PSA level. Further investigations revealed a localised prostate cancer with no evidence of spread. After discussion with the surgeon, a radical prostatectomy was performed. Bill was discharged with a catheter in situ and returned 2 weeks later for a trial removal. Pre-operatively, Bill had discussed PFMT and the possibility of some leakage post-operatively with the continence physiotherapist. After removal of the catheter Bill reported severe leakage with any movement but no post-void residual. Further verbal and written instruction on PFMT, bladder training, fluid balance and return to normal activities was provided. The urologist and specialist urology nurse also provided information and support. Bill made a good functional recovery and did not require additional MDT input.

At a review appointment 6 weeks later, Bill reported an improvement in continence with leakage only on coughing or bending, but still required pads. Frequency was now every 2 hours and urgency could be controlled, with no nocturia. The PFMT programme was reviewed and Bill was keen to comply with periodic reviews. Surgical margins were clear and PSA was monitored at 3-month and then 6-month intervals with no increase. At 9 months, Bill was satisfied with his quality of life and was discharged from physiotherapy.

Case study 3: Patient C – palliative

Ruth, a 45-year-old female, presented with a 3-kg weight loss in a 5-month period and lower abdominal pain. Investigations revealed what was thought to be a simple multi-loculated cyst. A laparotomy was performed, which revealed bilateral abnormal ovaries with tumour deposits throughout the pelvis, a solitary metastasis in the omentum and a large node in the left external iliac region. Optimal debulking was undertaken and pathology confirmed a poorly differentiated serous cystadenocarcinoma, Stage IIIC. Post-operative recovery was slow as she developed paralytic ileus, a rectovaginal fistula and required help and advice on mobilising, fatigue management and return to independent activities. Surgery for the fistula was postponed to allow commencement of chemotherapy.

Over the next 3 years, Ruth had three sessions of chemotherapy. During this period she complained of fatigue, arthralgia and myalgia. MDT input included advice on diet, energy conservation, relaxation, positioning and gentle exercises. Sadly, the final chemotherapy session was ineffective and Ruth started to show symptoms of rectovaginal fistula with vaginal bleeding. An MRI showed bulky tumour with early bladder invasion, infiltration around the S1 nerve root and extensive lymphadenopathy. Pelvic radiotherapy was commenced to try and control these symptoms.

One month after radiotherapy Ruth reported increasing left-leg pain and swelling. Doppler investigations were negative; lymphadenopathy was the cause of the oedema. She was referred to the community palliative care team for pain and lymphoedema assessment and management. Ruth, however, refused multi-layer lymphoedema bandaging (palliative) and so a compression garment was provided along with a leg exercise and skin care programme.

As the disease progressed, Ruth was admitted with bilateral leg oedema extending into the genitalia and abdomen with ascites and bilateral pleural effusions. Oxygen therapy was commenced and positions of ease and breathing control instigated. Made-to-measure low-grade compression garments were helpful for containment (not compression) and comfort in the short term. Community OT assessed for equipment and adaptations to facilitate independent living at home. Transfers were difficult due to lower limb and trunk oedema; therefore, the hoist and appropriate pressure-relieving seating became essential. An extra wide commode and other aids were provided as genital and leg oedema caused problems with toileting. At this stage, further medical management was no longer appropriate and a bed was secured in the hospice. Sadly, Ruth died prior to transfer, but she had achieved her wish of remaining at home for as long as possible.

Key learning points

- Gynaecological and prostate cancers are common and can occur at any age.
- If diagnosed early, treatment for most can be effective but may result in comorbid conditions, which decrease quality of life.
- Management must be holistic and include potential bladder, bowel and sexual dysfunction.

References

American Cancer Society (2007). *Cancer facts and figures*. Retrieved June 2007 from www.cancer.org

Aston, J. L., Lodoice, A. E. & Sharpio, N. L. (2006). Interaction between warfarin and cranberry juice. *Pharmacotherapy, 26* (9), 1314–1319.

Behtash, N., Ghaemmaghami, F., Ayatollahi, H., Khaledi, H. & Hanjani, P. (2005). A case-control study to evaluate urinary tract complications in radical hysterectomy. *World Journal of Surgical Oncology, 3* (1), 12.

Benedetti-Panici, P., Zullo, M. A., Plotti, F., Manci, N., Muzii, M. & Angioli, R. (2004). Long-term bladder function in patients with locally advanced cervical carcinoma treated with neoadjuvant chemotherapy and type-4 radical hysterectomy. *Cancer, 100,* 2110–2117.

Benoit, M. F. & Hannigan, E. V. (2006). A 10-year review of primary fallopian tube cancer at a community hospital: a high association of synchronous and metachronous cancers. *International Journal of Gynaecological Cancer, 16* (1), 29–35.

Berek, J. S. (2005). Epithelial ovarian cancer. In: J. Berek & N. Hacker (Eds.), *Practical gynaecological/oncology* (4th ed., pp. 443–511). Philadelphia: Lippincott Williams & Wilkins.

Berek, J. S. & Hacker, N. F. (2005). Nonepithelial ovarian and fallopian tube cancer. In: J. Berek & N. Hacker (Eds.), *Practical gynaecological/oncology* (4th ed., pp. 511–543). Philadelphia: Lippincott Williams & Wilkins.

Biglia, N., Mariani, L., Marenco, D., Robba, C., Peano, E., Kubatzki, F. & Sismondi, P. (2006). Hormonal replacement therapy after gynaecological cancer. *Gynakol Geburtshilfliche Rundsch, 46* (4), 191–196

Bø, K., Larsen, S., Oseid, S., Kvarstein, B., Hagen, R. & Jörgensen, J. (1988). Knowledge about and ability of correct pelvic floor muscle exercises in women with urinary stress incontinence. *Neurourology and Urodynamics, 7,* 261–262.

Bolderston, A., Lloyd, N., Wong, K., Holden, L. & Robb-Blenderman, L. (2006). The prevention and management of acute skin reactions related to radiation therapy: a systematic review and practice guideline. *Supportive Care in Cancer, 14* (8), 802–817.

Bump, R. C., Hurt, W. G., Fantl, J. A. & Wyman, J. F. (1991). Assessment of Kegel pelvic muscle exercise performance after brief verbal instruction. *American Journal of Obstetrics and Gynecology, 165* (2), 322–329.

Campion, M. J. (2005). Preinvasive disease. In: J. Berek & N. Hacker (Eds.), *Practical gynaecological/oncology* (4th ed., pp. 265–337). Philadelphia: Lippincott Williams & Wilkins.

Canavan, T. P. & Cohen, D. (2002). Vulvar cancer. *American Family Physician, 66* (7), 1269–1276

Cancer BACUP. (2006). Cervix, ovarian, prostate, uterus, vulva, womb (endometrium) cancers (Booklets). Retrieved March 2007 from www.cancerbackup.org.uk

Cheville, A. (2001). Rehabilitation of patients with advanced cancer. *Cancer Supplement*, 92 (4), 1039–1047.

Chiarelli, P. & Markwell, S. (1992). *Lets get things moving-over coming constipation*. Sydney, Australia: Health Books.

Clayton, N. L., Jaaback, K. S. & Hirschowitz, L. (2005). Primary fallopian tube carcinoma – the experience of a UK cancer centre and a review of the literature. *Journal of Obstetrics and Gynaecology*, 25 (7), 694–702.

Cook, T. (2004). Gynaecological surgery. In: J. Mantle, J. Haslam & S. Barton (Eds.), *Physiotherapy in obstetrics and gynaecology* (2nd ed., pp. 309–333). Edinburgh: Butterworth Heinemann.

Decker, T. W., Cline-Elsen, J. & Gallagher, M. (1992). Relaxation therapy as an adjunct in radiation oncology. *Journal of Clinical Psychology*, 48 (3), 388–393.

Del Priore, G., Taylor, W. Y., Esdaile, B. A., Masch, R., Martas, Y. & Wirth, J. (2005). Urinary incontinence in gynecology patients. *International Gynecological Cancer*, 15, 911–914.

Denton, A. S., Clarke, N. W. & Maher, E. I. (2002a). Non-surgical interventions for late radiation cystitis in patients who have received radical radiotherapy to the pelvis. *Cochrane Database Systematic Review*, Art No: CD001773.

Denton, A. S., Forbes, A., Andreyev, J. & Maher, E. I. (2002b). Non-surgical interventions for late proctitis in patients who have received radical radiotherapy to the pelvis. *Cochrane Database Systematic Review*, Art No: CD003455.

Denton, A. S. & Maher, E. I. (2003). Interventions for the physical aspects of sexual dysfunction in women following pelvic radiotherapy. *Cochrane Database Systematic Review*, Art No: CD003750.

Devine, E. C. (1992). Effects of psychoeducational care for adult surgical patients: a meta-analysis of 192 studies. *Patient Education and Counselling*, 19, 129–142.

Donnellan, S. M, Duncan, H. J, Macgregor, R. J. & Russell, J. M. (1997). Prospective assessment of incontinence after radical retropubic prostatectomy: objective and subjective analysis. *Urology*, 49 (2), 225–230.

Donovan, K. A., Taliaferro, L. A., Alvarez, E. M., Jacobsen, P. B., Roetzheim, R. G. & Wenham, R. M. (25 September 2006). Sexual health in women treated for cervical cancer: characteristics and correlates. *Gynecology and Oncology*. (Epub ahead of print)

Dorey, G. (2006). *Pelvic dysfunction in men. Diagnosis and treatment of male incontinence and erectile dysfunction*. England: John Wiley and Sons Ltd.

Eifel, P. J. (2006). Concurrent chemotherapy and radiation therapy as the standard of care for cervical cancer. *Nature Clinical Practice. Oncology*, 3 (5), 248–255.

El Husseiny, G., Al Bareedy, N., Mourad, W. A., Mohamed, G., Shourkri, M., Sibji, J. & Ezzat, A. (2002). Prognostic factors and treatment modalities in uterine sarcoma. *American Journal of Clinical Oncology*, 25 (3), 256–260.

Floratos, D. L., Sonke, G. S., Rapidou, C. A., Alivizatos, G. J., Deliveliotis, C., Constantinides, C. A. & Theodorou, C. (2002). Biofeedback vs verbal feedback as learning tools for pelvic muscle exercises in the early management of urinary incontinence after radical prostatectomy. *British Journal of Urology International*, 89 (7), 714–719.

Fontaine, E., Ben Mouellk, S., Thomas, L., Otmezguine, Y. & Beurton, D. (2004). Urinary continence after salvage radiation therapy following radical prostatectomy, assessed by a self-administered questionnaire: a prospective study. *British Journal of Urology International*, 94 (4), 521–523.

Fraunholz, I. B., Schopohl, B. & Bottcher, H. D. (1998). Management of radiation injuries of vulva and vagina. *Strahlentherapie und Onkologie*, 147 (Suppl 3), 90–92.

Gibstone, R. I. & Keefe, D. M. (2006). Cancer chemotherapy-induced diarrhoea and constipation: mechanisms of damage and prevention strategies. *Support Care Cancer*, 14 (9), 890–900.

Giovannucci, E. & Michaud, D. (2007). The role of obesity and related metabolic distur-bances in cancers of the colon, prostate, and pancreas. *Gastroenterology, 132* (6), 2208–2225.

Grant, P. (2006). Radical trachelectomy. *Australian and New Zealand Journal of Obstetrics and Gynaecology, 46* (5), 372–374.

Grumann, M., Robertson, R., Hacker, N. F. & Sommer, G. (2001). Sexual functioning in patients following radical hysterectomy for stage 1B cancer of the cervix. *International Journal of Gynaecological Cancer, 11* (5), 372–380.

Gunnell, A. S., Tran, T. N., Torrang, A., Dickman, O. W., Sparen, P., Palmgren, J. & Yli-talo, N. (2006). Synergy between cigarette smoking and human papillomavirus Type 16 in cervical cancer in situ. *Cancer Epidemiology Biomarkers & Prevention.* (Epub ahead of print).

Hacker, N. F. (2005a). Uterine cancer. In: J. Berek & N. Hacker (Eds.), *Practical gynaecolog-ical/oncology* (4th ed., pp. 397–443). Philadelphia: Lippincott Williams & Wilkins.

Hacker, N. F. (2005b). Vaginal cancer. In: J. Berek & N. Hacker (Eds.), *Practical gynaecolog-ical/oncology* (4th ed., pp. 585–603). Philadelphia: Lippincott Williams & Wilkins.

Hacker, N. F. (2005c). Vulvar cancer. In: J. Berek & N. Hacker (Eds.), *Practical gynaecologi-cal/oncology* (4th ed., pp. 543–585). Philadelphia: Lippincott Williams & Wilkins.

Hacker, N. F. (2005d). Cervical cancer. In: J. Berek & N. Hacker (Eds.), *Practical gynaecolog-ical/oncology* (4th ed., pp. 337–397). Philadelphia: Lippincott Williams & Wilkins.

Hameed, A. (2006). PSA an overview of what we need to know. *Urology, 10* (6), 9–11.

Harris, R. P. & Lohr, K. N. (2002). Screening for prostate cancer: an update for the evidence for the US Preventative Services Taskforce. *Annals of Internal Medicine, 137* (11), 917–929.

Haslam, J. & Pomfret, I. (2002). Should pelvic floor muscle exercises be encouraged in peo-ple with and indwelling urethral catheter in situ? *Journal of the Association of Chartered Physiotherapists in Women's Health, 91,* 18–22.

Hatch, K. D. (2005). Laparoscopy. In: J. Berek & N. Hacker (Eds.), *Practical gynaecologi-cal/oncology* (4th ed., pp. 783–801). Philadelphia: Lippincott Williams & Wilkins.

Hatch, K. D. & Berek, J. S. (2005). Pelvic exenteration. In: J. Berek & N. Hacker (Eds.), *Practical gynaecological/oncology* (4th ed., pp. 801–819). Philadelphia: Lippincott Williams & Wilkins.

Heber, D. (2005). Cervical cancer. In: J. Berek & N. Hacker (Eds.), *Practical gynaecologi-cal/oncology* (4th ed., pp. 715–737). Philadelphia: Lippincott Williams & Wilkins.

Hopkins, M. P. & Nemunaitis-Keller, J. (2001). Carcinoma of the vulva. *Obstetrics and Gy-necology Clinics of North America, 28* (4), 791–804.

Irico, G., Escobar, H. & Marinelli, B. (2006). Cervical cancer prevention: a current status of the knowledge. *Revista de la Facultad de Ciencias Medicus (Cordoba, Argentina), 62* (2 Suppl 1), 37–47.

Jensen, P., Groenvold, M., Marianne, C., Thranov, I., Petersen, M. & Machin, D. (2003). Early-Sage cervical carcinoma, radical hysterectomy, and sexual function. *Cancer, 100* (1), 97–106.

Jepson, R. G., Mihalijevic, L. & Craig, J. (2004). Cranberries for preventing urinary tract infections. *The Cochrane Database of Systematic Reviews (Complete Reviews),* Issue 1, Art No: CD001321.

Kadmon, D. (2002). Radiation therapy after radical prostatectomy: strike early, strike hard! The case for adjuvant radiation therapy. *Urology, 4* (2), 87–89.

Keskar, V., Mohanty, P. S., Gemeinhart, E. J. & Gemeinhart, R. A. (2006). Cervical cancer treatment with a locally insertable controlled release delivery system. *Journal of Controlled Release, 115* (3), 280–288.

Koelbl, H. (2006). The effect of hysterectomy (simple and radical) on the lower urinary tract. In: L. Cardozo & D. Staskin (Eds.), *Textbook of female urology and urogynaecology* (2nd ed., pp. 1363–1367). England: Informa Healthcare.

Kohn, M. (2003). The state of CAM in UK cancer care: advances in research, practice and delivery. *Invited speaker at The National Cancer's Institute's Office of Cancer Complementary and Alternative Medicine*. Retrieved November 2006 from www.cancer.gov.cam

Krishnan, C. S., Grant, P. T., Robertson, G. & Hacker, N. F. (2001). Lymphatic ascites following lymphadenectomy for gynecolgical malignancy. *International Journal of Gynaecological Cancer, 11* (5), 392–396.

Lee, F. & Patel, H. R. (2002). Prostate cancer; management and controversies. *Hospital Medicine, 63,* 465–470.

Long, L. E. (2001). Being informed: undergoing radiation therapy. *Cancer Nursing, 24* (6), 462–468

Lynch, H. T., Watson, P., Lynch, J. F., *et al.* (1993). Hereditary ovarian cancer, heterogeneity in age at onset. *Cancer, 71* (2 Suppl), 573–523.

Lukaszuk, K., Liss, J., Nowaczuyk, M., Sliwinski, W., Maj, B., Wozniak, I., Nakoniecznhy, M. & Barwinska, D. M. (2007). Survival of 231 cervical cancer patients, treated by radical hysterectomy, according to clinical and histopathological features. *European Journal Gynaecology Oncology, 28* (1), 23–27.

Macnab, J. C., Walkinshaw, S. A., Cordiner, J. W. & Clements, J. B. (1986). Human papillomavirus in clinically and histologically normal tissue of patients with genital cancer. *Northern England Journal of Medicine, 315* (17), 1052–1058.

Markwell, S. J. & Sapsford, R. R. (1995). Physiotherapy management of obstructed defaecation. *Australian Journal of Physiotherapy, 41,* 279–283.

Mazar, D. & Waxman, J. (2002). Prostate cancer. *Postgraduate Medical Journal, 78,* 590–595.

McLeod, G. L. (2004). Success and failure of single-modality treatment for early prostate cancer. *Reviews in Urology, 6* (Suppl 2), S13–S19.

Naik, R., Nwabinelli, J., Mayne, C., Nordin, A., de Barros, Lopes, A., Monaghan, J. M. & Hilton, P. (2001). Prevalence and management of (non-fistulous) urinary incontinence in women following radical hysterectomy for early stage cervical cancer. *European Journal of Gynaecology Oncology, 22* (1), 26–30.

National Institute for health and Clinical Excellence (NICE) (2002). *Improving outcomes in urological cancers.* N0138. Retrieved March 2007 from www.nice.org

National Institute for health and Clinical Excellence (NICE) (2006). *High dose rate brachytherapy for carcinoma of the cervix.* N0996. Retrieved March 2007 from www.nice.org.uk

Neises, M. (2002). Sexuality and sexual dysfunction in gynaecological psycho oncology. *Onkologie, 25* (6), 571–574.

Omura, G. A., Brady, M. F., Homesley, H. F., Yordan, E., Major, F. J., Buchsbaum, H. J. & Park, R. C. (1991). Long-term follow-up and prognostic factor analysis in advance ovarian carcinoma: the Gynecologic Oncology Group Experience. *Journal of Clinical Oncology, 9* (7), 1138–1172

Pessini, S. A., Zettler, C. G., Wender, M. C., Pellanda, L. C. & Silvera, G. P. (2007). Survival and prognostic factors of patients treated for Stage I to Stage III endometrial carcinoma in a reference cancer center in Southern Brazil. *European Journal of Gynaecology Oncology, 28* (1), 448–450.

Porru, D., Campus, G., Caria, A., Madeddu, G., Cucchi A., Rovereto, B., Scarpa, R. M., Pili, P. & Usai, E. (2001). Impact of early pelvic floor rehabilitation after transurethral resection of the prostate. *Neurourology and Urodynamics, 20,* 53–39.

Raz, R., Chazan, B. & Dan, M. (2004). Cranberry juice and urinary tract infections. *Clinical Infectious Diseases, 38,* 1413–1419.

Reed, K. L. & Sanderson, S. (1992). *Concepts of occupational therapy*. Philadelphia: Lippincott, Williams & Wilkins.

Richardson, J. & Sabanathan, S. (1997). Prevention of respiratory complications after abdominal surgery. *Thorax*, *52* (Suppl 3), S31–S42.

Robinson, J. W., Faris, P. D. & Scott, C. B. (1999). Psychoeducational group increased vaginal dilation for younger women and reduces sexual fears for women of all ages with gynaecologic carcinoma treated with radiotherapy. *International Journal of Radiation Oncology Biological Physiological*, *44*, 47–506.

Roden, R. & Wu, T. C. (2006). How will HPV vaccines affect cervical cancer? *Nature Reviews: Cancer*, *6* (10), 753–763.

Saadat, M., Truong, P. T., Kader, H. A., Speers, C. H., Berthelet, E., McMurtrie, E. & Olivotto, I. A. (2007). Outcomes in patients with primary breast cancer and a subsequent diagnosis of endometrial cancer: comparison of cohorts treated with and without tamoxifen. *Cancer*, *110* (1), 31–37. (Epub ahead of print)

Sharpe, R. (1998). Physiotherapy and gynaecological surgery. In: R. Sapsford, J. Bullock-Saxton & S. Markwell (Eds.), *Women's health. A textbook for physiotherapists* (pp. 466–478). London: W. B. Saunders Company Ltd.

Shearsmith-Farthing, K. (2001). The management of altered body image: a role for occupational therapy. *British Journal of Occupational Therapy*, *64* (8), 387–389.

Singhal, P., Odunsi, K., Rodabaugh, K., Driscoll, D. & Lele, S. (2006). Primary fallopian tube carcinoma: a retrospective clinicopathologic study. *European Journal of Gynecology Oncology*, *27* (1), 16–18.

Sueppel, C., Kreder, K. & See, W. (2001). Improved continence outcomes with preoperative pelvic floor muscle strengthening exercises. *Urologic Nursing*, *21* (3), 201–210.

Sundquist, K. & Yee, L. (2003). Sexuality and body image after cancer. *Australian Family Physician*, *32* (1–2), 19–23.

Symonds, P. & Foweraker, K. (2006). Principles of chemotherapy and radiotherapy. *Current Obstetrics and Gynaecology*, *16* (2), 100–106.

Trabulsi, E. J. & Guillonneau, B. (2005). Laparoscopic radical prostatectomy. *Journal of Urology*, *173* (4), 1072–1079.

Watanabe, S. & Bruera, E. (1996). Anorexia and cachexia, asthenia, and lethargy. *Medical Clinics of North America*, *10*, 18–206.

Watson, T. (2007). *Electrotherapy and Cancer*. Powerpoint presentation ACPOPC Belfast 2007. Retrieved May 2007 from www.electrotherapy.org

Wille, S., Sobottka, A., Heidenreich, A. & Hofman, R. (2003). Pelvic floor exercises, electrical stimulation and biofeedback after radical prostatectomy: results of a randomized trial. *The Journal of Urology*, *179* (2), 490–493.

Wright, E. P., Kiely, M. A., Lynch, P., Cull, A. & Selby, P. J. (2002). Social problems in oncology. *British Journal of Cancer*, *87*, 1099–1104.

Websites and further reading

For health care professionals

Dorey, G. (2006). Pelvic dysfunction in men. *Diagnosis and treatment of male incontinence and erectile dysfunction*. England: John Wiley and Sons Ltd.

Laycock, J. & Haslam, J. (Eds.) (2002). *Therapeutic management of incontinence and pelvic pain*. London: Springer.

Mantle, J., Haslam, J. & Barton, S. (Eds.) (2004). *Physiotherapy in obstetrics and gynaecology* (2nd ed.). Edinburgh: Butterworth Heinemann.

For patients, carers and health care professionals

Living and Loving After Prostate Surgery
Author Professor Grace Dorey
Old Hill Farm, Portmore, Barnstaple, Devon, EX32 0HR. E-mail: grace.dorey@virgin.net.

Prostate Cancer: A Comprehensive Guide for Patients
Jane Smith, Raj Persaud & Kieran Jefferson
TFM Publishing.
Website: www.amazon.com

Hysterectomy Association. Tel: 0871 7811141.
Website: www.hysterectomy-association.org.uk.

The Daisy Network (Premature Menopause Support Group)
PO Box 392, High Wycombe, Bucks, HP15 7SH. Tel: 01628 473446/01628 625071. Email: dkhurst@btinternet.com.
It offers support, group meetings and workshops for women affected by premature menopause.

Ovacome
St Bartholomew's Hospital, West Smithfield, London, EC1A 7BE. Tel: 07071 781861. Email: ovacome@dial.pipex.com.
Website: www.ovacome.org.uk.
A national support group for all those involved with ovarian cancer.

Association of Chartered Society of Physiotherapists in Women's Health (ACPWH)
C/o CSP, 14 Bedford Row, London, WC1R 4ED.
Website: www.womensphysio.org.uk.

The Prostate Cancer Charity
3 Angel Walk, Hammersmith, London, W6 9HX.
Website: www.prostate-cancer.org.uk.

The Continence Foundation
307 Hatton Square, 16 Baldwin Gardens, London, EC1N 7RJ.

SECTION 3
SYMPTOM MANAGEMENT

Chapter 11

LYMPHOEDEMA

Rhian Davies and Sue Desborough

Learning outcomes

Having read this chapter the reader should be able to:

- Discuss the difficulties around establishing prevalence figures for lymphoedema
- Relate the management of lymphoedema to current understanding of the anatomy and physiology of the lymphatic system
- List the elements required in assessment
- Justify the content of a rehabilitation programme for these patients based on the patient's general health status

---

Introduction

As cancer treatment increases in volume and complexity, some patients are experiencing side effects that are a lasting legacy of their survivorship. Allied health professionals (AHPs) have specific and appropriate skills that can help reduce the impact of one such side effect, lymphoedema.

Lymphoedema is a chronic oedema caused by failure of the lymphatic drainage system. It is often noted in one or more limbs, but may involve the face, genitalia or trunk. It arises from congenital malformation of the lymphatic system or damage to the lymphatic vessels and/or lymph nodes, e.g. in patients being treated for cancer when the lymph nodes are removed (International Society of Lymphology [ISL], 2003). It can have a significant effect on health-related quality of life in physical, psychological and social aspects (Franks *et al.*, 2006; Velanovich & Szymanski, 1999). Despite the presence of congenital lymphoedema, many services have developed within cancer and voluntary services as the specialist skills have developed to meet the complexities of rehabilitating this patient group (MacLaren, 2003). Morgan *et al.* (2005) demonstrated that many community nurses assessed their current knowledge and skill in the care of patients with lymphoedema as only 'adequate or poor'.

It is important that the needs of the patient with lymphoedema are identified and that appropriate skills, education and information are available to facilitate a seamless journey through the acute, community and voluntary sectors. It is appropriate, therefore, that lymphoedema should have a fully integrated and multidisciplinary pathway of care.

Epidemiology and planning services

The aetiology is the result of accumulation of fluid and other elements, such as protein in the tissue spaces, due to an imbalance between interstitial fluid production and transport, usually low-output failure (ISL, 2003).

Lymphoedema is manageable but incurable; therefore, both incidence and prevalence (burden) figures are important in service planning. Whether the patient's cancer status is palliative, 'in active disease', 'in remission' or the lymphoedema is non-cancer related, management is aimed at minimising the impact of the condition and increasing independence (British Lymphology Society [BLS], 2001a). Similar to many long-term conditions, the needs of the lymphoedema patient can fluctuate greatly.

There should, therefore, be local and timely access to the appropriate level of care in all settings (Department of Health [DH], 2005). Service design will need to allow for a care pathway that crosses different providers to meet the need appropriately. Historically, coordination of such services at strategic level has not always been evident (MacLaren, 2003); however, the recent publication of The Lymphoedema Framework (best practice document) (Lymphoedema Framework [LF], 2006) will aim to improve future planning of these services.

Incidence and prevalence

Figures for lymphoedema can be varied and conflicting. The difficulties lie largely in variances in definition and research and diagnostic methodology. In breast-cancer-related lymphoedema (BCRL), for example, the incidence figures have varied depending on whether the critical factor is a volume difference in the affected arm of 200 mL, volume excess of 10% or a circumferential difference of 2 cm at a given point. Williams *et al.* (2005) reviewed epidemiological figures for lymphoedema from which the following have been taken:

- Breast cancer treatment – overall incidence 30% (combination of surgery and radiotherapy).
- Malignant melanoma treatment – groin dissection/ilioinguinal lymph node dissection 21–80%; this has been reduced by the use of sentinel lymph node biopsies (SLNB) and fascia-preserving techniques.
- Genitourinary cancer treatment – penile carcinoma treated by inguinal dissection 100%, by inguinal lymphadenectomy 16.0–28.5%. Carcinoma of bladder treated by radical radiotherapy 20%, by radical cystoscopy 10%.
- Gynaecological cancer treatment – cervical and vulval overall incidence of 20%, but where infection follows radical vulvectomy including groin dissection 48%. Improvements in technique described to reduce the risk of lymphoedema include preservation of the saphenous vein during inguinal lymphadenectomy and omentoplasty in treating cervical cancer.

- Sarcoma treatment – incidence following wide local excision and radiotherapy 30–50%.
- Lymphoedema secondary to non-cancer factors (trauma, infection, chronic inflammatory conditions, hypertension and venous insufficiency). Figures are varied and often include patients with primary lymphoedema. A recent survey of vascular consultants in the UK demonstrated higher incidence among their referrals following arterial reconstructions than from cellulitis, venous disease and venous surgery (Tiwari *et al.*, 2006). Worldwide the commonest cause of secondary lymphoedema is filariasis, transmitted by mosquito, affecting as many as 120 million people in 80 countries; 40 million suffering disability and disfigurement (World Health Organization [WHO], 2000).
- Primary lymphoedema is due to a congenital lymphatic dysplasia (ISL, 1995). There are no published figures to confirm prevalence and incidence, although small UK studies have been reported (Williams *et al.*, 2005).
- Both the preceding non-cancer-related categories were included in a UK study which used the clinical classification of oedema being present for 3 months or more and defined as 'chronic oedema'. This found a prevalence of 1.33/1000 population (Moffatt *et al.*, 2003) rising to 5.4/1000 in those aged over 65. This compares to the 1.44/1000 prevalence reported in Norway (Petlund, 1990).

It is hoped that incidence will reduce with developments in cancer treatment techniques; e.g. the use of SLNB alongside improved understanding of the effects of radiotherapy delivery (Nardone *et al.*, 2005; Senekus-Konefka & Jassem, 2006). Karakousis (2006) reviewed his own surgical work for indicators leading to lymphoedema and found certain practices that lead to an increased risk of lymphoedema. These include excessively thin flaps in axillary dissections. In the lower limb, lymphoedema was more likely with thin flaps, wide resection of a primary melanoma below the knee, post-operative cellulitis, obesity and failure to follow a prophylactic regimen of leg elevation and compression stockings. Other improvements may come from greater use of preventative protocols which include lymphoscintigraphy (Campisi *et al.*, 2006).

Physiology and anatomy of the lymphatic system

Key events in cancer development and progression occur in the lymphatic system; this forms the basis for evaluation, prognosis and treatment. It also plays an important part in infection and inflammation, asthma and transplant rejection, as well as lymphoedema. Recent developments in genetics, recognition of endothelial growth factors, molecular biology and broader physiology are transforming our understanding of this previously poorly understood system (Ji, 2006; Mortimer & Levick, 2006; Witte *et al.*, 2006). It is anticipated that this new evidence, combined with the international lymphoedema management consensus work (ISL, 2003; LF, 2006), will lead to improved lymphoedema treatment and outcomes. This is already evident in some areas of care, such as advice on exercise, which will be discussed later in this chapter (Lane *et al.*, 2005b).

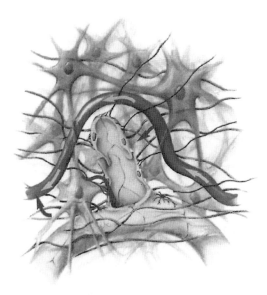

Figure 11.1 The lymphatic loop. [Reproduced by permission of Medi (UK) Ltd.]

The lymphatic system is designed to return fluid and proteins to the vascular circulation via a network of unidirectional vessels, many running parallel to the venous system. The lymph passes through a series of lymph nodes to eventually reach the subclavian veins where the filtered lymph rejoins the blood system. This system has an essential role in maintaining fluid balance, transporting fats and proteins and also providing an immune response. Traditionally, Starling's principle of fluid exchange has been taught as an explanation of the fluid dynamics. This describes the forces affecting capillary filtration and the movement of fluid into the interstitial tissues, with the venous end reabsorbing most of this filtrate. Evidence now suggests that the majority of interstitial fluid is returned to the blood circulation via the lymphatics and not by reabsorption into venous capillaries (Karlsen *et al.*, 2006; Mortimer & Levick, 2004).

Areas of skin territories (lymphotomes) are drained through superficial initial lymphatics, via pre-collector and collector lymphatics, into superficial lymph node groups and then into deeper lymphatics (Figure 11.1). Collateral routes across the skin into neighbouring skin territories and towards alternative lymph nodes can be established when lymph nodes are absent or damaged. This forms the basis of lymphatic massage, which is commonly known as manual lymphatic drainage (MLD). Recent investigations with breast cancer patients propose that there may be some women that are predisposed to hand swelling and others protected, which may explain why some women develop lymphoedema in the hand, whilst others who have apparently undergone the same treatment do not (Stanton *et al.*, 2006a). Pain *et al.* (2005) found uptake of protein into local blood and/or proteolysis increased after axillary surgery and suggest that this may protect against BCRL. Recent studies have also shown an increase in incidence of cellulitis in this patient group (Mallon *et al.*, 1997; Mortimer, 2000). Soo *et al.* (2006) audited objective signs of lymphoedema in patients admitted to hospital with cellulitis. Clinical, serological and microbiological factors were used in the diagnosis: 47% had skin changes consistent with lymphoedema, 87% had abnormal lymphoscintigraphic scans and 62% had abnormal lymphatics in the non-cellulitic leg, which may suggest that the lymphatic changes predate the cellulitic event.

Local arterial pulsation, body movements causing variations in tissue pressure and massage may all influence the uptake of fluid and proteins from the tissues into the thin-walled initial lymphatic networks. This increased uptake stimulates contractions in collector lymphatics. Movement of lymph through deeper, larger vessels to the thoracic duct and right lymphatic duct is further enhanced by changes in intra-thoracic and intra-abdominal pressures produced by breathing and pulsation of adjacent vessels, such as the aorta (Vaqas & Ryan, 2003). The calf muscle pump (Parmar *et al.*, 2006) and the status of the vascular system as a whole (Tiwari *et al.*, 2006) play key roles in the effectiveness of the lymphatic system.

This developing understanding of the physiology of the lymphatic system in health and in pathological state forms the basis of effective lymphoedema management.

Assessment of lymphoedema

Historically, assessment and research has tended to rely heavily on volume or circumferential measurements of limbs, recording comparison with an unaffected contralateral limb and with changes over time. The limitations of using this as a single-outcome measure is being increasingly acknowledged (LF, 2006 p. 10; Stanton *et al.*, 2006b) and may lead to significant underdiagnosis. International consensus (LF, 2006) recommends a multi-modal assessment to include:

- Medical assessment
  - History
  - Physical examination
  - Specialist investigations – used only where differential diagnosis from the above has not been possible; e.g. ultrasound for skin thickening/tissue fibrosis, colour Doppler to exclude deep venous thrombosis (DVT) and venous anomalies, lymphoscintigraphy (especially if thought to be of non-cancer origin) to assess existing lymphatics, computerised tomography (CT)/magnetic resonance imaging (MRI) show distinctive honeycomb pattern in tissues or obstruction by tumour or excessive adipose tissue, bioimpedance (Hayes *et al.*, 2005) or genetic tests
- Lymphoedema assessment
  - ISL staging (ISL, 2003), where
    - 0 = subclinical state
    - 1 = fluid in tissues resolves on elevation and pitting may be seen
    - 2 = manifest pitting, no reduction with elevation
    - Late 2 = oedema firm, pitting may not be evident
    - 3 = hard thickened skin, no pitting, skinfolds, fat deposits, warty growths, hyperpigmentation
  - Severity
    - If unilateral: mild <20% excess limb volume, moderate 20–40%, severe >40% excess limb volume (BLS, 2001a)

- Skin condition
- Subcutaneous changes
- Shape distortion
- History of cellulitis/erysipelas (an acute form of cellulitis involving the dermal papillae)
- Movement or functional impairment of limb or effect on rest of the body
- Psychosocial morbidity
- Other associated complications or multi-pathology

Example documentation can be found in the best practice document (LF, 2006).

Limb volume measurement

Circumference measurement using a tape measure remains the routine measurement of arm or leg swelling. Circumferential (c) measurements are taken every 4 cm up the limb. Total limb volume is then calculated using the formula c^2/π. Various programmed calculators and electronic programmes are available for this calculation and some can additionally provide charts and graphs. The total volume is then expressed in millilitres and compared, where possible, to the unaffected limb. In specialist clinics, the limb may be measured optoelectronically using a perometer or the bioimpedance levels may be recorded. For volume measurement of hands or feet, water displacement is reliable but can be time consuming and messy.

Skin condition

Skin changes are more likely to occur in long-standing lymphoedema; however, the skin on the affected and adjacent areas, such as the trunk, should also be assessed for:

- Dryness, fragility, hyperkeratosis (thickened brown pigmentation/build up of proteins), dermatitis
- Redness, pallor, cyanosis, pigmentation
- Warmth, coolness, cellulitis, erysipelas, fungal infection
- Deepened skinfolds, Stemmer sign*, orange peel skin (dimpled)
- Lymphorrhoea (weeping skin), lymphangiectasia (blister-like), papillomatosis (warty growths), lipodermatosclerosis (on the lower leg, associated with chronic venous insufficiency)

Vascular assessment

As vascular status can have significant impact on lymphatic status (Tiwari *et al.*, 2006), and lymphoedema management involves compression therapy (compression

---

* Stemmer sign is said to be positive when the skinfold at the base of the second toe or the middle finger cannot be raised.

hosiery, bandaging or machines), a vascular assessment is required. A general assessment taken from the colour and condition of the skin, along with a history relating to activity (e.g. intermittent claudication) or pain/discomfort (e.g. restless legs), may give sufficient cause for concern relating to the vascular status and necessitate Doppler screening. Of particular concern with cancer patients is the high risk of venous thrombus associated with metastases. Similarly, arm oedema associated with superior vena cava obstruction needs distinguishing from pure breast-cancer-related arm lymphoedema, as the management and implications are quite different.

In lower limb oedema, it is common practice to carry out an objective assessment using ankle brachial pressure index (using a 4- or 5-Hz head) or toe brachial pressure. Pulse oximetry or pulse oscillography may also be used. However, these methods are subject to error in the presence of oedema and should be checked by further vascular tests if inconsistent with previous observations.

Pain assessment

Historically, there has been an impression that lymphoedema does not cause pain. This may be because non-cancer lymphoedema patients are not routinely assessed for pain. Pain is however a feature of varying significance in quality-of-life studies (Moffatt et al., 2003; Sitzia & Sobrido, 1997) – one study showing 50% of patients taking regular analgesia. Pain charts and visual analogue scores can be useful adjuncts to a general assessment.

Movement and functional impairment

A baseline assessment of function in activities of daily living and specific measurement of range of movement, strength and fine/gross movements will provide both objective and subjective markers for both lymphoedema and related treatment progression. Pain et al. (2003) argue that physical function may be a more appropriate measure than volume excess in BCRL and emphasise that manual dexterity appears to have greater impact than arm volume excess on overall psychological morbidity. For lower limb oedema, it may be relevant to use a disability scale such as the WHO Disability Assessment Scale (WHO, 2006). Generalist physiotherapists and occupational therapists have a great deal to offer these patients over and above the exercises discussed later when specific impairments are identified. The specialist knowledge of the oncology and palliative care physiotherapist or occupational therapist may also be required during the period of active or palliative cancer care.

Diet and weight

Obesity may be a risk factor regarding lymphoedema development especially after breast cancer. However there is no evidence to substantiate this at present (Werner et al., 1991). One study noted that those who maintained their weight following mastectomy had a greater reduction in lymph volume after treatment than those who had gained weight (Bertelli et al., 1992). Body mass index (BMI) can be used as an assessment component, except in the palliative setting as weight gain or loss in this setting can be from a multitude of causes. Dietary advice is recommended for patients with a BMI >30 (LF, 2006).

Psychosocial assessment

The association of lymphoedema with cancer, and its chronic and incurable nature, can lead to significant psychosocial effects (McWayne & Heiney, 2005). These may include anxiety, depression, altered body image, reduced self-esteem and problems with relationships. Assessment should be sufficiently sensitive to identify patients who require onward referral for psychological or social support. Lack of motivation or ability to understand the management of the condition can be significant factors negatively affecting outcome.

Management of lymphoedema

The management plan is drawn from the outcomes of the holistic assessment and is not dependent on the size of the swelling alone. The main cornerstones of care are:

- Education of patient/carers
- Skin care
- Exercise and function
- Manual lymphatic drainage (MLD)/simple lymphatic drainage (SLD)
- Compression/containment via multi-layered lymphoedema bandaging (MLLB) or hosiery

Together these treatment techniques are known as decongestive lymphatic therapy (DLT) or complex decongestive therapy (CDT).

Additionally, some patients benefit from intermittent pneumatic compression or periods of elevation of the swollen limb. In rare cases, surgery is recommended of which there are three categories – surgical reduction (Browse *et al.*, 2003), procedures that bypass lymphatic obstruction (Campisi *et al.*, 2006) and liposuction (Brorson, 2006). Novel treatments which have yet to establish a sound evidence base include laser therapy, hyperbaric oxygen, lymphoedema taping, transcutaneous electrical nerve stimulation (TENS), pulsed magnetic field, thermal therapy, ultrasound, cryotherapy and complementary therapy (LF, 2006).

Packages of care are based on a self-care model and fall broadly into four categories of need (BLS, 2001a):

- At risk – appropriate education and advice for level of risk.
- Mild to moderate – education, skin care, compression garments, exercise, SLD/MLD. Some in this group may also need bandaging (MLLB).
- Moderate to severe – education, may need complex skin care, exercise and functional advice, up to 6 weeks daily MLLB (followed by long-term use of compression garments), MLD.

- Palliative – a package of care as above, tailored to the tolerance of the patient and their condition at any particular time.

DLT/CDT management is divided into two phases: the initial, intensive professional-led treatment phase, which can last for up to 6 weeks, and the maintenance phase, which aims to gradually facilitate the patient to assume control of the condition, yet receive 6-monthly, or as needed, professional reviews and new garment provision.

Education

It is essential that the patient with lymphoedema is empowered to manage their condition (National Institute for Clinical Excellence [NICE], 2004). Patients can be frightened by the unknown potential of the swelling, made worse by a general lack of knowledge among health care professionals. Early strategies to achieve personal responsibility are imperative for long-term success. Many related charities and hosiery manufacturers produce useful patient information leaflets to support the professional. The Lymphoedema Support Network (LSN), for example, provides a helpline, advice leaflets and instructional DVDs. In some geographical areas there are local support groups.

Precautions recommended to patients with lymphoedema or identified as being 'at risk' include:

- Avoid skin damage, and hence the potential for infection, by wearing protective clothing on the 'at-risk' limb(s) when handling sharp or hot materials, not walking barefoot if the legs are at risk, preventing insect bites and sunburn.
- Avoid injections, drips and acupuncture on the 'at-risk' limb, if other treatments can be given via another limb without detriment. Similarly, blood pressure readings should be done on the contralateral side whenever possible.
- The limb should be used as normally as possible (Hayes *et al.*, 2005) but avoid lifting excessively heavy weights (arms) or standing still for long periods (legs).
- Incorporate aerobic exercise such as swimming, dancing, walking and cycling into the daily routine or as appropriate to the patient's general health.
- Maintain a healthy weight range; reduce weight if obese (as appropriate to health status).

Skin care

Skin care is arguably the most important cornerstone in the management of lymphoedema. Anything that is placed on or in the skin, e.g. cosmetics or injections, has to be cleared by the lymphatic system and can impact on the management of the swelling. If good skin care is not achieved, the person with lymphoedema is at risk of developing conditions which are predisposing factors for recurrent cellulitis. Factors can include:

- Penetrating skin injury (Clark *et al.* 2005)
- Lymphorrhoea
- Fungal skin infection (tinea pedis)
- Elephantiasis skin changes (Mortimer 2000)

Daily skin care aims to maintain a healthy, hydrated skin and to reduce the risk of infective episodes. Patients are encouraged to moisturise twice daily with appropriate emollients, observe their skin for any damage (cuts, scratches or insect bites) and treat promptly to reduce their risk of cellulitis. Patients with lymphoedema of the toes are at increased risk of developing ingrown toenails and should be encouraged to observe for this. Appropriate treatment for an ingrown toenail is essential in order to prevent infection and pain; referral to a podiatrist may be necessary. Emollients are used in varying intensity depending on the condition of the skin and are subdivided into three groups:

- Bath oils
- Creams
- Ointments
    (Linnitt, 2000)

Healthy-looking skin may only need to be moisturised daily with a bland cream, whereas chronic skin changes may need the use of bath oil along with a soap substitute and twice daily oil. Most creams contain preservatives, some of which are known to cause sensitivities in inflamed skin (Ryan & Mallon, 1995). Parabens and lanolin (wool alcohols) are examples of common sensitising ingredients in emollients. If there are concerns that a patient has an allergy to these ingredients, bland oils should be used. Skin that is poorly hydrated over a period of time can itch (pruritus), causing the patient to scratch, thereby damaging the epidermis and increasing the risk of cellulitis. Some emollients include an anti-itch component.

Immunosuppression within the lymphoedema limb means a patient may react suddenly to an emollient they have been using for many years (Cameron, 1998). Referral to a dermatologist for patch testing to identify the allergen(s) will improve their care and reduce the risk of recurrent cellulitis. Once lymphoedematous tissue has had a bacterial infection, anecdotal evidence suggests that it can be reactivated at times from overexercise, long journeys and even treatment with MLLB (Mortimer, 2000). In this instance, long-term antibiotic therapy may be necessary in conjunction with good skin care. Guidance on antibiotic prescription for this patient group is available on the BLS website.

Exercise and function

Recent studies have improved our understanding of lymphoedema and exercise. Lane *et al.* (2005b) summarise the evidence and claim that during exercise both intrinsic and extrinsic mechanisms of lymphatic propulsion are enhanced. Current evidence does not support the notion that there is a relationship between vigorous upper body exercise and the occurrence of BCRL (Unruh & Elvin, 2004). This is supported by a study in which women participating in a graduated exercise programme, including dragon boat racing, showed an increase in both affected and unaffected arm volume consistent with increased arm strength, not oedema (Lane *et al.*, 2005a). Hayes *et al.* (2005) found that women were more likely to develop lymphoedema in their non-dominant arm than their dominant arm, again supporting activity rather than inactivity as a preventative measure. Isotonic exercises, which lengthen and shorten the muscle, are recommended rather than isometric (static exercise), in order to open the initial lymphatics permitting interstitial fluid to enter by means of the moving connective tissue, as described in the experiments of Mazzoni *et al.* (1990, cited by Lane *et al.*, 2005b).

This group of patients often has a combination of problems, including weakness, stiffness, poor posture, pain and lack of confidence (due to poor body image). It is therefore essential that a holistic programme is individually tailored, rather than exercise prescribed on the basis of lymphoedema diagnosis alone. Plans should include exercises for posture and breathing before working on proximal muscle groups and then moving onto more distal limb muscle groups, e.g. shoulder and upper arm before forearm and hand. An example of a simple exercise routine for BCRL can be seen on a DVD available from the Charity Breast Cancer Haven (www.breastcancerhaven.org.uk). This routine needs individual adaptation by the therapist in response to assessment outcomes and may need supplementary physiotherapy, occupational therapy or alternative therapy techniques to achieve maximal function.

Lymphatic massage – MLD and SLD

MLD is a very gentle, specific technique of massage which aims to improve lymphatic flow from compromised to uncompromised areas. Traditional, heavy or sport massage is avoided as it may exacerbate oedema by increasing capillary filtration. Robust, unbiased evidence of the effectiveness of MLD is lacking, although some studies have been conducted (McNeely *et al.*, 2004; Williams *et al.*, 2002) and a wealth of clinical opinion advocates the benefits of MLD. It has particular benefits for lymphoedema of the head and neck, genitalia or breast, where appropriate garment compression is harder to achieve. A health care professional must receive specific training for MLD from a recognised school prior to practising (LF, 2006; see BLS website).

As MLD requires a significant time resource (1–2 h per session) from a trained therapist, the use of self-massage (SLD), with/without assistance from carers/relatives, is often advocated (BLS, 2001b; Casley-Smith & Casley-Smith, 1997). Self-massage may be described with simple diagrams (Williams, 2006) or on DVD (see LSN website).

Compression/containment: multi-layered lymphoedema bandaging and hosiery

Compression and containment of the swollen limb are described in almost all forms of lymphoedema management (ISL, 2003; LF, 2006), although the evidence base has

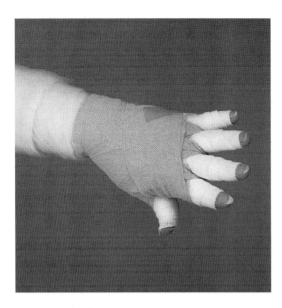

Figure 11.2 A bandaging technique for the hand. [Reproduced by permission of Medi (UK) Ltd.]

largely been extrapolated from other disciplines (Partsch & Junger, 2006). A period of short-stretch MLLB (intensive treatment phase) has been shown to produce a greater, and more sustained, reduction in limb volume (Badger *et al.*, 2000) prior to the use of compression hosiery. A period of 2–4 weeks is usual (BLS, 2001c), but may be longer, and involves the use of shaped foam, pads and specific bandaging techniques (Figures 11.2 and 11.3). This again requires specialist training and has heavy time and resource requirements.

Compression hosiery used in the management of lymphoedema is often of a higher compression value and stiffer construction than that used in venous conditions, unless the patient has a specific contraindication to its use (Clark & Krimmel, 2006). There are three compression classification standards in the UK, which can cause confusion for garment supply. Prescribers therefore need to understand the strength being described by each standard; e.g. 'class 2' in the traditionally used German standard (RAL-GZ 387:2000) gives a compression of 23–32 mm Hg at the ankle; however, the British standard class 2 (BS 6612:1985) provides only 18–24 mm Hg and French standard class 2 (ASQUAL) only 15–20 mm Hg. A lack of familiarity with the differences between the classifications used by various manufacturers can lead to undertreatment. Many lower-limb patients require RAL class 3 or 4.

Additional to the compression strength required to treat the condition, the selection of the garment used must take into account the area of limb that must be contained (usually the whole limb in lymphoedema), the ability of the patient to apply the garment and the patient's potential compliance level. Many styles and colours of garments, as well as 'donning and doffing' aids, are available from most specialist compression garment manufacturers (Figure 11.4).

The patient must be assessed for their suitability for compression by bandages or garments prior to treatment and on a regular ongoing basis for life-long management.

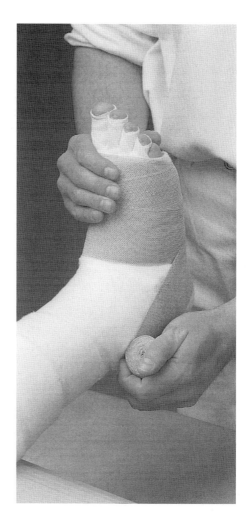

Figure 11.3 A bandaging technique for the foot. [Reproduced by permission of Medi (UK) Ltd.]

A regular and adequate supply of garments must be provided to each patient to ensure effective containment.

Intermittent pneumatic compression

This is another form of compression that may be used, although there is considerable debate over its effectiveness (LF, 2006). When applying intermittent pneumatic compression (IPC), a mechanical pump fills a multi-chambered garment, worn on the limb, to specific pressures in timed cyclical pulsations, e.g. 30 mm Hg in 45-s pulsations for a period of 30 min or more per day. IPC may be used as part of an intensive phase of treatment to reduce volume, usually being combined or preceded with MLD (Bray & Barrett, 2000) or other modalities. It may also be used on selected patients for long-term management. Caution should be taken with its use in palliative care or when used on bilaterally oedematous legs simultaneously (Boris *et al.*, 1998).

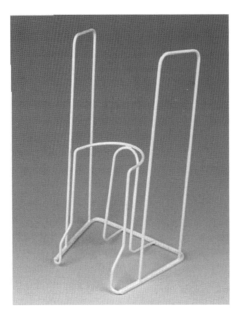

Figure 11.4 A stocking donning aid.
[Reproduced by permission of Medi (UK) Ltd.]

Summary

Lymphoedema is a chronic condition which can be managed but not cured. The recognised model of treatment has a non-invasive two-phase format. AHPs have a great deal to offer to this group of patients at various levels. By working with their professional basic knowledge principles and appreciating the chronic nature of the condition, a rehabilitation package of either uni- or multi-professional care, depending on need, can be tailored for rewarding results. Specialist postgraduate training, from a recognised lymphoedema school, is necessary to provide the specialised intensive management phase; however, other AHPs can provide advice and monitor 'at-risk' patient groups. Associated conditions, such as obesity, joint dysfunction and reduced mobility, can be managed by AHPs working in the cancer speciality. Whether the patient is undergoing curative treatment, palliation or is in remission, there is a basic need for health care professionals to have a working knowledge of lymphoedema management.

As cancer management strategies improve, more patients are surviving their cancer or living longer with active, but controlled, disease. The incidence of cancer-related lymphoedema is therefore likely to increase alongside the disease prevalence rates. This has significant implications for service providers.

Case study 1: Unilateral lower limb oedema

Lily, a 71-year-old widow, lives alone has two married children and school-age grandchildren. A brother and sister-in-law live nearby and are in good health and very supportive, along with a network of friends.

Relevant medical history

- Age 67 years: ovarian carcinoma diagnosed resulting in surgery (laparotomy, bilateral salpingo-oophrectomy and omentectomy) and chemotherapy
- Age 69 years: disease recurrence followed by a further excision, chemotherapy and radiotherapy to the left inguinal nodes
- Age 70 years: further recurrence in the right inguinal nodes and subsequent chemotherapy and radiotherapy
- Age 71 years: disease progression to left external iliac and left para-aortic nodes and mesentery

Onset of oedema

Seven months ago swelling was noted in left foot and ankle with progression to the lower leg after 1 month and upper leg after 3 months. Lily was referred to the lymphoedema practitioner who initiated a daily self-care regime comprising skin care, thigh-length graduated compression hosiery, simple exercises and SLD. Lily was informed of the LSN and joined her local group.

Cancer progression caused further worsening of the lymphoedema, and Lily was referred to the lymphoedema specialist. Concurrently, the oncologist arranged a colour Doppler ultrasound which excluded deep vein thrombosis as a possible cause for the increased leg swelling.

Lymphoedema progression

Lymphoedema was now noted in the left groin and lower abdomen. The subcutaneous tissues in the oedematous areas were predominantly thickened, firm and non-pitting, but there were no sensory changes or lymphoedema in the genital area or right leg. The percentage excess total limb volume in the left leg (compared to the right) was 38%. Lymphangiectasia was noted in the anterolateral aspect of the left lower leg. Lily described 'heaviness of the left leg', 'feels solid and stocky' and 'the skin feels tight'. The 'leg is tender and aches after being on my feet for a while'.

Lily was now experiencing disturbed sleep, which she attributed to anxiety about cancer progression and difficulty moving to get comfortable in bed. She was unable to fit into her preferred style of footwear and clothing and felt self-conscious of her altered body presentation. She avoided contact with her grandchildren as she did not want them to be frightened of her large foot and leg. Other activities also took longer, with Lily feeling exhausted after each task. She struggled to lift the left leg into and out of bed, lost confidence getting in and out of the bath and felt unsteady on the stairs. Standing to prepare a meal or do the ironing resulted in increased leg discomfort. Lily also developed a pronounced limp, accompanied by intermittent lower backache. Whereas she usually played bridge two or three times weekly, Lily stopped when it became too uncomfortable to sit at the bridge table.

Interventions

After an assessment and discussion with the lymphoedema specialist, Lily thought about her future objectives and agreed to the following interventions:

Lymphoedema specialist

Ten days reduced compression MLLB to the left leg, which improved comfort, treated the lymphangiectasia, prevented lymphorrhoea and improved limb shape and size. The skin care regime was continued during MLLB. MLD concurrent with MLLB was used to treat and prevent increased oedema proximal to the left leg and also soften the thickened tissues.

Lily was then provided with graduated compression one-legged pantyhose, which was to be worn each day. The panty section aimed to prevent further oedema proximal to the left leg. She continued daily skin care and SLD.

Physiotherapist
Lily was provided with a walking stick and gait correction which also increased her confidence. She was given appropriate flexibility and gentle resisted exercises to maintain range of movement and aid muscle development in the left leg.

Occupational therapist
A home visit was carried out and Lily was given advice regarding techniques to assist with moving about in bed, plus assistive devices to improve transfers. A perching stool was issued to prevent long periods of standing and for use when playing bridge. Advice was given regarding positioning of a stair rail, which Lily then had fitted. At this stage, Lily declined any other equipment for the bath or toilet but was aware that it was available if she wanted it.

Voluntary sector
Volunteer hospital transport enabled Lily to attend the intensive course of treatment with the lymphoedema specialist. The hospice equipment loan service was able to provide Lily with a reclining armchair, so that she could rest during the day with legs elevated, and benefits advice was provided by Macmillan Cancer Support. Lily attended the day hospice once a week, where touch therapy sessions alongside relaxation techniques helped to settle her mood. She also benefited from counselling, which enabled her to interact with the grandchildren again and cope with end-of-life issues.

Case study 2: Unilateral arm lymphoedema

Lynda, a 58-year-old lady, is married with one adult daughter living locally. Prior to a diagnosis of breast cancer, Lynda worked full time as a finance audit officer.

Relevant medical history

Lynda was diagnosed with Grade III right-sided inflammatory breast cancer at age 57.

Surgery
Right mastectomy with axillary node clearance; 25 nodes were removed, of which 24 were positive for cancer spread.

Prior to discharge from hospital, she was seen by the surgical physiotherapist who taught her appropriate post-mastectomy exercises, provided an exercise booklet and gave advice on posture and how to reduce the risk of developing lymphoedema.

Chemotherapy
Four weeks post-operatively Lynda commenced chemotherapy treatment.

Radiotherapy
Seven months post-operatively, on completion of chemotherapy, Lynda received 15 fractions of adjuvant radiotherapy to the right chest wall, axilla and supraclavicular fossa.

Presenting problems

Seven weeks post-operatively, Lynda developed pain and severe limitation of movement in the right shoulder and was referred by the breast surgeon for physiotherapy.

During radiotherapy Lynda developed swelling of the right arm. She had previously been referred by the surgical physiotherapist to the lymphoedema clinic due to her increased risk of developing lymphoedema as a result of the axillary node clearance and reduced movement and function of the right arm. At this stage, bilateral circumferential arm measurements and assessment of the subcutaneous tissues did not indicate any lymphoedema; however, further advice was given on how to reduce her risk. When arm swelling did develop during the later stages of radiotherapy, Lynda immediately recognised the changing symptoms and contacted the clinic. Her oncologist was aware of the new symptom and was monitoring Lynda closely for early local disease recurrence, which can be identified by the onset of lymphoedema.

Interventions

Physiotherapist

Initially, interventions included the use of TENS for shoulder pain management, advice on appropriate activity and reassurance, fascial release techniques, scar mobilisation, gentle stretches and range of movement exercises, all re-enforced by a handout. Steady progress was made during chemotherapy, with reduced stiffness of the right shoulder and improved range of movement and function. Weekly physiotherapy continued with a progressive exercise regime, postural work and normal movement/core control activities.

One week into radiotherapy, Lynda complained of increased stiffness of the right shoulder and onset of oedema. By the second week, range of movement and function had started to decline. Physiotherapy was continued to compliment the lymphoedema management regime, resulting in continuing functional progress. Lynda's husband was also taught to help with the stretches in supine and side lying and scar massage.

Post-surgery/radiotherapy, a residual sensory impairment was noted in the right axilla. Function in the dominant right arm was affected; however, Lynda remained determined and positive, with regard to her rehabilitation. Lynda's main goal was to return to work on a phased basis, alongside her Herceptin treatment. She was keen to reduce the arm oedema and retain the functional improvements.

Lymphoedema specialist

Following radiotherapy, Lynda presented with 25% excess limb volume in the right arm compared with the unaffected left arm. This was evenly distributed throughout the arm, and the overall 'shape' remained good. Lynda was already applying a pH-neutral moisturiser to the whole arm, axilla and chest wall, as recommended by the radiotherapy department, and her skin was soft, supple and intact. The tissues in the right arm were non-pitting and firmer when compared to the left arm.

In order to reduce the oedema, Lynda consented to a lymphoedema management regime of:

- Continued daily skin care and avoidance of venepuncture/blood pressure monitoring and trauma to the right arm and upper quadrant.
- Daily SLD.
- Continued exercise regime, under the guidance of the physiotherapist.
- Daily use of a Class 2 flat-knit lymphoedema arm sleeve with hand piece. MLLB was inappropriate at this point because it could have exacerbated her pain, stiffness and reduced range of movement.

Six weeks later, the excess limb volume in the right arm had reduced to 18% and new measurements were taken for replacement hosiery. Lynda felt encouraged to continue with her self-care regime and began to plan for her return to work. Three months later, the excess limb volume had reduced to 8%. The lymphoedema hosiery was replaced with circular-knit lymphoedema arm sleeves, and Lynda continued with her self-care regime and physiotherapy.

She was reviewed 3 months later, following her return to work, and had maintained the 8% excess limb volume. However, Lynda was now experiencing muscle and bone pain secondary to Herceptin. As a result, her progress with right shoulder movement plateaued before she regained full range and continued exercise was needed to ensure maintenance of the previous improvements.

Having achieved her goal of returning to work, Lynda continues to plan for the future. She has accepted that this involves an independent, daily lymphoedema management regime consisting of skin care, hosiery, SLD and exercise and a series of life-long reviews.

Key learning points

- Some groups of cancer patients are particularly 'at risk' of developing lymphoedema, e.g. breast cancer treated with surgery and radiotherapy and sarcoma treated with wide local excision and radiotherapy.
- Education and good skin care are essential for all 'at-risk' patients.
- A full assessment must take place before any form of treatment (including the provision of compression garments).
- The patient must be reviewed regularly (on average 6-monthly) and supplied with a minimum of two appropriate compression garments. The patient should have a local contact point to facilitate an unscheduled review if the condition deteriorates.
- Compression garments need to be specifically manufactured for this purpose (anti-embolism stockings will not adequately control lymphoedema) and must fit the patient properly. Garments can be made-to-measure or off-the-shelf. Poorly fitted or damaged garments will worsen the condition.
- Most lymphoedema patients can learn to be self-caring with a basic understanding of the condition and self-management techniques.

References

Badger, C. M., Peacock, J. L. & Mortimer, P. S. (2000). A randomized controlled parallel-group clinical trial comparing multilayer bandaging followed by hosiery versus hosiery alone in the treatment of patients with lymphoedema of the limb. *Cancer*, 88 (12), 2232–2237.

Bertelli, G., Venturini, M., Forno, G., Macciavello, F. & Dini, D. (1992). An analysis of prognostic factors in response to conservative treatment of postmastectomy lymphoedema. *Surgery, Gynaecology and Obstetrics*, 175 (5), 455–460.

Boris, M., Weindorf, S. & Lasinski, B. B. (1998). The risk of genital edema after external pump compression for lower limb lymphedema. *Lymphology*, 31 (1), 15–20.

Bray, T. & Barrett, J. (2000). Pneumatic compression therapy. In: R. Twycross, K. Jenns & J. Todd (Eds.), *Lymphoedema*. Oxford: Radcliffe Medical Press.

British Lymphology Society [BLS] (2001a). *Chronic oedema population and needs* [online]. Sevenoaks, Kent, UK: British Lymphology Society. Retrieved 22 August 2006 from www.lymphoedema.org/bls/membership/definitions.htm

British Lymphology Society [BLS] (2001b). *Guidelines for the use of manual lymphatic drainage (MLD) and simple lymphatic drainage (SLD) in lymphoedema* [online]. Sevenoaks, Kent, UK: British Lymphology Society. Retrieved 25 October 2006 from www.lymphoedema.org/bls/membership/guidelines.htm

British Lymphology Society [BLS] (2001c). *Strategy for lymphoedema care.* Sevenoaks, Kent, UK: British Lymphology Society.

Brorson, H. (2006). Quality of life following liposuction and conservative treatment of arm lymphedema. *Lymphology*, 39, 8–25.

Browse, N., Burnand, K. G. & Mortimer, P. (2003). *Diseases of the lymphatics* (pp. 179–204). London: Arnold.

Cameron, J. (1998). Red card for allergies. *Nursing Standard*, 13 (3), 23–24.

Campisi, C., Davini, D., Bellini, C., Taddei, G., Villa, G., Fulcheri, E., Zilli, A., Da Rin, E., Eretta, C. & Boccardo, F. (2006). Is there a role for microsurgery in the prevention of arm lymphedema secondary to breast cancer treatment? *Microsurgery*, 26 (1), 70–72.

Casley-Smith, J. R. & Casley-Smith, J. R. (1997). *Modern treatment for lymphoedema* (5th ed.). The Lymphoedema Association of Australia Inc. Adelaide: Terrace Printing.

Clark, B., Sitzia, J. & Harlow, W. (2005). Incidence and risk of arm oedema following treatment for breast cancer: a three year follow up study. *Quarterly Journal of Medicine*, 98, 343–348.

Clark, M. & Krimmel, G. (2006). Lymphoedema and the construction and classification of compression hosiery. In: *Lymphoedema framework template for practice: compression hosiery in lymphoedema.* London: MEP Ltd.

Department of Health [DH] (2005). *Supporting people with long term conditions* (p. 10). London: Department of Health.

Franks, P. J., Moffatt, C. J., Doherty, D. C., Williams, A. F., Jeffs, E. & Mortimer, P. S. (2006). Assessment of health-related quality of life in patients with lymphoedema of the lower limb. *Wound Repair and Regeneration*, 14, 110–118.

Hayes, S., Cornish, B. & Newman, B. (2005). Comparison of methods to diagnose lymphoedema amongst breast cancer survivors: 6-month follow up. *Breast Cancer Research & Treatment*, 89 (3), 221–226.

International Society of Lymphology [ISL] (1995). The diagnosis and treatment of peripheral lymphedema. A consensus document of the International Society of Lymphology Executive. *Lymphology*, 28, 113–117.

International Society of Lymphology [ISL] (2003). The diagnosis and treatment of peripheral lymphedema. Consensus document of the International Society of Lymphology. *Lymphology*, 36 (2), 84–91.

Ji, R.-C. (2006). Lymphatic endothelial cells, lymphangiogenesis, and extracellular matrix. *Lymphatic Research & Biology*, 4 (2), 83–100.

Karakousis, C. P. (2006). Surgical procedures and lymphedema of the upper and lower extremity. *Journal of Surgical Oncology*, 93 (2), 87–91.

Karlsen, T. V., Karkkainen, M. J., Alitalo, K. & Wiig, H. (2006). Transcapillary fluid balance consequences of missing initial lymphatics studied in a mouse model of primary lymphoedema. *Journal of Physiology*, 574 (2), 583–596.

Lane, K., Jespersen, D. & McKenzie, D. C. (2005a). The effect of a whole body exercise programme and dragon boat training on arm volume and arm circumference in women treated for breast cancer. *European Journal of Cancer Care*, 14, 353–358.

Lane, K., Worsley, D. & McKensie, D. (2005b). Exercise and the lymphatic system – implications for breast cancer survivors. *Sports Medicine*, 35 (6), 461–471.

Linnitt, N. (2000). Skin management in lymphoedema. In: R. Twycross, K. Jenns & J. Todd (Eds.), *Lymphoedema* (pp. 118–129). Oxford: Radcliffe Medical Press.

Lymphoedema Framework [LF] (2006). *Best practice document for the management of lymphoedema international consensus*. London: Medical Education Partnership Ltd.

MacLaren, J. (2003). Models of lymphoedema service provision across Europe: sharing good practice. *International Journal of Palliative Nursing*, 9 (12), 538–543.

Mallon, E., Powell, S., Mortimer, P. & Ryan, T. J. (1997). Evidence for altered cell-mediated immunity in postmastectomy lymphoedema. *British Journal of Dermatology*, 137, 928–933.

Mazzoni, M. C., Skalak, T. C. & Schmid-Schonbein, G. W. (1990) Effects of skeletal muscle fiber deformation on lymphatic volumes. *American Journal of Physiology* 259 (6 Pt 2), 1860–1868.

McNeely, M. L., Magee, D. J., Lees, A. W., Bagnall, K. M., Haykowsky, M. & Hanson, J. (2004). The addition of manual lymphatic drainage to compression therapy for breast cancer related lymphedema: a randomized controlled trial. *Breast Cancer Research and Treatment*, 86 (2), 95–106.

McWayne, J. & Heiney, S. P. (2005). Psychologic and social sequelae of secondary lymphedema: a review. *Cancer*, 104 (3), 457–466.

Moffatt, C. J., Franks, P. J., Doherty, D. C., Williams, A. F., Badger, C., Jeffs, E., Bosanquet, N. & Mortimer, P. S. (2003). Lymphoedema: an underestimated health problem. *Quarterly Journal of Medicine*, 96, 731–738.

Morgan, P. A., Franks, P. J. & Moffatt, C. J. (2005). Health-related quality of life with lymphoedema: a review of the literature. *International Wound Journal*, 2 (1), 47–62.

Mortimer, P. S. (2000). Acute inflammatory episodes. In: R. Twycross, K. Jenns & J. Todd (Eds.), *Lymphoedema*. Oxford: Radcliffe Medical Press.

Mortimer, P. S. & Levick, J. R. (2004). Chronic peripheral oedema: the critical role of the lymphatic system. *Clinical Medicine*, 4 (5), 448–453.

Mortimer, P. S. & Levick, J. R. (2006). Of mice and men: the translational physiology of a genetic form of lymphoedema. *The Journal of Physiology*, 574 (2), 331.

Nardone, L., Palazzoni, G., D'Angelo, E., Deodato, F., Gambacorta, M. A., Micciche, F. & Morganti, A. G. (2005). Impact of dose and volume on lymphedema. *Rays*, 30 (2), 149–155.

National Institute for Clinical Excellence [NICE] (2004). *Improving supportive and palliative care for adults with cancer: the manual*. London: National Institute for Clinical Excellence.

Pain, S. J., Barber, R. W., Solanki, C. K., Ballinger, J. R., Britton, T. B., Mortimer, P. S., Purushotham, A. D. & Peters, A. M. (2005). Short-term effects of axillary lymph node clearance surgery on lymphatic physiology of the arm in breast cancer. *Journal of Applied Physiology*, 99 (6), 2345–2351.

Pain, S. J., Vowler, S. L. & Purushotham, A. D. (2003). Is physical function a more appropriate measure than volume excess in the assessment of breast cancer-related lymphoedema (BCRL)? *European Journal of Cancer*, 39, 2168–2172.

Parmar, J. H., Aslam, M. & Standfield, N. J. (2006). Calf muscle pump failure in lower limb lymphoedema. *Phlebology*, 21 (2), 96–99.

Partsch, H. & Junger, M. (2006). Evidence for the use of compression hosiery in lymphoedema. In: *Lymphoedema framework template for practice: compression hosiery in lymphoedema*. London: MEP Ltd.

Petlund, C. F. (1990). Prevalence and incidence of chronic lymphoedema in western European country. In: M. Nishi, S. Uchina & S. Yabuki (Eds.), *Progress in lymphology XII* (pp. 391–394). Amsterdam: Elsevier Science Publishers BV.

Ryan, T. J. & Mallon, E. C. (1995). Lymphatics and the processing of antigens. *Clinics in Dermatology*, 13, 485–492.

Senekus-Konefka, E. & Jassem, J. (2006). Complications of breast-cancer radiotherapy. *Clinical Oncology*, 18, 229–235 .

Sitzia, J. & Sobrido, L. (1997). Measurement of health-related quality of life of patients receiving conservative treatment for limb lymphoedema using the Nottingham Health Profile. *Quality of Life Research*, 6, 373–384.

Stanton, A., Modi, S., Mellor, R., Levick, R. & Mortimer, P. (2006b). Diagnosing breast cancer-related lymphoedema in the arm. *Journal of Lymphoedema*, 1 (1), 12–15.

Stanton, A. W. B., Modi, S., Mellor, R. H., Peters, A. M., Svensson, W. E., Rodney, L. J. & Mortimer, P. S. (2006a). A quantitative lymphoscintigraphic evaluation of lymphatic function in the swollen hands of women with lymphoedema following breast cancer treatment. *Clinical Science*, 110 (5), 553–561.

Soo, J. K., Bicanic, T. A. & Mortimer, P. S. (2006). A study of the prevalence of lymphoedema in patients with cellulitis: R-2. *British Journal of Dermatology*, 155 (Suppl 1), 10.

Tiwari, A., Myint, F. & Hamilton, G. (2006). Management of lower limb lymphoedema in the United Kingdom. *European Journal Vascular and Endovascular Surgery*, 31, 311–315.

Unruh, A. M. & Elvin, N. (2004). In the eye of the dragon: women's experience of breast cancer and the occupation of dragon boat racing. *Canadian Journal of Occupational Therapy – Revue Canadienne d'Ergotherapie*, 71 (3), 138–149.

Vaqas, B. & Ryan, T. J. (2003). Lymphoedema: pathophysiology and management in resource-poor settings – relevance for lymphatic filariasis control programmes [online]. *Filaria Journal*. BioMed Central. Retrieved 22 August 2006 from www.filariajournal.com/content/2/1/4

Velanovich, V. & Szymanski, W. (1999). Quality of life of breast cancer patients with lymphoedema. *American Journal of Surgery*, 177, 184–187.

Werner, R. S., McCormick, B., Petrek, J., Cox, L., Cirrincione, C., Gray, J. R. & Yahalom, J. (1991). Arm edema in conservatively managed breast cancer: obesity is a major predictive factor. *Radiology*, 180 (1), 177–184.

Williams, A. F. (2006). Patient self-massage for breast cancer-related lymphoedema. *Journal of Community Nursing*, 20 (6), 24–29.

Williams, A. F., Franks, P. J. & Moffatt, C. J. (2005). Lymphoedema: estimating the size of the problem. *Palliative Medicine*, 19, 300–313.

Williams, A. F., Vadgama, A., Franks, P. J. & Mortimer, P. S. (2002). A randomised controlled crossover study of manual lymphatic drainage therapy in women with breast cancer related lymphoedema. *European Journal of Cancer Care*, 11 (4), 254–261.

Witte, M. H., Jones, K., Wilting, J., Dictor, M., Selg, M., McHale, N., Gershenwald, J. E. & Jackson, D. G. (2006). Structure function relationships in the lymphatic system and implications for cancer biology. *Cancer Metastasis Reviews*, 25 (2), 159–184.

World Health Organization [WHO] (2000). *Lymphatic filariasis* [online]. Retrieved 21 August 2006 from www.who.int/mediacentre/factsheets/fs102/en/

World Health Organization [WHO] (2006). *WHO disability assessment scale* [online]. Retrieved 21 September 2006 from www.who.int/icidh/whodas

Sources of further information

Lymphoedema Framework. *Template for Management: developing a lymphoedema service.* London: MEP Ltd, 2007. (Copies available from the offices of The British Lymphology Society or from Medi (UK) Ltd.)

British Lymphology Society, Wheatstone, 2 North Upton Lane, Barnwood, Gloucester GL4 3TA. Tel: 01452-613391.
Email: info@thebls.com; Website: www.thebls.com.

Lymphoedema Support Network, St Luke's Crypt, Sydney Street, London, SW3 6NH. Tel: 020 73514480. Website: www.lymphoedema.org/lsn.

Chapter 12

MANAGEMENT OF CANCER-RELATED FATIGUE

Catriona Ogilvy, Karen Livingstone and Dr Gillian Prue

Learning outcomes

After studying this chapter the reader should be able to:

- Understand the multi-dimensional nature of cancer-related fatigue
- Discuss the causes and symptoms of cancer-related fatigue
- Have knowledge of allied health professionals roles in the treatment and management of cancer-related fatigue
- Recognise the importance of multi-professional collaboration in the management of cancer-related fatigue
- Discuss how management techniques for cancer-related fatigue may vary when considering active treatments versus palliative care

---

Introduction

Excessive tiredness is a common complaint of today's society, with some level of fatigue found in nearly all of the population (Aaronson *et al.*, 1999; Bultmann *et al.*, 2002; David *et al.*, 1990; Pawlikowska *et al.*, 1994; Shen *et al.*, 2006). For most individuals fatigue is an acute experience, a protective response to physical and psychological stress (Ahlberg *et al.*, 2003) and is easily remedied by rest. Cancer-related fatigue (CRF) is dissimilar from the fatigue experienced by the general population. It has been hypothesised that CRF may have a different aetiology, severity and course than everyday fatigue (Cella *et al.*, 2002).

CRF is an almost universal symptom in patients receiving anti-cancer therapy (National Comprehensive Cancer Network [NCCN], 2006). It has a profound effect on the whole person and can persist for months or even years following completion of treatment (Ahlberg *et al.*, 2003). As a result CRF can have a phenomenal impact on a patient's life with devastating social and economic consequences (Flechtner & Bottomley, 2002), as well as the potential to hinder a patient's chance of remission or even cure, owing to the direct influence it can have on the desire to continue with treatment (Morrow *et al.*, 2002).

In a UK multi-centre survey of 576 cancer patients with varying diagnoses, half of which were currently receiving anti-cancer treatment, fatigue was reported to affect the subjects significantly more than any other symptom, with over 50% reporting fatigue as their biggest problem. It was concluded that fatigue had a much greater effect on individuals with cancer than any other physical or mental consequence of the disease or its treatment (Stone *et al.*, 2000b).

Specific pharmacological intervention for potentially reversible medical conditions known to present with fatigue, such as anaemia, hypothyroidism, pain, depression and anxiety, should be initiated as the first line of treatment and be evaluated as to their effectiveness. Non-pharmacological interventions are discussed in this chapter.

Definition

CRF is reported to be multi-dimensional in nature (Cella *et al.*, 1998; Fawcett & Dean, 2004; Nail, 2002; Portenoy & Itri, 1999; Servaes *et al.*, 2002; Stone *et al.*, 1998; Visovsky & Schneider, 2003), consisting of physical, psychological and cognitive components (Glaus, 1993). This was further demonstrated in a survey of cancer patients in Ireland where participants were asked to describe their fatigue. The most commonly reported phrases were 'no energy', 'tired' and 'exhausted'; however, phrases such as 'poor concentration', 'memory loss' and 'irritable' underscored the cognitive and emotional aspects of the experience (Dillon & Kelly, 2003).

The subjective and multi-dimensional character of CRF indicates that it is impossible to take a single view of the phenomenon (Piper, 1986). Its definition is largely influenced by an individual's perception and experiences of his/her own CRF, and creating a definition for all is difficult. The National Comprehensive Cancer Network (NCCN), an alliance of 20 of the leading cancer centres in the USA, attempts to define CRF as:

> *A distressing, persistent, subjective sense of tiredness or exhaustion related to cancer or cancer treatment that is not proportional to recent activity and interferes with usual functioning (NCCN, 2006).*

Aetiology

The aetiology of CRF remains to be fully explained, but its multi-factorial nature is widely documented (Ahlberg *et al.*, 2003; Fawcett & Dean, 2004; Lucia *et al.*, 2003; Morrow *et al.*, 2002; Portenoy & Itri, 1999; Stone *et al.*, 1998; Wagner & Cella, 2004). Identifying the factors associated with the development of CRF is complicated by the fact that multiple causes frequently coexist and may have additive effects (Wagner & Cella, 2004).

CRF may be a direct result of the cancer itself, i.e. the site and stage of the tumour. For example, in a baseline assessment before initiation of anti-cancer therapy, Stone *et al.* (2000a) observed that non-small-cell lung cancer produced significantly higher fatigue prevalence than breast or prostate cancer. Furthermore, it is plausible that fatigue severity increases with advancing stage of the disease (Ahlberg *et al.*, 2003).

As a result of the interaction between the tumour and the host's defence system, cytokines such as TNF, IL-1 and IL-6 are released in greater amounts in cancer patients (Lucia *et al.*, 2003). Morrow *et al.* (2002) proposed a hypothesis linking the release of cytokines and the perception of fatigue known as the hypothalamic–pituitary axis, cytokines and 5HT hypothesis. This states that cytokines such as TNF can alter central serotonin (5HT) levels. This serotonin dysregulation may help explain the development of CRF. The issue of cytokine release contributing to CRF does, however, remain controversial (Ahlberg *et al.*, 2003).

CRF as a consequence of the anti-cancer therapy

Fatigue is a common side effect of most chemotherapy regimes. Approximately 80% of patients receiving radiotherapy report symptoms of fatigue, which may be influenced by factors such as radiation dose, target field and radiation quality (Manzullo & Escalante, 2002). The severity of CRF experienced by patients is not consistent across all anti-neoplastic therapies and there appears to be a lack of consensus (Stone, 2002). Lucia *et al.* (2003) stated that in the breast cancer population fatigue following bone marrow transplantation and chemotherapy was more severe than that following chemotherapy alone. This in turn was more severe than the fatigue associated with radiotherapy. Dimeo (2002), however, suggested that radiotherapy-induced fatigue is greater than the fatigue in patients undergoing chemotherapy.

Many authors have indicated anaemia as a cause of CRF (Ahlberg *et al.*, 2003; Lucia *et al.*, 2003; Morrow *et al.*, 2002; Portenoy & Itri, 1999; Stone *et al.*, 1998). Ahlberg *et al.* (2003) stated that fatigue is the most frequent manifestation of anaemia in patients with cancer. In addition, the progressive muscle wasting resulting from cancer-related cachexia is often sited as a contributory factor to CRF (Fawcett & Dean, 2004; Stone *et al.*, 1998).

Lucia *et al.* (2003) described the pathophysiology of fatigue, suggesting that fatigue is a complex process originating from one or more steps in a chain of interactions between the central nervous system and the skeletal muscle fibre. The cancer and treatment may lead to insufficient blood and therefore oxygen being transported to muscles and impairment of skeletal muscle functioning from muscle mass atrophy; thus, the patient requires an increased effort to accomplish normal activities of daily living, leading to the perception of fatigue (Lucia *et al.*, 2003).

Psychosocial factors as well as physical factors are said to play a role in the development of CRF. CRF has been associated with mood disturbance (Fawcett & Dean, 2004), anxiety and depression, altered sleep and activity patterns (Portenoy & Itri, 1999). Furthermore, personality type and stress can also lead to a greater perception of fatigue severity (Stone *et al.*, 1998).

To summarise, CRF has been related to:

1. The direct effects of the tumour
2. Treatment side effects
3. Comorbid medical conditions such as anaemia
4. Exacerbating comorbid symptoms, e.g. pain or deconditioning
5. Psychosocial factors such as anxiety and depression
   (Wagner & Cella, 2004.)

Theoretical frameworks

Piper's integrated fatigue model is one of the most frequently referenced theoretical frameworks for CRF (Piper *et al.*, 1987; Winningham *et al.*, 1994). The framework identifies subjective (perception) and objective (physiological, biochemical and behavioural) signs of fatigue (Piper *et al.*, 1987; Winningham *et al.*, 1994). It incorporates the patterns most frequently reported in the literature to influence CRF, e.g. the disease and its subsequent treatment, symptoms, the environment, psychological factors, social and life events, changes in energetics and activity and rest patterns (Piper *et al.*, 1987). The model draws attention to the importance of individual perception of CRF and summarises the many possible causes of CRF emphasising its multi-factoral and multi-dimensional nature (Winningham *et al.*, 1994). It has been criticised, however, for not including a weighting of the variables that may contribute to the development of CRF (Winningham *et al.*, 1994).

An alternative, the Winningham psychobiological-entropy model defines fatigue as an energy deficit (Winningham *et al.*, 1994). This model relates fatigue to the disease, anti-neoplastic treatment, any other symptoms as well as activity and functional status (Nail & Winningham, 1993). There are four propositions inherent to the model; too much or too little rest can lead to fatigue, too much or too little activity can lead to fatigue, a balance between rest and activity can promote restoration, but an imbalance can cause deterioration, and finally a reduction in activity caused by any symptom, not necessarily fatigue, will lead to an increase in fatigue and a subsequent decline in function (Nail & Winningham, 1993; Winningham & Barton-Burke, 2000). The model suggests that fatigue can not only be a primary symptom of cancer but also occur as a secondary symptom as a result of the individual's response to other symptoms (Winningham, 1992).

Assessment

To aid the diagnosis of CRF, Cella *et al.* (1998) developed a set of four diagnostic criteria for the International Classification of Diseases – 10 (ICD-10), proposing 11 symptoms of CRF:

- Significant fatigue, diminished energy or increased need to rest, disproportionate to any recent change in activity level
- Complaints of generalised weakness or limb heaviness
- Diminished concentration or attention
- Decreased motivation or interest to engage in usual activities
- Insomnia or hypersomnia
- Experience of sleep as unrefreshing or non-restorative
- Perceived need to struggle to overcome inactivity
- Marked emotional reactivity (e.g. sadness, frustration and irritability) to feeling fatigued
- Difficulty in completing daily tasks attributed to feeling fatigued
- Perceived problems with short-term memory
- Post-exertional malaise lasting several hours
  (Cella *et al.*, 1998.)

To meet the diagnostic criteria, 6 of these 11 symptoms must be present almost every day for 2 weeks over the period of 1 month. One of the symptoms must be 'significant fatigue, diminished energy, or an increased need to rest, disproportionate to any recent change in activity levels' (Cella *et al.*, 1998). The second, third and fourth criteria suggest that the fatigue must interfere with usual functioning, be linked to cancer or cancer treatment and not be a consequence of a comorbid psychiatric disorder (Cella *et al.*, 1998).

The experience of fatigue is unique to each individual; therefore, the clinician cannot provide an accurate objective report on an individual's personal experience (Ahlberg *et al.*, 2003; McColl, 2004). The most effective method to assess this subjective sensation is with a self-report tool (Piper *et al.*, 1987).

To date, there is no universally accepted self-report tool for the measurement of CRF (National Cancer Institute [NCI], 2003). This has led to inconsistencies in the measurement of symptoms and a variety of assessment tools are reported in the literature (Jacobsen, 2004; Jacobsen & Thors, 2003; Sadler & Jacobsen, 2001; Wu & McSweeney, 2001). A number of CRF instruments exist that assess fatigue as a unidimensional construct; they measure only one aspect of fatigue and therefore cannot provide an accurate assessment of the full spectrum of CRF (Stein *et al.*, 1998). The most comprehensive approach would be to assess CRF using a multi-dimensional measure (Jacobsen & Thors, 2003). A few examples of multi-dimensional measures are currently available for use. These are:

- The revised Piper fatigue scale (Piper *et al.*, 1998)
- The multi-dimensional fatigue inventory (Smets *et al.*, 1995)
- The fatigue symptom inventory (Hann *et al.*, 1998)
- The multi-dimensional fatigue symptom inventory-short form (Stein *et al.*, 2004)

The multiprofessional management of CRF

The multi-dimensional nature of CRF requires assessment which focuses on the psychological as well as the pathophysiological and biochemical causes and management using both pharmacological and non-pharmacological techniques. Whilst these interventions have shown to individually improve the management of CRF for patients, a multi-professional team approach creating a programme of treatment is more likely to be effective than offering the treatment in isolation (Barsevick, 2002; Escalante, 2003; NCCN, 2006; Richardson, 1998).

Whilst specific professions have their own core skills, the roles of heath care professionals in this area may become blurred as many aspects of CRF overlap and interlink (refer to Chapter 15). Effective communication skills and collaborative working with all members of the multi-professional team is imperative in the effective management of CRF.

The role of physiotherapy in the management of CRF

Muscle atrophy and decreased stamina are marked components of CRF. In patients with cancer, toxic treatments and a decreased level of activity during treatment are presumed to reduce physical performance. Therefore patients must use greater effort and expend more energy to perform their usual activities leading to symptoms of fatigue (NCCN, 2006).

Exercise has the strongest evidence base and is reported as the most effective non-pharmacological intervention, though patients with CRF may struggle with exercise (Mock, 2004; Tomkins Stricker *et al.*, 2004).

Prescriptive exercise for CRF

Following an extensive literature review (Watson and Mock, 2004) the following recommendations were made:

1. The exercise programme begins when the patients start their adjuvant therapy and lasts throughout the treatment.
2. It is of low-to-moderate intensity (50–70% of maximum heart rate, or 11–13 Borg scale rating for perceived exertion).
3. It is progressive, based on cardiovascular conditioning, building from 15–30 min, 3–5 days a week.
4. It is predominantly aerobic in nature, although interval training has been tested and found to be effective.
5. It should stress the importance of an exercise diary, documenting the session mode, intensity, duration, target heart rate, symptoms experienced etc.

The CRF Clinical Practice Guidelines (NCCN, 2006) suggest that treatment for CRF should be offered at three main stages of the cancer journey. Physiotherapy and exercise advice is appropriate at each of these stages.

During active treatment. High levels of fatigue following chemotherapy are often reported during the first 72 h, which commonly deteriorates with subsequent treatments (Tomkins Stricker *et al.*, 2004), and fatigue also increases over the course of radiotherapy (Irvine *et al.*, 1998).

General malaise following exercise is a common symptom of CRF (Wagner-Raphael & Cella, 2001) and this should be avoided. Recovery time should be monitored and it is advisable that it should not take longer than 30 min before the patient feels his/her energy levels returning.

Patients may become immunosuppressed during their treatment and resistance to infection will be lowered. Therefore some types of exercise such as swimming may be contraindicated at this time.

When active treatment if completed and on long-term follow-up. When treatment is completed patients can often feel isolated and struggle to return to their previous levels of activity. CRF can be at its peak post-treatment when the patient is often physically very weak, especially if he/she has had no exercise advice during treatment. Only a minority of patients report engaging in regular physical activity during treatment and in general, provision of exercise within cancer care in the UK is currently rare (Stevenson & Fox, 2005).

Following assessment, the physiotherapist can agree to short- and long-term goals over a 3- to 6-month period. Starting with low-to-moderate intensity, exercise, including aerobic, and resistive work, targeting weakened areas, gradually increasing in intensity, duration and frequency are dependent on the levels of fatigue. There will be some patients who require help with motivation and for these patients exercising within a group situation may be extremely beneficial (Kolden *et al.*, 2002). However there are always patients who are extremely familiar with the notion of exercise and see the best way of getting better as pushing through the pain and fatigue barrier. These patients are challenging for the physiotherapist in a different way and good communication skills are required to educate and prevent overexertion.

At end of life. There will be many causes of fatigue, including progression of disease, pain, medication, depression, anaemia, poor nutrition and sleep disturbance, and management of these symptoms should be the focus of care (NCCN, 2006).

Fatigue is the most prevalent symptom in patients with advanced cancer (Barnes & Bruera, 2002). The effectiveness and safety of exercise at this stage has only begun to be evaluated (Tomkins Stricker *et al.*, 2004). Porock *et al.* (2000) showed that stretching, dancing, chair or bed exercise performed several times a day, at an intensity and duration equalling half of what they could comfortably perform, increased activity levels without compounding levels of fatigue (Ream & Stone, 2004). Exercise as an intervention at the end of life should be little and often as energy allows. The physiotherapist's aim is to maintain mobility and independence; intervention should be goal specific, e.g. getting up from a chair.

It is important to note that extreme caution should be taken when working with this group of patients and close consultation with the medical team is advised.

The role of occupational therapy in the management of CRF

It is widely reported that one major effect of CRF is the consequence it has on a person's ability to function in his/her usual roles and activities of daily life (Barsevick, 2002; Curt *et al.*, 2000).

To date, there remains little evidence published on the specific role of occupational therapy (Lowrie, 2006) in the treatment and management of CRF; however, the core skills of the occupational therapist (OT) in assessing and treating difficulties in attending to activities of daily living lend themselves ideally to the assessment of and treatment of CRF. Patients have reported a loss or decrease in function in areas such as household chores, employment, social or leisure activities with family or friends and the ability to carry out personal care activities. In a study by Curt *et al.* (2000), 91% of patients reported fatigue preventing them from leading a 'normal' life and 88% indicated an alteration to their daily routine as a result of fatigue (Figure 12.1).

Not having the energy or strength to carry out everyday activities that are so important to a person's daily life can lead to a loss of roles, a sense of isolation and thus have a negative impact on a persons over all quality of life (Curt *et al.*, 2000; Davidson *et al.*, 2002; Glaus, 1993).

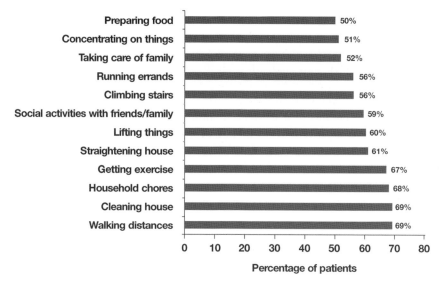

Figure 12.1 Daily activities that were 'a lot' or 'somewhat' more difficult in cancer patients when experiencing CRF. [Reproduced with permission from Watson and Mock, 2003.]

In the assessment and management of CRF, the OTs must take a holistic and creative approach if difficulties resulting from CRF are to be managed effectively, a philosophy which sits well within the client-centred framework and philosophy of occupational therapy practice (Lowrie, 2006).

Energy conservation

Barsevick (2002, p. 16) describes the act of energy conservation as 'the deliberate planned management of one's personal energy resources' as a way of preventing the further depletion of already low-energy resources. Energy-conserving strategies can include prioritising, pacing, labour-saving devices, delegating, rest periods and routine (Barsevick, 2002). OTs are specialised in the area of activity analysis and occupational performance and, therefore, ideally suited to educate patients in the principles of energy-conserving strategies. It is imperative that these strategies deployed by OTs are taught not as routine or as a recipe book approach. Patients should be assessed on an individual basis and energy-conserving strategies discussed with them. Changes to daily routine can sometimes result in decreased self-esteem; the decision to implement suggestions must be an individual choice (Lowrie, 2006).

Rest and relaxation

Anxiety and sleep disturbance are frequently reported in patients with CRF (Berger & Walker, 2001; Portenoy & Itri, 1999). Davidson *et al.* (2002) reported that approximately one-third of patients with cancer reported difficulty in sleeping, which in turn interfered with their daytime functioning. The relationship between sleep disturbances and fatigue is complex; for example, lack of sleep at night-time may lead to daytime fatigue, in turn leading to habits such as daytime napping and 'sleeping in'. These habits perpetuate night-time sleep disturbances (Dale, 2004). In a study by Curt *et al.* (2000), the most commonly recommended therapy by health care professionals for reducing fatigue, as reported by 37% of patients, was bed rest or relaxation. There remains little evidence demonstrating the benefits of relaxation as a therapy in managing CRF and conflicting evidence supporting the use of rest in the alleviation of CRF.

Refer to Chapter 15 for more detail of the allied health professional (AHP) role in anxiety management.

Education and information giving

There is a clear need for health care professionals to provide clear, concise and well-timed information when educating patients and carers (Jakel, 2002). Information given to patients and families aims to facilitate their understanding of their fatigue and offers coping strategies. Patients receiving timely information, for example, prior to commencing anti-cancer therapies have reported a less negative overall experience of fatigue (Ream *et al.*, 2003). However, each case must be judged individually by the OT with regard to the level of information provided and its timing. Lowrie (2006) recommends that it might not be appropriate to provide information about potential difficulties prior to patients commencing treatment as this may cause them added stress and anxiety and potentially contribute to their CRF.

Rehabilitation versus compensatory approach

The occupational therapy approach will vary depending on stage of disease, treatment and prognosis. For example, a patient in the early stages of treatment or a patient who has completed treatment will benefit more from an educational and rehabilitative approach. Adopting a rehabilitation approach by using energy-conserving strategies such as pacing and prioritising (Barsevick *et al.*, 2002; Lowrie, 2006) during heightened periods of fatigue will enable a person to continue with meaningful everyday activities. This maintains independence and quality of life and prevents the minimisation of overall activity levels during this time, which could in turn lead to further fatigue.

Patients with advanced disease, on the other hand, are likely to benefit more from energy-conserving strategies, such as labour-saving devices, e.g. bathing equipment or delegation of tasks to family or social services, therefore adopting a more compensatory/adaptive approach.

OTs have a unique and valuable role within the assessment and management of CRF. Due to the nature of occupational therapy as a profession, OTs are well equipped in this particular area of cancer care and are skilled in adopting the holistic approach needed to effectively manage the multi-dimensional nature of CRF (Lowrie, 2006).

The role of the dietitian in the management of CRF

Prior to treatment, a comprehensive assessment of patients is carried out regarding their diet, weight history and body mass index (BMI) alongside social aspects. The aim is to restore optimum nutritional status in preparation for treatment and to address underlying fatigue. During treatment, nutritional support can address the possible influencing factors identified as causing CRF in the individual. As part of palliative care, the focus is to maintain quality of life and minimise discomfort caused by CRF.

There is no single means to eliminate taste or saliva alterations, which affect CRF, but may be minimised by encouraging good oral hygiene, use of artificial saliva, spray bottle of water, soft moist foods and sugar-free chewing gum. Small frequent snacks and fluid intake should be encouraged. Nausea and vomiting can be severely debilitating and may be the result of psychological factors, such as anxiety or stress, or may be a conditioned response where the patient expects to be sick. These issues need to be addressed appropriately with psychological support. Irritation of the upper gastrointestinal (GI) tract, chemotherapy, GI obstruction or constipation, delayed gastric emptying, hypercalcaemia and antibiotics can also affect CRF, all of which illustrate the multi-factorial issues which have to be considered.

Case study 1

Shaun, a 57-year-old retired mechanic, was diagnosed with adenocarcinoma of the stomach 5 months ago. Following his third cycle of chemotherapy, Shaun has been reporting increasing symptoms of fatigue and expressing concerns at how he will manage at home. Shaun lives with his wife (also in her late 50s) in a two-bedroomed semi-detached house.

Shaun was referred to OT for functional assessment prior to discharge home, physiotherapy for reduced mobility and both addressed his increasing anxiety.

The ward OT conducted a thorough functional assessment regarding all aspects of personal and domestic activities of daily living. Shaun was able to strip wash and dress independently on the ward if he was seated. Shaun was keen to bathe independently at home, something he had not been able to do for a while, explaining to the OT that he was simply 'too tired to be heaving myself in and out of the bath', and that 'I can't expect my wife to help me'. The OT recommended that showering required less energy; to which he agreed. Shaun was assessed using a showerboard safely over the bath in hospital and OT arranged provision of this equipment via his local social service OT to facilitate independent showering at home. The hospital OT also requested provision of a perching stool for Shaun to use in the bathroom to conserve energy during activities such as brushing his teeth and shaving.

Shaun's wife attended to all domestic needs at home; however, both she and Shaun were wanting to continue to carryout activities they had done together, such as shopping, since his retirement 2 years ago. With Shaun's consent, a referral was made to his local wheelchair service for provision of an attendant-propelled wheelchair for outdoor use. Due to a waiting list at his local wheelchair service, arrangements were made for his wife to collect an appropriate wheelchair from her local Red Cross Medical Loans branch for short-term use.

Working together with the physiotherapist, a graded exercise programme was introduced, starting with low-intensity aerobic exercise and resistive strength exercises for large muscle groups. The exercise programme was monitored closely by the physiotherapist during inpatient admissions and adapted as necessary.

Shaun was referred to the dietitian when his wife reported that she found it very difficult to encourage Shaun to eat as he complained that food tasted 'off'. The dietitian met with both Shaun and his wife and reassured them that taste changes were a very common side effect of chemotherapy. They were advised to avoid the offending foods but given suggestions of alternatives in each particular food group to try. A good oral hygiene regimen was encouraged and plenty of fluids recommended.

Outcomes of therapy intervention

As discussed before, there is no universally accepted self-report tool for the measurement of CRF (NCI, 2003). Formal outcome measures can also be very tiring for them to complete, which is contraindicated. Outcomes can be measured by patients' subjective feedback on their satisfaction of achieving goals such as successful and safe return home and satisfaction with the activity level they have achieved.

Case study 2

Caroline, a 27-year-old woman, was diagnosed with metastatic colon cancer 18 months ago. Following 1 year of treatment, including surgery and chemotherapy, Caroline had been admitted to an acute palliative care ward for management of symptoms including increased pain, weight loss, shortness of breath, anxiety and fatigue. Caroline and her family had been told by medical staff that they expected her prognosis to be less than 3 months.

On admission, Caroline reported a dramatic reduction in her mobility at home as well as weight loss over a number of weeks. As a result of her worsening symptoms, Caroline required the assistance of one person to transfer her from bed to chair and ward nursing staff reported helping Caroline with all personal care needs.

From discussions during the palliative care multi-professional meeting, Caroline was referred to dietetics, occupational therapy, physiotherapy and social work for full assessment of all her needs and planning for safe and timely discharge home. Caroline lived with her partner of 2 years in a rented first-floor flat with no lift. Her mother, father and younger brother Paul (23 years) all live nearby in the family house.

Following physiotherapy assessment, it was clear that Caroline would not manage to climb stairs on discharge due to generalised weakness, fatigue and shortness of breath. If she were discharged to her current accommodation, she would have no means of getting out of the flat once taken back there by ambulance staff.

During the occupational therapy assessment, Caroline expressed a wish to return to her parents' home where she could live downstairs and spend time with her family. Caroline declined provision of a hospital profiling bed, stating that her parents were planning to turn their diningroom into a downstairs bedroom (with double bed) for her and her partner. As her partner worked during the day, Caroline's mother was keen to take on the main carer's role, initially declining any help from social services. During further conversations with both the hospital OT and the social worker, Caroline agreed to accept support from social services having a morning care call to assist her with personal care needs. This would allow Caroline to conserve energy, enabling her to become engaged in meaningful activities during the rest of the day.

The dietitian took an initial diet history and found that, due to anxiety, Caroline's appetite had diminished significantly. This was further exacerbated by her changing bowel habits following surgery and chemotherapy leaving her with periods of diarrhoea. She was advised to follow a low-residue diet and also, to minimise further weight loss, to increase the energy and protein content of her diet. High-protein nutritional supplements were prescribed to help to boost her intake. Review appointments were planned to monitor her nutritional intake as compliance is often difficult to achieve without monitoring and encouragement.

Summary

CRF is the most prevalent symptom reported by individuals with cancer (Mock, 2004) and can affect patients at any stage of their illness causing significant distress and disability. Whilst this debilitating condition is often acknowledged and recognised by health care professionals, CRF is often not addressed (Ream & Stone, 2004) despite the growing evidence of effectiveness of many pharmacological and non-pharmacological interventions.

Understanding the impact of CRF for patients and their families and grasping their interpretation of its meaning is essential. Fatigue has historically been perceived as an indication of ongoing or deteriorating disease and thus time for education, explanation and information is an important task for all health care professionals working in oncology. This will help in the patients' understanding of their fatigue, their motivation and cooperation in working with their medical team and give the best possible results of their treatment.

The multi-dimensional nature of CRF is complex and before any treatment is offered an accurate assessment of all aspects of CRF is vital. Identification of likely causes of the fatigue is a critical factor before determining the best possible treatment. It is imperative that health care professionals adopt a flexible and holistic approach to the management of CRF in order to accommodate the many varied symptoms and consider all the treatment options available.

Specific pharmacological intervention for potentially reversible medical conditions known to present with fatigue, such as anaemia, hypothyroidism, pain, depression and anxiety, should be initiated as the first line of treatment and be evaluated as to their effectiveness. Should CRF still present as a problem, this chapter highlights evidence-based non-pharmacological treatments that have shown to be effective in managing this condition, such as physiotherapy, occupational therapy and importance of dietary advice.

Health care professionals treating patients with cancer should always be aware of CRF and be ready and able to discuss this fully with the patient. Referral for assessment and treatment interventions should be timely and involve a wider team approach. Early therapeutic intervention and education could minimise the impact of CRF described by the patient and give them guidance to control and manage this common and distressing symptom of cancer care.

Key learning points

1. There is a need for increased awareness and understanding of CRF in oncology. This will include further education for health care professionals working in oncology, highlighting importance of accurate diagnosis and assessment of CRF.
2. Where appropriate, advice given about CRF prior to cancer treatment commencing and early referral for intervention is most beneficial.
3. Further work in establishing systematic and integrative management programmes for CRF involving pharmacological and non-pharmacological management of CRF.
4. Clinicians need to constantly evaluate and reappraise effectiveness of interventions and adapt CRF management programmes accordingly.
5. Further research is required into the efficacy of treatments available involving randomised trials and larger numbers at all stages of cancer and its treatments.

References

Aaronson, L. S., Teel, C. S., Cassmeyer, V., Neuberger, G. B., Pallikkathayil, L., Pierce, J., Press, A. N., Williams, P. D. & Wingate, A. (1999). Defining and measuring fatigue. *Image: Journal of Nursing Scholarship*, *31*, 45–50.

Ahlberg, K., Ekman, T., Gaston-Johansson, F. & Mock, V. (2003). Assessment and management of cancer-related fatigue in adults. *The Lancet*, *362* (9384), 640–650.

Barnes, E. A. & Bruera, E. (2002). Fatigue in patients with advanced cancer: a review. *International Journal of Gynaecological Cancer*, *12*, 424–428.

Barsevick, A., Whitmer, K., Sweeney, C. & Nail, L. (2002). A pilot study examining energy conservation for cancer treatment-related fatigue. *Cancer Nursing*, *25* (5), 333–341.

Barsevick, A. M. (2002). Energy conservation and cancer-related fatigue. *Rehabilitation Oncology*, *20* (3), 14–17.

Berger, A. & Walker, S. N. (2001). An explanatory model of fatigue in women receiving adjuvant breast cancer chemotherapy. *Nursing Research*, *50* (1), 43–52.

Bultmann, U., Kant, I. J., Schroer, C. A. P. & Kasl, S. V. (2002). The relationship between psychosocial work characteristics and fatigue and psychological distress. *International Archives of Occupational and Environmental Health*, *75*, 259–266.

Cella, D., Lai, J.-S., Chang, C. H., Peterman, A. & Slavin, M. (2002). Fatigue in cancer patients compared with fatigue in the general United States population. *Cancer*, *94*, 528–538.

Cella, D., Peterman, A., Passick, S., Jacobsen, P. & Breitbart, W. (1998). Progress towards guidelines for the management of fatigue. *Oncology*, *12*, 369–377.

Curt, G. A., Breutbart, W., Cella, D., Groopman, J. E., Horing, S. J., Itri, L. M., Johnson, D. H., Miaskowski, C., Scherr, S. L., Portenoy, R. K. & Vogelzang, N. J. (2000). Impact of cancer-related fatigue on the live of patients: new findings from the fatigue coalition. *The Onocogist*, *5* (5), 353–360.

Dale, E. (2004). Cancer pain, fatigue, distress and insomnia in cancer patients. *Clinical Cornerstone*, *6* (1), 15–21.

David, A., McDonald, E., Mann, A., Pelosi, A., Stephens, D., Ledger, D., Rathbone, R. & Mann, A. (1990). Tired, weak or in need of a rest: fatigue among general practice attenders. *British Medical Journal*, *301*, 1199–1202.

Davidson, J. R., Maclean, A. W., Brundage, M. D. & Schulze, K. (2002). Sleep disturbances in cancer patients. *Social Science and Medicine*, *54*, 1309–1321.

Dillon, E. & Kelly, J. (2003). The status of cancer fatigue on the island of Ireland: AIFC professional and interim patient surveys. *The Oncologist*, 8, 22–26.

Dimeo, F. (2002). Radiotherapy related fatigue and exercise for cancer patients: a review of the literature and suggestions for future research. *Frontiers in Radiation Therapy Oncology*, 37, 49–56.

Escalante, C. P. (2003). Treatment of cancer-related fatigue: an update. *Support Cancer Care*, 11, 79–83.

Fawcett, T. N. & Dean, A. (2004). The causes of cancer-related fatigue and approaches to its treatment. *Professional Nurse*, 19, 503–507.

Flechtner, H. & Bottomley, A. (2002). Fatigue assessment in cancer clinical trials. *Expert Reviews in Pharmacoeconomics Outcomes Research*, 2, 67–76.

Glaus, A. (1993). Assessment of fatigue in cancer and non-cancer patients and in healthy individuals. *Supportive Care in Cancer*, 1, 305–315.

Hann, D. M., Jacobsen, P. B., Azzarello, L. M., Martin, S. C., Curran, S. L., Fields, K. K., Greenberg, H. & Lyman, G. (1998). Measurement of fatigue in cancer patients: development and validation of the fatigue symptom inventory. *Quality of Life Research*, 7, 301–310.

Irvine, D., Vincent, L., Graydon, J. & Bubela, N. (1998). Fatigue in women with breast cancer receiving radiation therapy. *Cancer Nursing*, 21 (2), 127–135.

Jacobsen, P. B. (2004). Assessment of fatigue in cancer patients. *Journal of the National Cancer Institute Monographs*, 32, 93–97.

Jacobsen, P. B. & Thors, C. L. (2003). Fatigue in the radiation therapy patient: current management and investigations. *Seminars Radiation Oncology*, 13, 372–380.

Jakel, P. (2002). Patient communication and strategies for managing fatigue. *Oncology*, 16 (9), 141–145.

Kolden, G. K., Strauman, T. J., Ward, A., Kuta, J., Woods, T. E., Schneider, K. L., Heerey, E., Sanborn, L., Burt, C., Millbrandt, L., Kalin, N. H., Stewart, J. A. & Mullen, B. (2002). A pilot study of group exercise training (GET) for women with primary breast cancer: feasibility and health benefits. *Psycho-Oncology*, 11, 447–456.

Lowrie, D. (2006). Occupational therapy and cancer-related fatigue. Chapter 6 in J. Cooper (Ed.), *Occupational therapy in oncology and palliative care* (2nd ed.). Chichester: Wiley.

Lucia, A., Earnest, C. & Perez, M. (2003). Cancer-related fatigue: can exercise physiology assist oncologists. *The Lancet Oncology*, 4, 616–625.

Manzullo, E. F. & Escalante, C. P. (2002). Research into fatigue. *Hematology-Oncology Clinics of North America*, 16, 619–628.

McColl, E. (2004). Best practice in symptom assessment: a review. *Gut*, 53 (4), 49–54.

Mock, V. (2004). Evidence-based treatment for cancer-related fatigue. *Journal of the National Cancer Institute Monographs*, 32, 112–118.

Morrow, G. R., Andrews, P. L. R., Hickok, J. T., Roscoe, J. A. & Matheson, S. (2002). Fatigue associated with cancer and its treatment. *Supportive Care in Cancer*, 10, 389–398.

Nail, L. M. (2002). Fatigue in patients with cancer. *Oncology Nursing Forum*, 29, 537–544.

Nail, L. M. & Winningham, M. L. (1993). Fatigue. In: S. L. Groenwald, M. Hansen Frogge, M. Goodman & C. H. Yarbo (Eds.), *Cancer nursing: principles and practice* (3rd ed., pp. 609–617). London: Jones and Bartlett.

National Cancer Institute (NCI) (2003). *Fatigue*. National Cancer Institute [online]. Retrieved 8 July 2003 from http://www.cancer.gov/

National Comprehensive Cancer Network [NCCN] (2006). *Clinical practice guidelines in oncology: cancer related fatigue*, v.1.2006 [online]. Retrieved 10 October 2006 from http://www.nccn.org/professionals/physician_gls/PDF/fatigue.pdf/

Pawlikowska, T., Chadler, T., Hirsch, S. R. & Wessely, S. C. (1994). Population based study of fatigue and psychological distress. *British Medical Journal*, 308, 763–770.

Piper, B. F. (1986). Fatigue. In: V. K. Carrieri, A. M. Lindsey & C. W. West (Eds.), *Pathophysiological phenomena in nursing: human responses to illness* (pp. 219–234). Philadelphia: W.B. Saunders.

Piper, B. F., Dibble, S. L., Dodd, M. J., Weiss, M. C., Slaughter, R. E. & Paul, S. M. (1998). The revised Piper fatigue scale: psychometric evaluation in women with breast cancer. *Oncology Nursing Forum, 25,* 677–684.

Piper, B. F., Lindsey, A. M. & Dodd, M. J. (1987). Fatigue mechanisms in cancer patients: developing nursing theory. *Oncology Nursing Forum, 14,* 17–23.

Porock, D., Kristjanson, L. J., Tinnelly, K., Duke, T. & Blight, J. (2000). An exercise intervention for advanced cancer patients experiencing fatigue: a pilot study. *Journal of Palliative Care, 16* (3), 30–36.

Portenoy, R. K. & Itri, L. M. (1999). Cancer-related fatigue: guidelines for evaluation and management. *The Oncologist, 4* (1), 1–10.

Ream, E., Browne, N., Glaus, A., Knipping, C. & Frei, I. A. (2003). Quality and efficiency of educational materials on cancer-related fatigue: views of patients from two European countries. *European Journal of Oncology Nursing, 7* (2), 99–109.

Ream, E. & Stone, P. (2004). Clinical interventions for fatigue. In: J. Armes, M. Krishnasamy & I. Higginson (Eds.), *Fatigue in cancer.* Oxford: Oxford University Press.

Richardson, A. (1998). Measuring fatigue in patients with cancer. *Support Cancer Care, 6* (2), 94–100.

Sadler, I. J. & Jacobsen, P. B. (2001). Progress in understanding fatigue associated with breast cancer treatment. *Cancer Investigations, 19,* 723–731.

Servaes, P., Verhagen, C. & Bleijenberg, G. (2002). Fatigue in cancer patients during and after treatment: prevalence, correlates and interventions. *European Journal of Cancer, 38* (1), 27–43.

Shen, J., Barbera, J. & Shapiro, C. M. (2006). Distinguishing sleepiness and fatigue: focus on definition and measurement. *Sleep Medicine Reviews, 10,* 63–76.

Smets, E. M. A., Garssen, B., Bonke, B. & De Haes, J. C. J. M. (1995). The multidimensional fatigue inventory: psychometric qualities of an instrument to assess fatigue. *Journal of Psychometric Research, 39,* 315–325.

Stein, K. D., Jacobsen, P. B., Blanchard, C. M. & Thors, C. (2004). Further validation of the multidimensional fatigue symptom inventory-short form. *Journal of Pain and Symptom Management, 27,* 14–23.

Stein, K. D., Martin, S. C., Hann, D. M. & Jacobsen, P. B. (1998). A multidimensional measure of fatigue for use with cancer patients. *Cancer Practice, 6,* 143–150.

Stevenson, C. & Fox, K. R. (2005). Role of Exercise for cancer rehabilitation in UK hospitals: a survey of oncology nurses. *European Journal of Cancer Care, 14,* 63–69.

Stone, P. (2002). The measurement, causes and effective management of cancer-related fatigue. *International Journal of Palliative Nursing, 8,* 120–128.

Stone, P., Richards, M., Ahern, R. & Hardy, J. (2000a). A study to investigate the prevalence, severity and correlates of fatigue among patients with cancer in comparison with a control group of volunteers without cancer. *Annals of Oncology, 11* (5), 561–567.

Stone, P., Richards, M. & Hardy, J. (1998). Review: fatigue in patients with cancer. *European Journal of Cancer, 34,* 1670–1676.

Stone, P., Richardson, A., Ream, E., Smith, A. G., Kerr, D. J. & Kearney, N. (2000b). Cancer-related fatigue: inevitable, unimportant and untreatable? Results of a multicentre patient survey. *Annals of Oncology, 11* (8), 971–975.

Tomkins Stricker, C., Drake, D., Hoyer, K. & Mock, V. (2004). Evidence-based practice for fatigue management in adults with cancer: exercise as an intervention. *Oncology Nursing Forum, 31* (5), 963–976.

Visovsky, C. & Schneider, S. M. (2003). Cancer-related fatigue. *Online Journal of Issues in Nursing* [online], *8* (3), Retrieved September 2006 from http://www.nursingworld.org

Wagner, L. I. & Cella, D. (2004). Fatigue and cancer: causes, prevalence and treatment approaches. *British Journal of Cancer*, *91* (5), 822–828.

Wagner-Raphael, L. & Cella, D. F. (2001). ICD-10 International classification of diseases: 10th Revision, clinical modification. Cancer-related fatigue: assessment and management. In: M. Marty & S. Pecorelli (Eds.), *Fatigue and cancer ESO scientific update* (Vol. 5). Amsterdam, The Netherlands/Melville, NY: Elsevier Science and Oncology.

Watson, T. & Mock, V. (2003). Exercise and cancer-related fatigue: a review of current literature. *Rehabilitation Oncology*, *21* (1), 23–32.

Watson T. & Mock, V. (2004). Exercise as an intervention for cancer-related fatigue. *Physical Therapy*, *84* (8), 736–743.

Winningham, M. L. (1992). How exercise mitigates fatigue: implications for people receiving cancer therapy. In: R. M. Johnson (Ed.), *The biotherapy of cancer V* (pp. 16–20). Pittsburgh: Oncology Nursing Press.

Winningham, M. L. & Barton-Burke, M. (Eds.) (2000). *Fatigue in cancer: a multidimensional approach*. Massachusetts: Jones and Bartlett.

Winningham, M. L., Nail, L. M., Barton-Burke, M., Brophy, L., Cimprich, B., Jones, L. S., Pickard-Holley, S., Rhodes, V., St Pierre, B., Beck, S., Glass, E. C., Mock, V. L., Mooney, K. H. & Piper, B. (1994). Fatigue and the cancer experience: the state of the knowledge. *Oncology Nursing Forum*, *21*, 23–36.

Wu, H.-S. & McSweeney, M. (2001). Measurement of fatigue in people with cancer. *Oncology Nursing Forum*, *28*, 1371–1384.

Chapter 13

CANCER PAIN

Dr Karen Robb and Charlie Ewer-Smith

Learning outcomes

After studying this chapter the reader should be able to:

- Discuss the key principles of pain management in patients with cancer
- Highlight the possible causes of pain in the cancer patient and the main pharmacological and non-pharmacological approaches to management
- Implement and evaluate an evidence-based approach to the management of pain in patients with cancer

---

Introduction

Worldwide incidence of cancer has increased and great advances in medicine and technology have resulted in significantly more patients living with their disease. For this reason, the management of pain problems associated with cancer and/or its treatment is gaining increasing recognition and significance. Patients with cancer may present with a range of pain problems, many of which can be complex and multi-dimensional. The concept of 'total pain' was first introduced by Dame Cicely Saunders in 1967 to address the various dimensions of cancer-related pain, i.e. emotional, psychosocial and spiritual components of pain, and highlight that addressing only the physical aspects of pain is unlikely to bring about pain relief (Saunders, 1967).

As key members of the multi-professional team, allied health professionals (AHPs) play an important role in the management of patients with cancer pain and may encounter these patients at various stages in the 'cancer journey'. It is universally acknowledged that 'no one individual can possess the range of skills necessary to provide a comprehensive programme of pain management' (O'Brien, 1993) and therapists must recognise the important contribution they can make to patient care through comprehensive assessment and implementation of treatment based on best available evidence. Pain management for cancer patients needs to be comprehensive to address the multiple factors affecting the patient's quality of life (Ventafridda, 1989). This management plan should be holistic, patient centred and flexible to allow for changes.

Pain has often been quoted as one of the most dreaded aspect of cancer and there is a wealth of literature examining the psychological impact of cancer pain and the detrimental effect it can have. It has been suggested that 'emotional distress is the most consistent psychological variable associated with pain in the cancer population' (Syrjala & Chapko, 1995). Unrelieved pain is incapacitating and can interfere with physical functioning and activities of daily living often resulting in psychological distress.

The International Association for the Study of Pain (IASP) has declared that freedom from pain should be a basic human right (International Association for the Study of Pain [IASP], 2004). When we consider that the World Health Organization has estimated that 4 million people have cancer pain (Simpson, 2000), and when we also consider the lack of pain control methods available in many developing countries, we start to appreciate the global scale of cancer pain and the significance of the problem.

Prevalence, definitions and characteristics

There are many excellent textbooks and publications which address cancer pain in great detail and these are listed under 'Further reading' at the end of this chapter.

The prevalence of pain associated with cancer varies enormously and is dependent on many factors including stage of disease and treatments undergone. Pain from cancer tends to increase in severity as disease progresses, and Hearn and Higginson (1999) suggest that pain is prevalent in between 58 and 84% of patients with advanced disease. Untreated cancer pain has been described as an 'enormous and truly unfortunate problem' (Krames, 2004).

The IASP has defined pain as 'an unpleasant sensory and emotional experience associated with actual or potential tissue damage, or described in terms of such damage' (Merskey & Bogduk, 1994). This definition highlights some important aspects of the pain experience, in summary that pain is a physiological and psychological experience, may be a warning sign of actual or perceived tissue damage and also that pain can occur in the absence of tissue damage (Unruh et al., 2002). It clearly also identifies the multi-dimensional experience of pain highlighting the sensory, affective and cognitive dimensions.

Cancer pain has been described as 'a nociceptive mosaic composed of acute pain, chronic pain, tumour-specific pain and treatment-related pain, cemented together by ongoing psychological responses of distress and suffering' (Goudas et al., 2001). To classify pain, we use acute, chronic or cancer pain as the main categories; however, cancer pain has features of both acute and chronic pain and can be considered in the following way:

1. Pain directly due to the cancer, e.g. bony metastatic disease
2. Pain indirectly due to the cancer, e.g. spinal nerve root compression by a tumour
3. Pain secondary to cancer treatment, e.g. peripheral neuropathy secondary to chemotherapy
4. Pain not related to cancer or its treatment but which coexists, e.g painful osteoarthritic joint

Cancer-related pain describes all pains due to cancer and/or its treatment.

One attempt to systematically describe cancer-related pain characteristics and syndromes involved a prospective, cross-sectional, multi-centre survey of 58 pain specialists and over 1000 patients (Caraceni & Portenoy, 1999). Results suggested that over 93% of patients had >1 pain caused by cancer and 21% of patients had >1 pain caused by cancer treatments. A staggering 67% of patients reported a worst pain >7/10, which we know is representative of severe pain (Serlin et al., 1995) and is likely to interfere with activities of daily living (Cleeland & Ryan, 1994; Twycross et al., 1996).

It has been hypothesised that cancer-related pain and non-cancer pain are fundamentally different (Turk et al., 1998). Cancer-related pain is often due to an identifiable pathology, e.g. tumour infiltration, and as such patients can be seen as suffering from a 'real disease' (Turk et al., 1998). This is in contrast to many of the benign chronic pain syndromes, e.g. low back pain, where the cause of pain is not readily identifiable and much of the cause can be placed on psychological factors.

Chronic cancer-treatment-related pain is becoming increasingly recognised as many more patients are now surviving and living with the effects of treatment (Jung et al., 2003; Macrae, 2001). Some of these pain problems are similar in presentation to many benign pain syndromes and for this reason it has been suggested that they are managed in a similar way.

Cancer-related pain can be nociceptive, neuropathic or a mixed clinical picture and it is important to identify the aetiology and pathophysiology of the pain when planning treatment. Patients with cancer often have multiple pains and multiple causes of pain. Cancer pain can coexist with a wide range of other symptoms, which may include fatigue, nausea and vomiting, breathlessness, deconditioning, anxiety, fear and depression. The presentation of the patient will vary depending on a range of other factors, including stage of disease, treatment(s) undergone and general medical status of the patient. Therapists need to be aware of the full clinical picture and this will be discussed in more detail under 'Assessment'.

Responses to cancer-related pain

When considering therapy interventions with an individual experiencing cancer-related pain it is essential to first explore the meaning of the pain to that person and to those closest to them. An individual's ethnocultural affiliation, spiritual, religious and philosophical beliefs all impact on perception and response to cancer pain (Bates et al., 1993).

Research into the beliefs, thoughts and emotional responses of these patients with pain highlights a common response as one of fear (Zaza & Baine, 2002). This can be fear of the pain experience, fear of the pain indicating further damage or a worsening of disease (Cleeland, 1985, Coluzzi, 1996) and even fear of others' reactions to their pain (National Council for Hospice and Specialist Cancer Services, 2003; Ward et al., 1993). Patients and carers often believe that cancer-related pain is inevitable and to be tolerated (Wallace et al., 1995). They may be reluctant to report it for fear of further treatments, side effects to pain medication or for concern of being 'a nuisance' (Speck, 2002). In a study to clarify the relationship between pain and cancer, Mitsuko (1997) notes that over half the subjects assumed that an increase in pain signified progression of the disease and Ward *et al.* (1993) report similar attitudes in caregivers.

Thoughts and emotional responses regarding pain can contribute to the intensity of a person's pain experience (Bates *et al.*, 1993). Those associated with higher levels of pain intensity experienced may include anxiety, depression, fear of the future, hopelessness, negative perceptions of personal and social competence, decreased social activity/social support and lack of control over pain (Breitbart *et al.*, 2004).

Impact of cancer-related pain

The experience of pain is multi-dimensional, impacting cognitive, emotional, physical, social, spiritual and behavioural components of a person. It affects concentration, the ability to solve problems and make decisions. Pain can cause reduced appetite, insomnia, irritability, low mood, feelings of despair and hopelessness, anger and low self-esteem as well as reduce a person's interest and pleasure in what is usually important to him or her. It can also reduce strength, vitality, activity tolerance and mobility (Cancerbackup, 2005; Gamlin & Lovel, 2002).

Cancer patients with pain report significantly lower levels of performance status than those without pain (Lin *et al.*, 2003). In a study investigating adaptation to pain, Turk *et al.* (1998) demonstrated that pain due to cancer was associated with higher levels of perceived disability and a lower degree of activity. It is clear that pain may affect a person's ability to care for him- or herself, to work or to participate in fulfilling activities. Loss of independence, isolation, disempowerment, reduced sense of personal competency, changes in relationships and roles, changes in body image, changes in communication, the ability to manage concurrent life events and social difficulties are all reported (Zaza & Baine, 2002). A common response to pain is the development of 'pain behaviour'. This includes maladaptive behaviours such as guarding the painful area, pain watching (hypervigilance), developing an overly sedentary lifestyle and avoiding activities. This inactivity can result in further problems, such as deconditioning, increased muscular tension on movement and increased attention to pain.

In a study of palliative patients' perspectives of rehabilitation, Belchamber & Gousy (2004) quote that 'pain was described as terrifying, frightening and devastating. This emotional pain also had an effect on the participants immediate family, social circle of friends and neighbours, often causing high levels of anxiety and feelings of isolation.' The experience of cancer pain may result in disruption to family caregivers' quality of life in the areas of physical, psychological, social and spiritual well-being (Ferrell *et al.*, 1999).

Cancer-related pain is extremely complex and influenced by a plethora of factors. The resulting distress of patients and carers makes each experience unique, and an individualised assessment by a skilled multi-professional team is essential for optimal management (National Council for Hospice and Specialist Palliative Care Services, 2003).

Assessment and measurement

General principles

For a broad overview of a therapies' approach to pain assessment and measurement the reader is directed to Strong *et al.* (2002), Strong and Bennett (2002) and main and Spanswick (2001) (Chapters 7–12). The terms 'assessment' and 'measurement' sometimes get confusing but it is important to distinguish between them. Assessment is 'the broader examination of the relationship between different components of the pain experience for a given patient', whereas measurement is 'the quantification of each component' (Strong *et al.* 2002).

It is clear that assessment of cancer-related pain should be multi-professional, multi-dimensional and timely, but there may be aspects of assessment which are profession- or discipline specific. Assessment may require some detailed examination of physical or psychosocial factors, e.g. joint range of movement or anxiety, but should always focus on a patient's functional ability, as this is the key concern for therapists. Assessment is rarely possible over one interaction; it is an information gathering exercise and is a continual process which guides initial and ongoing treatment. The multi-professional team must liaise closely to ensure that assessment is systematic and accurate.

Assessment will be guided by the cause and nature of the pain and the context in which it is present, e.g. the format of assessment for a hospitalised patient with terminal disease and severe intractable pain will differ from that of an outpatient with no evidence of cancer but chronic cancer-treatment-related pain. The former will require an urgent and accurate assessment which will be chiefly medically led (with input from others) and will aim to provide effective pain relief as quickly as possible. The latter may involve a comprehensive, multi-professional assessment and may focus on a non-pharmacological approach (e.g. cognitive–behavioural therapy) to improve function. Regardless of the nature of the problem, the patient must remain at the heart of the assessment process and listening carefully to the patient appears to be central to a good outcome.

History taking is a vital component of pain assessment and should include medical and psychosocial history (including recognition of spiritual, cultural and religious aspects). A detailed pain history is vital to assess the background to, and development of, the pain problem. Therapists must be alerted to the possibility that a new pain report may be an indication of progressive disease and be aware of the relevant 'red flags' when completing their individual assessment. An excellent knowledge of cancer and its treatment will facilitate a thorough pain assessment.

For example, a patient with a history of left breast cancer is being seen by a community physiotherapist, she was recently hospitalised for 5 fractions of radiotherapy for management of spinal metastatic disease, she now reports a new pain in her left hip when mobilising, it is severe in intensity and not relieved by simple analgesia: this finding is suggestive of a further metastatic deposit in her femur and the relevant oncology team should be alerted urgently.

There are three components of assessment that must be considered in all patients:

- A description of the pain (including severity, irritability and nature)
- Responses to the pain
- The impact of pain on the person's life (Strong & Bennett, 2002b)

These have all been discussed in some detail in this chapter. When assessing the impact of pain on an individual, clinical reasoning may be guided by consideration of two broad movement-related categories devised for physiotherapists: activity limitation (or functional limitation) and physical impairments (Jones & Rivett, 2004). Activity restrictions relate to what patients are reporting they are having difficulties with functionally, e.g. climbing stairs. Physical impairments relate to physical signs which patients may not be aware of until physical examination, e.g. muscle weakness or increased sensitivity of tissues around a painful joint. Therapists must be aware of the dangers of placing too much attention on correction of physical impairments at the expense of function (Simmonds, 1999). For many cancer patients, especially those with advanced disease, it will be more important to complete a task than to focus on correction of individual impairments.

Measurement tools

It is commonly recognised that 'exploring and monitoring outcomes is central to ethical and high-quality clinical practice' (Long & Fairfield, 1996). For this reason, it is important to utilise reliable and valid outcome measures. A great variety of tools are now available but there are no clear guidelines for selecting one or more measures over others. There has been a wealth of literature examining the psychometric properties of cancer pain measures and research findings support the multi-dimensional nature of cancer-related pain as well as the validity of the most commonly used measures of pain intensity and pain interference (Jensen, 2003).

Outcome measures for use in clinical practice must be feasible (i.e. practical, inexpensive and easy to use), provide extra clinical information and be responsive to changes over time. Many measures are self-report in style and these include single-item rating scales of pain intensity, such as visual analogue scale (VAS) or numerical ratings scale (NRS). Both are commonly used in clinical practice and have consistently shown good reliability and validity. A VAS consists of a 10-cm line which can be horizontal or vertical with 'no pain' at one end and 'pain as bad as you can imagine' at the other end. Patients are asked to make a mark on the line which represents their pain intensity at that time. An NRS is similar but is numbered from 0 to 10 and patients are asked to score their pain accordingly. Previous research has suggested cut-off points for mild, moderate and severe pain on an NRS (Figure 13.1). This is useful to consider when assessing whether improvements in pain report are clinically

Mild   **Moderate**   **Severe pain**

0   1   2   3   4   5   6   7   8   9   10

No pain   **Pain as bad as**
                                                           you can
                                                         imagine

Figure 13.1 Mild, moderate and severe pain as represented on NRS. 0–4, mild; 5–6, moderate; 7–10, severe. [Reprinted with permission from Serlin *et al.* (1995). Copyright 1995, with permission from Elsevier.]

significant. As severity of pain is the primary factor in determining the impact of pain on the patient (Serlin *et al.*, 1995), lowering pain scores should be a priority. A drop in pain report from 9/10 to 7/10 may be less clinically significant than a drop from 7/10 to 5/10, although the incremental change is the same. This is because the latter represents a fall from a severe to a moderate pain category whereas the former does not.

The Brief Pain Inventory (BPI) (Cleeland & Ryan, 1994) has been extensively used in cancer pain research and is a useful clinical tool as it reports both pain intensity and pain interference using NRS. The BPI has four questions addressing current pain and past worst, least and average pain alongside seven items referring to the extent with which pain interferes with activities of daily living. Responses to the final seven items are averaged to form a pain interference score.

The importance of the patient remaining at the heart of the treatment process has been previously emphasised. A standardised, client-centred, individualised measure which can be used to detect the impact of therapy intervention on the patient's self-perception of occupational performance is the Canadian Occupational Performance Measure (Baptiste *et al.*, 1993). This measure has also been demonstrated to empower and actively encourage patient participation in therapy interventions.

Other tools which can be used include pain drawings (which are often simple body charts) or descriptive questionnaires such as the McGill Pain Questionnaire (Melzack, 1975).

Management of cancer-related pain

The priorities will have been identified at assessment and wherever possible, management should begin with a clear explanation of the goals of treatment, the interventions to be utilised (including the health care professionals involved), the likely outcomes of treatment, with timescales, and any possible adverse effects of treatment. Good communication is vital both within the multi-professional team and with the patient and their family/carers. Close liaison between team members is important especially when different interventions are started concurrently; in some circumstances this may not be recommended as success of individual treatments may be difficult to establish.

The alternative approach is to evaluate the success of the overall approach and this may be more appropriate when pain is particularly severe and difficult to manage.

Palliative care patients have expressed a need for open and honest dialogue with health care professionals (HCP) about all aspects of pain management but research suggests that this is often not possible until contact is made with a palliative care team (Bostrom *et al.*, 2003). This suggests a need for education in pain management for all HCPs caring for cancer patients. This must be recognised by educational establishments, managers and commissioners to ensure the cancer workforce is adequately trained.

Medical approaches

A broad summary of pharmacological interventions will be followed by a brief introduction to other interventions including invasive techniques.

Pharmacological approaches

Over two decades ago, the World Health Organization (WHO) initiated a programme to improve the management of cancer-related pain worldwide. An international panel of experts was convened and the first guidelines, entitled 'Cancer Pain Relief', were published in 1986 (WHO, 1986). Central to these guidelines was the use of a three-step analgesic ladder which progressed from the use of simple analgesics to strong opioids depending on pain severity. Other therapeutic interventions (including adjuvant drugs) can be integrated at any step on the ladder (Figure 13.2).

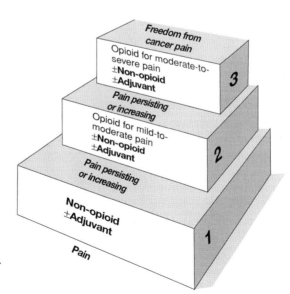

Figure 13.2 The WHO analgesic ladder (reproduced with permission). Analgesics are classified as Group 1–3 as indicated on the steps.

Table 13.1 The key principles of the WHO method of cancer pain relief.

Number	Principles
1	Cancer pain can and should be treated
2	Evaluation and treatment of cancer pain are best achieved by a team approach
3	The first steps are to take a detailed history and to examine the patient carefully to determine the cause of pain and nature of the pain
4	Treatment begins with an explanation and combines physical and psychological approaches, using both non-drug and drug treatments
5	It is useful to have a sequence of specific aims, such as to increase the hours of pain-free sleep, to relieve the pain at rest, to relieve the pain when standing or active
6	Drugs alone usually give adequate relief from pain caused by cancer, provided that the right drug is administered in the right dose at the right time
7	'By mouth': the oral route is the preferred route for analgesics including morphine
8	'By the clock': for persistent pain, drugs should be taken at regular time intervals and not 'as needed'
9	'By the ladder': (a) unless the patient is in severe pain, begin by prescribing a non-opioid and adjust the dose, if necessary, to the maximum recommended dose, (b) if or when the non-opioid no longer adequately relieves pain, an opioid drug should be prescribed in addition to the non-opioid, (c) if or when the non-opioid for mild to moderate pain (e.g. codeine) no longer adequately relieves pain, it should be replaced by an opioid for moderate to severe pain (e.g. morphine)
10	'For the individual': the right dose of an analgesic is the dose that relieves the pain. The dose of oral morphine may range from as little as 5 mg to more than 1000 mg
11	Adjuvant drugs should be prescribed as indicated
12	For neuropathic pain, a tricyclic antidepressant or an anticonvulsant is the drug of choice
13	'Attention to detail': it is essential to monitor the patient's response to the treatment to ensure that they obtain maximum benefit with as few adverse effects as possible

Reproduced with permission.

The three main categories of drugs used to treat cancer-related pain are non-opioids, opioids and adjuvants. Non-opioids comprise paracetamol and non-steroidal anti-inflammatory drugs (NSAIDs). Adjuvants are a miscellaneous group of drugs which relieve pain in certain circumstances. They include corticosteroids, antidepressants, antiepileptics, NMDA (N-methyl-D-aspartate) receptor channel blockers, antispasmodics and muscle relaxants. Opioids can be weak or strong and are described in more detail in the next section. The WHO analgesic ladder is now recognised worldwide and the key principles of the WHO method of cancer pain relief are shown in Table 13.1.

There have been numerous case series over the years evaluating the effectiveness of the analgesic ladder and it has been reported to adequately control cancer-related pain in the vast majority of cases (Zech *et al.*, 1995). In recognition that some patients fail to respond to the three-step approach it has been suggested that a fourth rung is added to the ladder to represent 'interventional techniques' (see next section). The WHO analgesic ladder allows considerable flexibility in drug choices and is not a rigid protocol. It must however be utilised as part of a comprehensive strategy for pain management; it is not the panacea for all cancer-related pains.

For AHPs working in cancer care, one of the most important groups of drugs to develop a deeper understanding of is opioids, e.g. morphine. Individuals' responses to opioids vary greatly and can be affected by such factors as pain severity, previous drug use, age, extent of disease and past medical history. Common side effects include constipation and nausea (for this reason laxatives and antiemetics are routinely prescribed), drowsiness, hallucinations and myoclonic tremor.

'The correct dose of an analgesic is the dose that relieves the pain', and for opioids there are no standard doses; dosage can range from as little as 5 mg to more than 1000 mg every 4 h (Foley, 2006). Morphine is considered the gold-standard 'step 3' analgesic and is the most widely available in a range of oral formulations for normal release (for dose titration) and modified release (for maintenance treatment). It is worth noting that some patients may develop intermittent flare-ups of pain called 'breakthrough pain' whilst having their morphine dose monitored or titrated. Note that breakthrough pain also occurs in patients on a fixed analgesic schedule. For these patients, morphine preparations which are fast acting and easily administered are most appropriate. The preferred alternative route for patients unable to take morphine orally is subcutaneous and for patients with more advanced cancer, portable battery-powered syringe drivers are often used.

It is occasionally necessary to switch strong opioids due to poor response, poor compliance and/or adverse effects. This is called 'opioid rotation/switching' and some examples of alternative strong opioids include buprenorphine, fentanyl, hydromorphone, methadone and oxycodone. Hanks *et al.* (2001) provide an extensive summary of evidence-based guidelines on opioid use in cancer.

Other medical approaches

A range of other options are also open to the medical team. Breivik (2000) provides an overview of interventional techniques such as nerve blocks. Spinal (epidural or intrathecal) administration of opioids, in conjunction with local anaesthetics or clonidine, can be considered when intolerable side effects occur or when pain is particularly difficult to manage, e.g. movement-related incident pain (Hanks *et al.*, 2001).

Where bony metastatic disease is present, radiotherapy and bisphosphonates are commonly used and both have shown good efficacy in clinical trials.

Therapy interventions

General principles of practice. When considering a therapies' approach to patient management the main aims are to relieve pain (wherever possible) and to improve function and quality of life using treatments based on the available evidence. Management should be patient centred, collaborative and restorative and involve family and carers to ensure a timely and coordinated approach to treatment planning and goal setting. The patient's engagement in the therapy partnership is one of the most important aspects of therapy. This relationship can be used to assist the person and those close to them to identify and retain valued activities and roles and, when appropriate, to adjust to role changes (College of Occupational Therapists [COT], 2004).

Early referral to therapies is especially important with palliative care patients but also, with others, to prevent chronicity and help anticipate future problems. We now know that high levels of acute pain are consistent predictors for the development of chronic pain and for this reason, AHPs need to liaise closely with medical colleagues to ensure that acute pain (e.g. post-operative pain) is well managed.

Therapists are often first to establish that pain is not optimally managed due to the nature of rehabilitation and the time that is spent with individual patients. Patients may appear to have good pain control at rest but may complain of increased pain on movement, e.g. when transferring bed to chair. This is sometimes known as 'incident pain' (which is an example of breakthrough pain) and is particularly difficult to manage. There are a range of interventions which can be employed by therapists in these circumstances (to be discussed in the next section), but patients may require increases in, or changes to, their analgesia to allow them to fully participate in rehabilitation. It is the responsibility of the therapist to communicate fully with the multi-professional team to enable this to happen.

Therapists are generally good listeners and take time to understand patients and when armed with the appropriate skills, are in an excellent position to help patients return to meaningful activity. It is important that both patients and other HCP recognise the value and range of therapy interventions for cancer patients and know how to access services (in a range of care settings) in a timely manner. Coordination of services is important to ensure proper handover of information and onward referral when patients move from one setting to another, e.g. hospital to hospice.

Much can be learnt from therapists who work with musculoskeletal pain and there is a plethora of literature examining the role of physiotherapy and occupational therapy for patients with benign pain. Some key messages include:

- Basic science research has shaped the development of physiotherapy practice; e.g. it is now recognised that changes within the central nervous system can contribute to pain states.
- 'Hurt' may not necessarily equate with harm – this suggests that a pain response may not be localised to the site of damage.
- Ongoing pain is unlikely to be easy to cure.
- Behaviours such as focusing on pain, worrying about it and getting distressed by it all seem to help 'imprint pain' and establish it permanently.
- Maladaption to pain may be prevented with the implementation of effective early pain management strategies (Gifford *et al.* 2005)

Therapists working with cancer patients may find some of these messages helpful but must recognise that the bulk of this work has focused on a non-cancer population.

Therapy interventions

There is currently a lack of evidence for the use of therapy interventions for patients with cancer-related pain. Current guidelines on the control of cancer pain do not adequately address therapy interventions (Scottish Intercollegiate Guidelines Network [SIGN], 2002) and research is urgently required in this field.

As discussed, AHP interventions focus on relieving pain, reducing physical limitations and improving functional ability whilst addressing psychosocial, spiritual and cultural aspects of the pain experience. Interventions can be classified as physical, psychosocial, lifestyle adjustment or educational approaches.

Physical approaches

A range of interventions are employed and include:

- Therapeutic exercise
- Graded and purposeful activity
- Postural re-education
- Massage and soft-tissue mobilisation
- Transcutaneous electrical nerve stimulation (TENS)
- Heat and cold

Some of these are traditionally administered by physiotherapists, e.g. therapeutic exercise and TENS, but other HCPs may have sufficient skills in this area, e.g. occupational therapist and clinical nurse specialists. Graded activity for return to function is inextricably linked with therapeutic exercise but may traditionally be considered the domain of the occupational therapist. When utilising these approaches, a certain amount of manual handling is required and therapists must pay special attention to patient comfort and position at all times. For this reason, position and handling are not formally discussed but therapists must always be aware of factors such as careful handling of limbs and special care of areas where sensation is altered, e.g. allodynia and the use of supports such as pillows or custom-made splints/orthoses.

An extensive review of the use of exercise is beyond the scope of this chapter but the main goal of exercise is to address the problems associated with inactivity/immobility (specific or general) and fear of movement and tackle the 'vicious cycles' that are set up (Figure 13.3). The detrimental effects of immobilisation are well documented and include muscle wasting/weakness, joint stiffness, reduced motor control, mood changes, decreased self-efficacy, reduced coping capacity and cardiovascular deconditioning. Exercise programmes must be tailored to the individual needs of the patient and should start cautiously, build up gradually and be within patients' tolerance levels. Douglas (2005) provides a review of exercise in cancer patients, which includes guidance on specific precautions. For a systematic review of exercise in cancer, see Stevinson *et al.* (2004).

Engagement in meaningful activities (which may include craft, recreation or work) has been shown to assist patients with cancer pain to improve their self-concept and attain task mastery (Kennett, 2000). Involving patients in activities that are

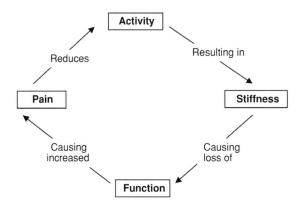

Figure 13.3 Effects of chronic pain on lifestyle, highlighting the vicious cycle that develops.

purposeful can promote movement, alter mood and act as a diversion from pain. Appropriately prescribed and graded activities, either individually or in groups, can be used to increase activity tolerance, autonomy, social integration, self-esteem and competency and decrease pain behaviours (Heck, 1988).

Postural re-education may be appropriate in patients who have altered posture or kinematics secondary to pain. For example, patients who develop chronic post-surgical pain following breast cancer treatment often adopt protective postures resulting in shoulder girdle protraction, elbow flexion, a poking chin and associated muscle spasm and muscle imbalances. It is important to attempt correction of such postural abnormalities early in rehabilitation to avoid further dysfunctional movement patterns. In head and neck patients there is growing evidence for the use of progressive resistive exercise training to manage shoulder dysfunction and pain secondary to spinal accessory nerve damage and the importance of correcting posture and scapular stability prior to resistance exercise has been documented (McNeely et al., 2004).

Soft-tissue mobilisation is widely practised in the management of pain and includes techniques such as scar mobilisation/massage, myofascial techniques and connective-tissue massage. Massage techniques are also commonly practised by complementary therapists – discussed later. An extensive review is beyond the scope of this chapter, but a wealth of information is available on such approaches (Hunter, 1994; Mannheim, 2001). There is extensive anecdotal evidence to support the use of connective-tissue techniques in a range of cancer-treatment-related musculoskeletal problems (Fourie, 2006).

TENS is a non-invasive form of electrical stimulation which has been used for many years to treat a wide range of pain problems. It is commonly used in a variety of settings and is the only form of electrotherapy which can be safely administered in cancer patients. Conventional TENS is the most common mode of delivery used in practice and should be the first treatment option in most situations. It is generally recommended to start with TENS electrodes in the painful area or an adjacent dermatome. The intensity should be 'strong but comfortable' and patients can safely increase treatment time up to several hours as long as no side effects or accommodation to treatment (i.e. the patient gets used to the sensation and benefits diminish) occur.

Although there are several systematic reviews addressing TENS use in benign pain, there is only one review available on TENS for cancer pain (Pan *et al.*, 2000). Although experts suggest that TENS has an important role, there are currently no formal guidelines on the use of TENS in cancer patients. Readers are directed to standard textbooks or online resources for full guidance on TENS use (Walsh, 1997; www.electrotherapy.org). A Cochrane review on the use of TENS in cancer pain is anticipated in Summer 2008 and may further current thinking as well as stimulate research in this field (Robb *et al.*, submitted). Only two randomised controlled trials (RCTs) evaluating TENS use in cancer-related pain have been identified (Gadsby *et al.*, 1997; Robb *et al.*, 2007) and the effectiveness of TENS remains inconclusive.

Both heat and cold have been used for centuries to manage pain and there are an increasing number of methods available for the therapist. Application of heat can be achieved from simple approaches, e.g. a hot bath to aid relaxation or more local applications such as hot packs. Cold can be delivered via ice packs and home remedies can be devised using, e.g., frozen peas. All standard contraindications and precautions must be followed and choice of treatment will depend on pain presentation and the therapeutic effects needed.

Psychosocial approaches

There is substantial evidence to suggest that psychosocial interventions are effective in the management of cancer pain (Meyer & Mark, 1995; Thomas & Weiss, 2000). Common interventions include distraction, anxiety management, relaxation and guided imagery; more sophisticated techniques such as hypnosis can be taught to patients, although specialist training is required to implement this safely. Cognitive–behavioural therapy is gaining increasing recognition amongst therapists working with cancer patients and its effectiveness for chronic (benign) pain patients is now widely recognised.

A recent pilot study investigated a cognitive–behavioural-led pain management programme for patients with chronic cancer-treatment related pain (Robb *et al.*, 2006). Although there were several limitations to this study, the findings were positive and demonstrated improvement in both physical and psychosocial functioning. Further research was recommended.

In a study using imagery and relaxation training with intermediate- to advanced-stage cancer patients, Sloman (1995) found significant improvements in intensity, severity and sensation of pain and non-opiod analgesia intake. In a similar trial considering psychological interventions for cancer pain relief, Syrjala and Chapko (1995) concluded that relaxation and imagery training and cognitive–behavioural training reduce cancer-treatment-related pain.

Educating the patient and their carers in anxiety management techniques and relaxation skills is also known to be effective in the management of pain and can assist the patient in taking control and modulating his or her own pain (Cooper, 1997).

Lifestyle adjustment. Therapists can identify and teach skills to enable a restoration of function without provoking painful episodes (Breitbart *et al.*, 2004).

Occupational therapists have a key role in teaching skills which include task adaptation, goal setting, work simplification, compensatory techniques, lifestyle management, time management, energy conservation and ergonomic principles, as well as identifying and working within pain tolerance parameters (COT, 2004; Strong & Bennett, 2002a, b).

Environment can influence occupational performance and it is essential for therapists to assess whether equipment or environmental adaptation are required. Such interventions can minimise exacerbations of pain and increase patient autonomy. Therapists may also provide advice on posture, seating, positioning and pressure care as well as the use of orthoses (e.g. collars, splints) (Cooper, 1997; COT, 2004).

Educational approaches. These include workshops or lectures targeted at HCP or patients and their caregivers. A systematic review of educational interventions for cancer pain control (Allard, 2001) included 33 studies, of which 6 were RCTs and 76% were directed as HCPs. This review concluded that educational interventions can improve pain knowledge of HCPs but do not necessarily decrease patients' pain levels. The use of pain diaries was recommended in ambulatory settings but further research was recommended to establish the effectiveness of approaches targeted at patients.

Other approaches

Patients may occasionally require advice and support for other symptoms related to pain, e.g. decreased appetite or nausea and vomiting as a result of analgesic preparations. In these instances, advice and guidance may be sought from a dietitian who can provide a full assessment and advice on nutritional intake, coping strategies etc.

Complementary and alternative medicine

There is growing interest in the use of complementary and alternative medicine (CAM) in the management of cancer-related pain. A systematic review of the use of CAM in terminally ill patients (Pan *et al.*, 2000) suggested that both acupuncture and massage may be beneficial in relieving pain in palliative care settings. An extensive overview of acupuncture for cancer pain management can be found in Filshie and Thompson (2000) and there is growing evidence for the use of acupuncture for a range of cancer-related pain conditions. Further research is required in this field but the difficulties of trial design and the importance of separating the active from the 'non-specific' effects of treatment must be recognised.

A Cochrane review (Fellowes *et al.*, 2004) concluded that massage may reduce symptoms of anxiety in cancer patients and this is important to recognise as anxiety and pain levels are often linked. An RCT by Soden *et al.*, (2004) investigated aromatherapy massage in a hospice setting and found that although there were no improvements in pain control or anxiety, sleep scores were significantly improved in the treatment group. Further research is needed to fully evaluate this intervention.

Case study 1

Mrs A was a 58-year-old woman who had undergone a wide local excision of her left breast with axillary node dissection followed by post-operative radiotherapy and tamoxifen. She developed recurrent disease and underwent a left mastectomy with latissimus dorsi flap reconstruction and implant. Mrs A lived with her partner and had given up work and all social activities due to the development of chronic cancer-treatment-related pain. She had a history of major depressive disorder but no other medical history of note. Prior to her surgery she had no pain but chest wall and breast pain started during her radiotherapy when she suffered a severe radiotherapy skin reaction. Until her second operation Mrs A had constant pain and noticed a further increase in her pain in the post-operative period. For pain control she used co-dydramol. See Table 13.2 for a summary of her clinical presentation and the resultant treatment.

Mrs A made excellent progress and after an intensive programme of rehabilitation with a multi-professional team enjoyed a return to meaningful activity with an increased capacity to manage her pain using a wide range of coping strategies.

Table 13.2 Summary of clinical presentation and the resultant treatment – Case study 1.

Main clinical findings	Treatment plan
Complete lack of understanding of the causes of her pain, confusion over explanations and advice given to her	Explanation of her reconstructive surgery, the side effects of radiation and the theory of chronic pain
General physical deconditioning secondary to depression, avoidance behaviour and underactivity	Introduction of an exercise regime with walking and pacing of activities previously enjoyed, e.g. line dancing
Decreased functional use of her left arm secondary to avoidance behaviour and underactivity	Graded exercise programme including stretches and strengthening exercises for left arm. Pacing of domestic chores
Altered posture secondary to pain and muscle spasm	Mobilisation of soft tissue and scarring. Postural advice and correction of muscle imbalance. Advice on relaxation
Strong feeling of frustration as a result of the way her pain had been managed and of the limitations pain imposed on her	Exploration and ventilation of her frustration
Clinical depression reducing self-esteem and self-confidence, limiting daily and social activities and reinforcing physical deconditioning	Introduction of goal setting and activity scheduling Identification of primary emotions and cognitive reconstructuring of underlying beliefs about her care and about her pain
Avoidance behaviour as a result of her pain and depression; daily tasks and activities, meeting people, driving her car, asking clarifications of medical information	Explanation of how these patterns contribute in maintaining her pain. Graded self-exposure
Use of analgesics as her only strategy to cope with the pain	Teaching of deep breathing relaxation, visualisation techniques and use of distraction activities

Case study 2

Mr B was a 70-year-old man with prostate cancer and bony metastatic disease in his spine and left femur. He was married and lived at home with his wife and his 25-year-old son. He had a comfortable lifestyle, a large house and a garden and his wife was his main carer. He had no community support. The Macmillan nurse referred the patient to the community physiotherapist with decreased mobility due to pain in his lumbar spine and left leg. He was taking regular morphine (orally) for his pain but had no self-management strategies in place. Managing daily tasks was becoming increasingly difficult due to pain. The main findings on assessment of Mr B were:

- Localised low back pain with associated tissue tenderness; referred (neuropathic) pain in his left leg
- Generalised muscle weakness in lower limbs
- Difficulties with sitting, standing and getting in/out of the bath
- Reduced enjoyment of previously enjoyed activities
- Increasing anxiety and low mood as a result of the above

Mr B's family was becoming increasingly upset with the deterioration in his condition. Mrs B was becoming more tired and their son was very anxious about leaving them to go back to university. When describing pain and its impact on his family, several emotions were abound, including frustration, disappointment, guilt, anxiety, loss of control and family roles.

Interventions were targeted at Mr B's main problems. An urgent referral was made to the community occupational therapist and joint sessions were organised to work on addressing the physical impairments and functional limitations. The physiotherapist taught Mr B how to use conventional TENS and recommended regular use in the painful areas. A graded exercise programme was implemented to address muscle weakness and pacing of activity was taught to address the problems sitting and standing. The physiotherapist also liaised with the community palliative care team to review Mr B's analgesic regime, in particular to consider the addition of an adjuvant drug, e.g. gabapentin to address the neuropathic pain. The occupational therapist worked with Mr. B to identify the areas of his life that he most valued and explored meaningful activities that he was keen to re-engage in. Education regrading activity, realistic goal planning, time management and prioritising valued activities was provided. Mr B worked with the occupational therapist to adapt his environment to suit his needs. Appropriate pieces of equipment were prescribed to facilitate independence, conserve energy and minimise pain on exertion. Several treatment sessions focused on the use of various relaxation and anxiety management techniques, and Mr B's family was closely involved in this. Over time, Mr B became aware of how to prioritise and plan activity and used cognitive techniques to start adapting to a different pace of lifestyle. These interventions enabled Mr B and his family to minimise his pain experience, adjust to his level of function and focus on enjoyable and valuable occupations.

Summary

Cancer-related pain is complex and multi-dimensional and requires a multidisciplinary team approach to address the many different dimensions of the pain experience. Comprehensive and timely assessment and clear communication between team members are both pivotal to a successful outcome. AHPs have an important role in patient management and have specific skills which enable them to be patient focused and holistic. AHPs utilise strategies which aim to improve patient functioning and quality of life but the challenge remains to practice in an evidence-based way.

Key learning points

- Cancer-related pain can only be effectively managed using a multi-professional approach.
- Assessment must be tailored to the individual but must include a description of the pain, responses to the pain and the impact of pain on both patient and caregivers.
- The pharmacological management of cancer-related pain is based on the WHO analgesic ladder.
- Therapy interventions should be collaborative, patient centred and should focus on improving patient function and quality of life.
- A range of therapy interventions have been utilised but there is limited evidence for many of the common treatments used.

References

Allard, P. (2001). Educational interventions to improve cancer pain control: a systematic review. *Journal of Palliative Medicine, 4* (2), 191–203.

Baptiste, S., Law, M., Pollock, N., Polatajko, H., McColl, M. A. & Carswell, A. (1993). The Canadian occupational performance measure. *World Federation of Occupational Therapy Bulletin, 28*, 47–51.

Bates, M. S., Edwards, W. T. & Anderson, K. O. (1993). Ethnocultural influences on variation in chronic pain perception. *Pain, 52*, 101–112.

Belchamber, C. A. & Gousy, M. H. (2004). Rehabilitative care in a specialist palliative day care centre: a study of patient's perspectives. *International Journal of Therapy and Rehabilitation, 11* (9), 425–434.

Bostrom, B., Sandh, M. & Lundberg, D. (2003). Cancer-related pain in palliative care: patient's perceptions of pain management. *Journal of Advanced Nursing, 45* (4), 410–419.

Breitbart, W., Payne, D. & Passik, S. D. (2004). Psychological factors in pain experience. In: D. Doyle, G. Hanks, N. Cherny & K. Calman (Eds.), *Oxford textbook of palliative medicine* (3rd ed., pp. 425–426). Oxford: Oxford Press.

Breivik, H. (2000). Nerve blocks – simple injections, epidurals, spinals and more complex blocks. In: K. H. Simpson & K. Budd (Eds.), *Cancer pain management* (pp. 84–99). Oxford: Oxford University Press.

Cancerbackup (2005). *Describing pain* [online]. Retrieved 1 November 2006 from http://cancerbackup.org.uk/resourcessupport/symptomssideeffects/pain

Caraceni, A. & Portenoy, R. K. (1999). An international survey of cancer pain characteristics and syndromes. *Pain, 82*, 263–274.

Cleeland, C. S. (1985). Measurement and prevalence of pain in cancer. *Seminars in Oncology Nursing, 1*, 87–92.

Cleeland, C. S. & Ryan, K. M. (1994). Pain assessment: global use of the brief pain inventory. *Annals of Academy of Medicine Singapore, 23* (2), 129–138.

College of Occupational Therapists [COT] (2004). HOPE: the specialist section of occupational therapists in HIV/AIDS, oncology, palliative care and education. *Occupational therapy intervention in cancer. Guidance for professionals, managers and decision makers.* London: College of Occupational Therapists.

Coluzzi, P. H. (1996). A model for pain management in terminal illness and cancer care. *The Journal of Care Management*, 2, 45–76.

Cooper, J. (Ed.) (1997). *Occupational therapy in oncology and palliative care*. Chichester: Whurr.

Douglas, E. (2005). Exercise in cancer patients. *Physical Therapy Reviews*, 10 (22), 71–88.

Fellowes, D., Barnes, K. & Wilkinson, S. (2004). Aromatherapy and massage for symptom relief in patients with cancer. *Cochrane Database of Systematic Reviews*, Issue 3.

Ferrell, B. R., Grant, M., Borneman, T., Juarez, G. & ter-Veer, A. (1999). Family caregiving in cancer pain management. *Journal of Palliative Medicine*, 2 (2), 185–195.

Filshie, J. & Thompson, J. W. (2000). Acupuncture and TENS. In: K. Simpson and K. Budd (Eds.), *Cancer pain management* (pp. 188–200). Oxford: Oxford University Press.

Foley, K. M. (2006). *Appraising the WHO analgesic ladder on it's 20th birthday: an interview with Kathleen Foley* [online]. Retrieved 16 March 2007 from http://www.whocancerpain.wisc.edu/eng/19_1/Interview.html

Fourie, W. (2006). *Understanding our connective tissue: an introduction*. Course handbook.

Gadsby, J. G., Franks, A., Jarvis, P. & Dewhurst, F. (1997). Acupuncture-like transcutaneous electrical nerve stimulation within palliative care. *Complementary Therapies in Medicine*, 5, 13–18.

Gamlin, R. & Lovel, T. (2002). *Pain explained*. Rugby: Altman.

Goudas, L., Carr, D. B., Bloch, R., Balk, E., Ioannidis, J. P. A., Terrin, N., Gialeli-Goudas, M., Chew, P. & Lau, J. (2001). *Management of cancer pain volume 1: evidence report/technology assessment* (chapter 1, p. 2) [online]. Retrieved 15 March 2007 from http://www.ncbi.nlm.nih.gov/books/bv.fcgi?rid=hstat1.section.49605

Gifford, L. Thacker, M. & Jones, M. A. (2005). Physiotherapy and pain. In: S. B. McMahon & M. Koltzenburg (Eds.), *Wall and Melzack's textbook of pain*. Edinburgh: Churchill Livingstone.

Hanks, G. W., de Conno, F., Cherny, N., Hanna, M., Kalso, E., McQuay, H. J., Mercadante, S., Meynadier, J., Poulain, P., Ripamonti, C., Radbruch, L., Roca, J., Casas, I., Sawe, J., Twycross, R. G. & Ventafridda, V. (2001). Morphine and alternative opioids in cancer pain: the EAPC recommendations. *British Journal of Cancer*, 84 (5), 587–593.

Heck, S. A. (1988). The effect of purposeful activity on pain tolerance. *The American Journal of Occupational Therapy*, 42 (9), 577–581.

Hearn, J. & Higginson, I. J. (1999). Epidemiology of pain: pain associated with cancer. In: *Task force on epidemiology*. Seattle, Washington, DC: International Association for the Study of Pain.

Hunter, G. (1994). Specific soft tissue mobilization in the treatment of soft tissue lesions. *Physiotherapy*, 80, 15–21.

International Association for the Study of Pain [IASP] (2004). *The relief of pain should be a human right* [online]. Retrieved 23 October 2006 from www.painreliefhumanright.com

Jensen, M. P. (2003). The validity and reliability of pain measures in adults with cancer. *The Journal of Pain*, 4 (1), 2–21.

Jones, M. & Rivett, D. (Eds.) (2004). *Clinical reasoning for manual therapists*. Oxford: Butterworth Heinemann.

Jung, B. F., Ahrendt, G. M., Oaklander, A. L. & Dworkin, R. H. (2003). Neuropathic pain following breast cancer surgery: proposed classification and research update. *Pain*, 104, 1–13.

Kennett, C. E. (2000). Participation in a creative arts project can foster hope in a hospice day centre. *Palliative Medicine*, 14 (5), 419–425.

Krames, E. S. (2004). Cancer pain demands an integrated approach. *Supportive Oncology*, 2 (6), 504–505.

Lin, C. C., Lai, Y. L. & Ward, S. E. (2003). Effect of cancer pain on performance status, mood states, and level of hope among Taiwanese cancer patients. *Journal of Pain and Symptom Management*, 25 (1), 29–37.

Long, A. F. & Fairfield, G. (1996). Confusion of levels in monitoring. outcomes and/or process. *Lancet*, 347, 1572.

Macrae, W. A. (2001). Chronic pain after surgery. *British Journal of Anaesthesia*, 87 (1), 88–98.

Main, C. J. & Spanswick, C. C. (2001). *Pain management: an interdisciplinary approach*. Edinburgh: Churchill Livingstone.

Mannheim, C. J. (2001). *The myofascial release manual* (3rd ed.). New Jersey: Slack Incorporated.

McNeely, M. L., Parliament, M., Courneya, C. S., Seikaly, H., Jha, N., Scrimger, R. & Hanson, J. (2004). A pilot study of a randomised controlled trial to evaluate the effects of progressive resistance exercise training on shoulder dysfunction caused by spinal accessory neurapraxia/neurectomy in head and neck cancer survivors. *Head and Neck*, 26 (6), 518–530.

Melzack, R. (1975). The McGill pain questionnaire: major properties and scoring methods. *Pain*, 1, 277–299.

Merskey, H. & Bogduk, N. (1994). Classification of chronic pain. In: *Definitions of chronic pain syndromes and definition of pain terms* (2nd ed.). Seattle, Washington, DC: International Association for the Study of Pain.

Meyer, T. J. & Mark, M. M. (1995). Effects of psychosocial interventions with adult cancer patients: a meta-analysis of randomised experiments. *Health Psychology*, 14 (2), 101–108.

Mitsuko, Y. (1997). A study of well-being and pain control in cancer patients. *Nihon Kango Kagakkaishi*, 17 (4), 56–63.

National Council for Hospice and Specialist Palliative Care Services (2003). *Guidance for managing cancer pain in adults*. London: The National Council for Palliative Care.

O'Brien, T. (1993). Symptom control. In: C. Saunders & N. Sykes (Eds.),*The management of terminal malignant disease*. London: Hodder and Stoughton.

Pan, C. X., Morrison, R. S., Ness, J., Fugh-Berman, A. & Leipzig, M. (2000). Complementary and alternative medicine in the management of pain, dyspnoea and nausea and vomiting near the end of life: a systematic review. *Journal of Pain and Symptom Management*, 20 (5), 374–387.

Robb, K., Benett, M., Johnson, M., Simpson, K. & Oxberry, S. (Submitted). TENS for cancer-related pain in adults. *Cochrane Database of Systematic Reviews*. London: Wiley-Blackwell.

Robb, K. Newham, D. & Williams, J. E. (2007b). Transcutaneous electrical nerve stimulation vs transcutaneous spinal electroanalagesia for chronic pain associated with breast cancer treatments. *Journal of Pain and Symptom Management*, 33 (4), 410–419.

Robb, K. A., Williams, J. E., Duvivier, V. & Newham, D. J. (2006). A pain management programme for chronic cancer-treatment related pain: a preliminary study. *The Journal of Pain*, 7 (2), 82–90.

Saunders, C. M. (1967). *The management of terminal illness*. London: Hospital Medical Publication.

Serlin, C., Mendoza, T. R., Nakamura, Y., Edwards, K. R. & Cleeland, C. S. (1995). When is cancer pain mild, moderate or severe? Grading pain severity by its interference with function. *Pain*, 61, 277–284.

Scottish Intercollegiate Guidelines Network [SIGN] (2002). *Control of pain in patients with cancer*. Edinburgh: Scottish Intercollegiate Guidelines Network.

Simmonds, M. (1999). Physical function and physical performance in patients with pain: what are the measures and what do they mean? In: M. Max (Ed.), *Pain 1999 – an updated review. Refresher course syllabus* (pp. 127–136). Seattle, Washington, DC: IASP Press.

Simpson, K. (2000). Philosophy of cancer pain management. In: K. Simpson and K. Budd (Eds.), *Cancer pain management: a comprehensive approach* (p. 2). Oxford: Oxford University Press.

Sloman, R. (1995). Relaxation and the relief of cancer pain. *Nursing Clinics of North America*, *30*, 697–709.

Soden, K., Vincent, K., Craske, S., Lucas, C. & Ashley, S. (2004). A randomised controlled trial of aromatherapy massage in a hospice setting. *Palliative Medicine*, *18* (2), 87–92.

Speck, P. (2002). The nature of non-physical pain. In: R. Hillier, I. Finlay & A. Miles (Eds.), *The effective management of cancer pain* (2nd ed.). London: Aesculapius Medical Press.

Stevinson, C., Lawlor, D. A. & Fox, K. R. (2004). Exercise interventions for cancer patients: a systematic review of controlled trials. *Cancer Causes Control*, *15* (10), 1035–1056.

Strong, J., Sturgess, J., Unruh, A. M., Vicenzino, B. (2002). Pain assessment and measurement. In: J. Strong, A. Unruh, A. Wright & G. Baxter (Eds.), *Pain: A textbook for therapists*. Edinburgh: Churchill Livingsstone.

Strong, J. & Bennett, S. (2002). Cancer pain. In: J. Strong, A. Unruh, A. Wright & G. Baxter (Eds.), *Pain: A textbook for therapists*. Edinburgh: Churchill Livingstone.

Syrjala, K. L. & Chapko, M. E. (1995). Evidence for a biopsychosocial model of cancer treatment-related pain. *Pain*, *61*, 69–79.

Thomas, E. M. & Weiss, S. M. (2000). Nonpharmacological interventions with chronic cancer pain in adults. *Cancer Control*, *7* (2), 157–164.

Turk, D. C., Sist, T. C., Okifuji, A., Miner, M. F., Florio, G., Harrison, P., Massey, J., Lema, M. L. & Zevon, M. A. (1998). Adaptation to metastatic cancer pain, regional/local cancer pain and non-cancer pain: role of psychological and behavioural factors. *Pain*, *74* (2–3), 247–256.

Twycross, R., Harcourt, J. & Bergl, S. (1996). A survey of pain in patients with advanced cancer. *Journal of Pain and Symptom Management*, *12* (5), 273–282.

Unruh, A. M., Strong, J. & Wright, A. (2002). Introduction to pain. In: J. Strong, A. M. Unruh, A. Wright & G. D. Baxter (Eds.), *Pain: a textbook for therapists*. Edinburgh: Churchill Livingstone.

Ventafridda, V. (1989). Continuing care a major issue in cancer pain management. *Pain*, *36*, 137–143.

Wallace, K., Reed, B., Pasero, C. & Olsson, G. L. (1995). Staff nurses' perceptions of barriers to effective pain management. *Journal of Pain and Symptom Management*, *10*, 204–213.

Walsh, D. (1997). *TENS: clinical applications and related theory* (1st ed.). London: Churchill Livingstone.

Ward, S. E., Goldberg, N., Miller-McCauley, V., Mueller, C., Nolan, A., Pawlik-Plank, D., Robbins, A., Stormoen, D. & Weissman, D. E. (1993). Patient related barriers to management of cancer pain. *Pain*, *52*, 319–324.

World Health Organization [WHO] (1986). *Cancer pain relief*. Geneva: World Health Organization.

Zaza, C. & Baine, N. (2002). Cancer pain and psychosocial factors. A critical review of the literature. *Journal of Pain and Symptom Management*, *24*, 526–542.

Zech, D. F., Grond, S., Lynch, J., Hertel, D. & Lehmann, K. A. (1995). Validation of WHO Guidelines for cancer pain relief: a 10 year prospective study. *Pain*, *63*, 65–76.

Further reading

Doyle, D., Hanks, G., Cherny, N. & Calman, K. (Eds.) (2004). *Oxford textbook of palliative medicine* (3rd ed.). Oxford: Oxford University Press.

Feuerstein, M. (Ed.) (2007). *Handbook of cancer survivorship* (chapters 9, 20). New York: Springer.

Hiller, R., Finlay, I. & Miles, A. (Eds.) (2000). *The effective management of cancer pain* (1st and 2nd ed.). London: Aesculapius Medical Press.

Simpson, K. & Budd, K. (Eds.) (2000). *Cancer pain management.* Oxford: Oxford University Press.

On-line patient resources

Cancerbackup (2005). *Describing pain* [online]. Retrieved 28 August 2007 from http://cancerbackup.org.uk/resourcessupport/symptomssideeffects/pain

National Cancer Institute (2000). *Understanding cancer pain* [online]. Retrieved 28 August 2007 from http://www.cancer.gov/PDF/d963687a-1401-43d4-a7c8-6753a3d60e1c/cancer_pain.pdf

Chapter 14

BREATHLESSNESS MANAGEMENT

Sarah Fisher and Daniel Lowrie

Learning outcomes

After reading this chapter the reader will be able to:

- Define and understand the construct of breathlessness
- Understand the causes of breathlessness in cancer
- Undertake comprehensive assessment of breathlessness
- Select and implement appropriate breathlessness interventions

---

Introduction

Breathlessness is a symptom frequently encountered by people with cancer, which often has an enormous impact on independence, confidence, self-esteem and quality of life (Hately *et al.*, 2003). It is crucial that therapists have a clear understanding of the nature of breathlessness in cancer and are confident in supporting patients to develop strategies to cope with this symptom.

There has been considerable interest over the last 15 years in the need to improve cancer-related breathlessness management, resulting in a correspondingly large volume of related published material. The emergence of non-pharmacological strategies in the management of cancer-related breathlessness has gained credence with all health professionals and has facilitated the development of breathlessness management clinics/services, often therapist led and utilising the skills of a range of multi-professional disciplines. This approach has developed the model first proposed by Corner *et al.* (1996) in which a group of lung cancer patients received weekly sessions with a nurse research practitioner over 3–6 weeks, using counselling, breathing re-training, relaxation and the teaching of coping and adaptation strategies to manage breathlessness. It was concluded that these patients benefited from this rehabilitative approach, and the strategies employed in this pilot study underwent further investigation by randomised controlled trial (Bredin *et al.*, 1999).

In cancer, breathlessness is interpreted as having a sinister significance and, therefore, may cause much more distress than the same degree of breathlessness in a non-cancer patient population. It is commonly held that in comparison with pain, breathlessness causes more anxiety in health professionals and is less easily managed.

Patients can detect this lack of professional confidence, which can contribute to their distress. This chapter presents an overview of the key themes related to the management of breathlessness for people with cancer. It considers the causes of breathlessness in cancer, the effective assessment of the breathless patient and a range of strategies that can assist in the management of this symptom.

Definition of breathlessness

Breathlessness is recognised as being a difficult construct to define, as an individual's experience is often unreflective of the apparent medical causes underlying the symptom (Regnard & Ahmedzai, 1990). A useful attempt at defining breathlessness is offered by the American Thoracic Society (1999, p. 322) that describes it as:

A term used to characterise a subjective experience of breathing discomfort that consists of qualitatively distinct sensations that vary in intensity. The experience derives from interactions among multiple physiological, psychological, social and environmental factors, and may induce secondary physiological and behavioural responses.

It is apparent from this definition that breathlessness is a multi-factorial symptom that will be interpreted uniquely by the individuals who experience it. It is also clear that the way in which people respond to an episode of breathlessness may vary in terms of their physiological response, feelings and behaviours. Because of this, for effective breathlessness management to occur, it is important that a holistic approach is adopted in which the emotional, sensory and biological elements of breathlessness are acknowledged and addressed in an integrated manner (Corner & O'Driscoll, 1999). The traditional biomedical model has its limitations; challenging this model allows a view of the total experience of breathlessness (Figure 14.1).

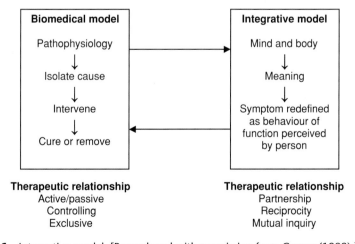

Figure 14.1   Integrative model. [Reproduced with permission from Corner (1998).]

In order to be able to manage breathlessness it is necessary to have an under-standing of the numerous phenomena that may cause or exacerbate the symptom. Whilst a unitary description of the precise mechanisms underlying breathlessness does not exist, a number of important potential mechanisms have been suggested. The American Thoracic Society (1999) states that the sensation of breathlessness results when there is an imbalance between respiratory motor activity and afferent feedback from chemoreceptors in the brain and arteries and/or mechanoreceptors or irritant receptors in the airways, lungs and chest wall. Research suggests that these different physiological mechanisms may give rise to qualitatively different sensations of breathlessness. For example receptors in the lung and parenchyma trigger a feeling of chest tightness; chemoreceptors cause a sensation of air hunger and information from the motor cortex or brain stem results in a sense of effort to breathe (Beach & Schwartzsein, 2006). Knowledge of the different mechanisms of breathlessness and the distinct sensations that result can be crucial to the recommendation of appropriate management strategies (Beach & Schwartzsein, 2006).

Causes of breathlessness in cancer

It is generally recognised that breathlessness is highly likely to occur in people with lung cancer; however, it should be remembered that large numbers of people with other cancer diagnoses also experience the symptom. This is often as a result of fac-tors such as lung or mediastinal metastases or radiotherapy fields overlapping the lung and causing pneumonitis leading to fibrosis (Dudgeon et al., 2001a). Estimates of the prevalence of breathlessness among people with cancer vary considerably de-pending on variables including diagnosis and disease stage. A study of 923 cancer outpatients conducted by Dudgeon et al. (2001b) found that breathlessness occurred in 49.1% of this group. Research suggests that as an individual's cancer progresses, the likelihood of breathlessness occurring increases (Potter et al., 2003). One investi-gation, examining the incidence of breathlessness in people with cancer during the last 6 weeks of life, identified breathlessness in 70.2% of this population (Reuben & Mor, 1986). Another study found breathlessness to occur in 78% of people with advanced lung cancer (Edmonds et al., 2001).

Breathlessness in the cancer patient has four main causal factors: the cancer itself; a result of cancer treatment; other concurrent conditions, e.g. chronic obstructive pulmonary disease (COPD), heart failure and general debilitation as a result of sys-temic illness; and the individuals perception of breathlessness including anxiety and behavioural response to the symptom (Manning & Schwartzstein, 1995). Figure 14.2 summarises the major causes of breathlessness and links them with the mechanism of pathophysiology on which they impact to produce a breathlessness response.

Assessment of breathlessness

The key to the successful management of breathlessness lies with skilled assessment and analysis of the assessment. Due to the complex nature of the mechanisms causing

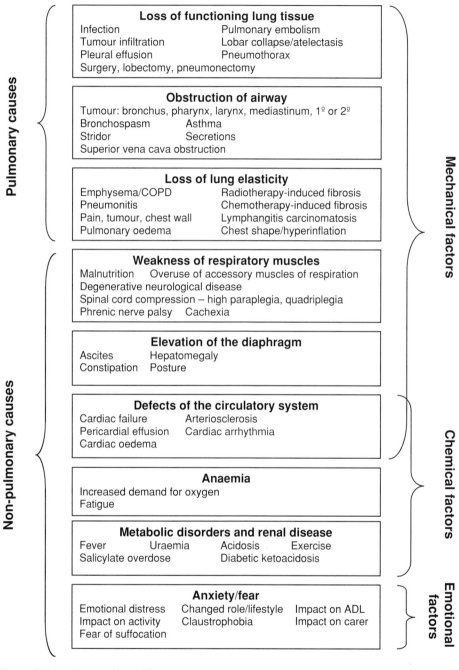

Pulmonary causes

Loss of functioning lung tissue
Infection   Pulmonary embolism
Tumour infiltration   Lobar collapse/atelectasis
Pleural effusion   Pneumothorax
Surgery, lobectomy, pneumonectomy

Obstruction of airway
Tumour: bronchus, pharynx, larynx, mediastinum, 1º or 2º
Bronchospasm   Asthma
Stridor   Secretions
Superior vena cava obstruction

Loss of lung elasticity
Emphysema/COPD   Radiotherapy-induced fibrosis
Pneumonitis   Chemotherapy-induced fibrosis
Pain, tumour, chest wall   Lymphangitis carcinomatosis
Pulmonary oedema   Chest shape/hyperinflation

Non-pulmonary causes

Weakness of respiratory muscles
Malnutrition   Overuse of accessory muscles of respiration
Degenerative neurological disease
Spinal cord compression – high paraplegia, quadriplegia
Phrenic nerve palsy   Cachexia

Elevation of the diaphragm
Ascites   Hepatomegaly
Constipation Posture

Defects of the circulatory system
Cardiac failure   Arteriosclerosis
Pericardial effusion   Cardiac arrhythmia
Cardiac oedema

Anaemia
Increased demand for oxygen
Fatigue

Metabolic disorders and renal disease
Fever   Uraemia   Acidosis   Exercise
Salicylate overdose   Diabetic ketoacidosis

Anxiety/fear
Emotional distress   Changed role/lifestyle   Impact on ADL
Impact on activity   Claustrophobia   Impact on carer
Fear of suffocation

Mechanical factors

Chemical factors

Emotional factors

Figure 14.2 Causes of breathlessness.

breathlessness, it is unlikely that any one professional will be able to undertake the whole assessment on his/her own. The broad scope of the multidisciplinary team is essential to gain full understanding of the patient's condition and breathlessness response.

Numerous unidimensional and multi-dimensional breathlessness assessment tools have been developed that may, in some instances, assist in investigating and monitoring the nature and intensity of breathlessness. Carrieri-Kohlman and Dudgeon (2006) present an analysis of the validity, reliability, responsiveness and clinical utility of a range of such instruments, including the visual analogue scale (VAS), modified Borg scale, numeric rating scale and cancer dyspnoea scale (CDS), that may be used with people with cancer. Therapists considering the use of formalised breathlessness assessment measures are directed to this reference for further reading.

Breathlessness assessment must be holistic and cover the key domains of physical, social and occupational, spiritual and psychological needs. Medical and physical assessment is essential to identify any reversible causes of breathlessness that will respond to appropriate medical intervention. Reversible causes of breathlessness such as congestive heart failure, exacerbation of COPD, cardiac arrhythmias, anaemia, pleural/pericardial effusion, bronchial infection and pulmonary emboli should be treated where appropriate.

Observation skills are extremely important when assessing the breathless patient. Initial observation of many aspects of respiratory function can be made before the patient is aware of the therapist's presence (Figure 14.3). This yields a rich source of information that can enable the skilled therapist to further investigate specific problems that will require more detailed assessment; e.g. the posture adopted by a patient may suggest fatigue, pain or respiratory distress.

Breathing rate	Breathing pattern	Rhythm	Use of pursed lip breathing	Use of accessory muscles
Chest wall movement	Chest shape	Bone metastases	Breath holding	Abdominal splinting
Breath sounds	Audible wheeze or rattle	Expectoration of secretions	Cough	Stridor
Posture including kyphosis and scoliosis	Positioning	Breathlessness at rest	Breathlessness on exertion	Exercise tolerance
Frequency of sighing or yawning	Fatigue	Sleep pattern	Level of restlessness or agitation	
Surgery	Pain	SVCO	Colour	

Figure 14.3 Physical factors to consider in respiratory assessment.

It is essential that the process of assessment incorporates an investigation of the potential psychological, spiritual and social dimensions of the symptom (Booth & Dudgeon, 2006). Corner and O'Driscoll (1999) propose a range of questions that should be included within a holistic breathlessness assessment for people with cancer. These include examination of the patterns of breathlessness (timing and frequency), the patient's perception of the severity and distress caused by their breathlessness, breathlessness triggers, impact on daily living and feelings associated with breathlessness. This information is crucial in helping a breathless person and his/her family to develop the strategies required to take increased control of the symptom. As such, these aspects of assessment constitute an intrinsic part of breathlessness management education (discussed later in this chapter).

Many patients will have pre-established coping mechanisms for their breathlessness, some of which may be helpful, whilst others are counterproductive. For example routine avoidance of particular activities due to the fear of breathlessness can result in anxiety, which may increase the frequency and severity of breathlessness episodes (Powell, 2000). It is an important part of assessment that therapists spend time with patients examining their coping strategies in order to determine which strategies are likely to be of ongoing benefit and which may have the potential to cause problems in the future.

It can be beneficial for the patient's family and carers to be actively involved in the breathlessness assessment process. The experience of watching a loved one struggle with breathlessness can result in feelings of fear, helplessness and guilt. Providing people close to the patient with the opportunity to discuss their own thoughts, feelings and experiences related to the patient's breathlessness can help to ensure that the needs of this vulnerable group are also acknowledged and addressed. Furthermore, the involvement of family and carers in the assessment and management process can increase the scope and reliability of information that is gathered and help to promote the recall of, and compliance with, recommended interventions.

Breathlessness management

A non-pharmacological approach to breathlessness management has emerged from the shift in understanding breathlessness as a symptom of physical dimension to one that is multi-dimensional. This has facilitated a change in the model of care from a drug-therapy-centred approach to a biopsychosocial and 'patient empowerment' approach. However, it is essential that all reversible causes of breathlessness be optimally managed by appropriate medical treatment.

Medical intervention

Medical intervention to provide symptomatic relief may include radiotherapy or chemotherapy, the effectiveness of which is determined by the histological type of lung cancer and its sensitivity to such treatment. The reader is referred to texts such as Souhami and Tobias (2003), who describe, in detail, the oncological management of lung cancer.

Other symptoms may be relieved by appropriate medical intervention and thereby assist in the holistic management of breathlessness. Common problems and their management are considered briefly:

- There may be an element of reversible bronchoconstriction, even in the absence of obvious wheeze and the use of bronchodilators via inhalers and nebulisers may be indicated.
- Reduction of peritumour oedema may improve breathlessness due to multiple lung metastases and lymphangitis carcinomatosa. To achieve this, corticosteroids may be used.
- Morphine reduces inappropriate and excessive respiratory drive and substantially reduces the ventilatory response to hypoxia and hypercapnia. By slowing respiration, breathing is made more efficient and the sensation of breathlessness is reduced. Nebulised morphine is used in some units, but its effects have been shown to be equal to that of nebulised saline (Boyd & Kelly, 1997).
- Panic with hyperventilation and the fear of suffocation will worsen breathlessness. The use of a benzodiazepine will assist in producing a sedative and muscle relaxant effect to combat this very distressing experience.
- Oxygen (O_2) is often helpful only if there is hypoxia and cyanosis. Ideally, pulse oximetry should be used to confirm hypoxia and an improvement in O_2 saturation with treatment. O_2 may help in sudden episodes of hyperventilation due, for instance, to panic, pulmonary oedema or pulmonary embolus and may be of benefit in COPD or lymphangitis. The risks of narcosis with O_2 in patients with COPD must not be forgotten. Carbon dioxide (CO_2) retention is a pathophysiological process in which too little CO_2 is removed from the blood by the lungs. The end result is hypercapnia, an elevated level of CO_2 dissolved in the bloodstream. Various diseases may lead to this state; disturbed gas exchange may lead to impaired excretion of the gas. The principal result of the increased amount of dissolved CO_2 is acidosis (respiratory acidosis, when caused by impaired lung function). As CO_2 levels increase, patients exhibit a reduction in overall level of consciousness as well as respiratory effort (narcosis). Severe increases in CO_2 levels can lead to respiratory arrest.
- Nebulised saline may be helpful in loosening secretions. Mucolytics can also aid expectoration; however, some patients find the increase in sputum distressing. Infection should be treated with the judicious use of antibiotics.
- A pleural effusion should be confirmed radiographically. The relative contribution of the pleural effusion to breathlessness needs to be assessed on an individual basis, the goal of drainage being to improve symptoms. The clinician needs to balance the possible benefits of pleural aspiration with the potential burden and risks of the procedure. At different points along the disease journey, the clinician may judge the appropriateness of intervention for drainage of a similar effusion volume differently. For the patient at an earlier stage in the course of the disease, pleurodesis or other surgical techniques may be appropriate for longer term control.

Non-pharmacological intervention

A wide variety of non-pharmacological breathlessness management strategies have been shown to be useful in supporting patients to manage their experience of breathlessness. These strategies are of particular importance when the physiological causes of breathlessness cannot be fully addressed through the use of pharmacological and/or medical interventions (Carrieri-Kohlman, 2006). The evidence supporting the use of non-pharmacological breathlessness interventions in cancer care will be explored in the remainder of this chapter.

Therapists should be aware that a 'recipe book' approach to non-pharmacological breathlessness management is unlikely to be effective and may, in some instances, be counterproductive. The specific interventions that are likely to be of most benefit to breathless patients may change over time, depending on factors such as stage of their illness, emotional state or social situation and, therefore, need to be customised to cater to individual patient's needs (Thompson et al., 2005).

It has been suggested that in the early stages of breathlessness, interventions focusing on education regarding personal coping strategies may be the most appropriate way of supporting patients, without overburdening them with concerns for their future. As disease progresses, the provision of support to adapt to loss of functioning, combined with strategies to improve comfort and independence through breathing retraining, activity modification and anxiety management, may become indicated. During the later stages of illness, existential issues may need to be explored with patients. At this time, increased attention to compensatory strategies, with the goal of promoting opportunities for fulfilment and maximising quality of life, may be beneficial (Thompson et al., 2005).

Non-pharmacological approaches can be used to reduce the sensation and impact of breathlessness in a number of different ways. Some strategies (such as breathing retraining, positioning and carefully graded exercise) are used to alter the physiological mechanisms that trigger or exacerbate breathlessness. Cognitive–behavioural approaches (including education, relaxation and improving symptom awareness) are hypothesised to improve the experience of breathlessness by reducing the cortical perception of the symptom. The impact of breathlessness on patient's lives can also be reduced by altering environments and routines through the use of interventions such as energy conservation, modifications to activities or routines and the provision of practical support with activities of daily living (Carrieri-Kohlman, 2006).

Strategies to alter the physiological mechanisms that trigger breathlessness

The aims of breathing retraining are to reduce the work of breathing and give patients confidence in their ability to control breathlessness episodes. A minimal approach should be adopted when intervening in a person's pattern of breathing. It is worth remembering that the patient has a pathophysiological reason to be breathless and that the goal of preventing a patient from ever being breathless is extremely unrealistic. Rather, the patient's goals should be around the development of coping strategies to manage and adapt to being breathless and the changes to lifestyle this might necessitate. An efficient breathing pattern will maximise lung capacity, and therefore oxygenation, reduce effort and anxiety and, as a consequence, facilitate a reduction in respiratory rate that occurs naturally and is not imposed. Careful use of language and instructions is essential to achieve a good result. If the patient has a high respiratory rate and shallow apical breathing pattern, being told to relax and take a slow, deep breath is likely to have the opposite effect to that desired. If the patient attempts to follow this instruction, he/she will override the physiologically driven respiratory rate and slow down the rate of breathing, reducing the availability of O_2 by reducing the volume of air available for gaseous exchange. The chemoreceptors will respond by re-establishing the fast respiratory rate in an attempt to increase oxygenation and the patient may well experience an increase in distress and breathlessness. The following steps can be followed to avoid this scenario (Figure 14.4).

During this sequence, breathing usually becomes slower and deeper naturally and there is a corresponding reduction in energy expenditure. This may take some time to achieve and the therapist must recognise the value of not rushing the process,

Step 1	Assist the patient to achieve a supported position of comfort, e.g. sitting upright in a chair or forward-lean sitting
Step 2	Encourage patients to become aware of their breathing by bringing their attention to their breathing pattern. Are they breathing apically, abdominally, with pursed lips and forced expiration? Are they using their nose or mouth? Also bring their awareness to the rate of their breathing. Do not attempt to change their respiratory rate, avoid use of words such as 'slow' or 'deep'
Step 3	Relaxation is then encouraged. Start by raising awareness of tense areas such as shoulder girdle, jaw, and hands. Remember at this point, patients may not be able to relax their shoulder girdle, as they need their accessory muscles to breathe. It is useful to demonstrate a relaxed posture and the therapist's own calm voice and breathing pattern will help reduce the patient's tension. Some patients find that gentle stroking of their back or shoulder girdle at the rate of their breathing can be helpful
Step 4	Comfortable, relaxed lower chest breathing can then be facilitated at the patient's rate of breathing by encouraging them to make expiration longer than inspiration. Breathing in gently through the nose and out through the mouth can assist this; however, mouth breathing is fine if the patient is unable to cope with breathing through their nose. It may be helpful for the patient to place their hands at the base of their ribs anteriorly in order to feel the diaphragmatic movement on inspiration and expiration. Patients may then be able to develop an abdominal pattern of breathing and/or raise their resting lung volume
Step 5	Relaxation is then rechecked. The shoulder girdle may now be able to relax as abdominal breathing has replaced the need for recruitment of accessory muscles. Give lots of positive feedback

Figure 14.4 A step-by-step approach to breathing retraining. [Adapted from Hough (1996).]

progressing at a pace comfortable to the patient and going back a step as required (Hough, 1996).

Positioning is fundamental to achieving a reduction in breathlessness and many breathless people automatically adopt a posture that eases their breathing. The following are examples of helpful positions:

- High side lying
- Sitting upright in a chair with feet, back and arms supported
- Forward lean sitting with arms resting on pillows on a table
- Standing relaxed, leaning forward with arms resting on a support such as a windowsill
- Standing relaxed, leaning backwards against a wall with the legs slightly apart, chest forward and relaxed, arms hanging

Individuals should experiment with different positions to find what suits them best and which to adopt for different situations. Some may find forward leaning positions claustrophobic (Hough, 1996).

Exercise is widely recognised as a beneficial tool in managing breathlessness for a variety of reasons. Patients will demonstrate improved cardiovascular fitness and muscle strength with regular specific exercise activity. Exercise also impacts positively on the sense of well-being, with reduced anxiety and depression being consistently reported and greater than any objective change. In addition, activity provides mechanical input that eases the perception of breathlessness. Improved posture and rhythmic coordination leads to a more efficient walking pattern. Exercise reduces blood pressure and risk of chest infection and promotes relaxation and sleep (Casaburi, 1992).

Patients should set their own goals and each exercise programme should be individually planned, acceptable to the patient, accessible, safe, show tangible benefits and be able to be maintained unsupervised at home. During activity patients should be discouraged from talking, rushing or breath-holding which can disturb the breathing pattern. They should be encouraged to maintain a rhythmic quality of movement, undertaking an aerobic type of exercise that should relate to their lifestyle, e.g. walking, stair climbing, static cycle or treadmill. A circuit of exercises, incorporating both mobility and strength, can be enjoyable and beneficial, utilising all the major muscle groups for maximum effect. Exercise can be increased gradually by maintaining breathlessness at a constant tolerable level while energy output gradually increases. It is important to avoid distress when progressing exercise and to set achievable goals (Hough, 1996).

Strategies to alter the central perception of breathlessness

People's perception of breathlessness will be affected by a number of factors, including their expectations, emotional state and behavioural response to the symptom. Individuals who feel unable to control breathlessness episodes and are constantly focused on, or in fear of, the symptom are likely to experience sensations of breathlessness disproportionate to the level of their actual physiological need (The

American Thoracic Society, 1999). Strategies aimed at improving the cognitive perception of, and behavioural response to, breathlessness can therefore be of considerable value.

The links between breathlessness and anxiety in people with cancer have been demonstrated in numerous studies (Bruera *et al.*, 2000; Chan *et al.*, 2005; Chiu *et al.*, 2004; Dudgeon *et al.*, 2001a; Dudgeon & Lertzman, 1998; Tanaka *et al.*, 2002). Anxiety can lead to increases in the fear and distress associated with breathlessness, thereby negatively effecting confidence in the ability to cope with the symptom (The American Thoracic Society, 1999). Given this, the incorporation of anxiety management strategies constitutes an important element of the breathlessness management advice provided by allied health professionals (AHPs). One of the most valuable approaches to anxiety management, associated with breathlessness, involves exploring the meaning and fears that patients associate with the symptom. Many people with cancer relate their breathlessness to negative phenomena such as loss of role, disease progression or even death (O'Driscoll *et al.*, 1999). Facilitating individuals with a history of breathlessness to explore their personal meanings associated with the symptom can help them to reduce feelings of isolation and offer a useful vehicle to vent fears.

Therapists can help patients to combat the effect of negative thought patterns that accompany a breathlessness episode, by working with them to develop 'safe' thoughts aimed at re-establishing a sense of control. Safe thoughts should be aimed at promoting a sense of positive re-enforcement and may include phrases such as 'I am relaxed', 'I can manage this' or 'I have got through this before' (Ewer-Smith, 2002, cited in Cooper, 2006).

For some patients, the presence of anxiety can exacerbate the physiological sensation of breathlessness, by triggering a state of overbreathing associated with the fight-or-flight response (known as hyperventilation syndrome). This 'overbreathing' leads to excessive expulsion of CO_2 from the body, which reduces arterial PCO_2 (partial pressure of CO_2) and increases the alkalinity of the blood plasma (Payne, 2000). These blood chemistry changes can result in a number of uncomfortable symptoms, including dizziness, headaches, paraesthesia, chest pain, palpitations and blurred vision. People frequently experiencing these symptoms become even more anxious and thus a vicious breathlessness, anxiety, breathlessness cycle ensues (Payne, 2000). For many patients this situation can be improved through the use of simple breathing exercises aimed at ensuring a gentle, controlled-out breath in order to restabilise the CO_2 concentrations in the blood. It is important to note that this approach to management should be adopted cautiously when working with patients with very advanced disease for whom rapid, shallow, apical breathing may constitute their ideal compensatory pattern to maximise respiration.

Relaxation is a useful tool in managing the perception of breathlessness. The body's physiological response to relaxation includes a reduction in respiratory rate, O_2 use and CO_2 production (Gosselink, 2003). Additionally, the use of relaxation can help in controlling unwanted, negative thoughts that would otherwise exacerbate anxiety and breathlessness (Payne, 2000). Research has demonstrated the potential benefit of relaxation techniques as part of a package of breathlessness management interventions for people with cancer. Both Corner *et al.* (1996) and Bredin *et al.* (1999) found progressive muscular relaxation assisted in the management of breathlessness. There are currently no published studies demonstrating the benefits of other relaxation techniques (such as guided visualisation, passive neuromuscular relaxation or autosuggestion) in reducing breathlessness in people with cancer; however, anecdotal evidence would suggest some benefit.

The use of distraction has also been proposed as a method of altering the perception of breathlessness. Strategies for distraction should be reflective of specific patient's interests and needs, such as watching television, listening to music, reading and praying (Carrieri-Kohlman, 2006). One study has demonstrated the short-term benefit of the use of music in reducing the sensation of breathlessness in people with COPD (Bauldoff *et al.*, 2002). No published research exists which demonstrates the specific efficacy of distraction techniques in cancer-related breathlessness. However, anecdotal evidence would again support their value.

It has been reported that exposure to cool flowing air on the face, e.g. through the use of a fan, can help to reduce the sensation of breathlessness. It is hypothesised that this occurs through the stimulation of the trigeminal nerve, which alters the afferent feedback processed in the brain (The American Thoracic Society, 1999). This can be of considerable value in that it is virtually cost free, can be easily implemented in almost any setting and is unlikely to cause unwanted side effects (Carrieri-Kohlman, 2006).

The provision of appropriately timed education in breathlessness management strategies can be of significant benefit by helping patients feel in control. A recent study found that people with lung cancer who received support and advice at a physiotherapy-led breathlessness clinic experienced reduced feelings of distress and a greater sense of control. This clinic offered education regarding breathing retraining, relaxation and activity pacing as well as the provision of psychosocial support (Hately *et al.*, 2003). Earlier research investigating nurse-led programmes also demonstrated positive benefits (Bredin *et al.*, 1999; Corner *et al.*, 1996). Based on the success of these programmes in helping to reduce psychosocial distress and improve functioning and quality of life, it is evident that the provision of education constitutes a key element of breathlessness management. Whilst it may not always be practical to establish clinics focused solely on breathlessness management (Johnson & Moore, 2003), positive outcomes can be gained by AHPs incorporating information and support as part of a holistic, person-centred approach to rehabilitation.

Assisting patients to develop an awareness of the factors that precipitate a breathlessness episode can enable them to develop increased feelings of control over their breathlessness and utilise personal coping strategies more efficiently and effectively (Bredin *et al.*, 1999). For example establishing an understanding of the patterns, duration and frequency of breathlessness episodes may help a patient to plan activities so as to minimise the functional impact of the symptom and ensure that adequate support is available when needed. Similarly, the identification of key breathlessness triggers (such as activities, thoughts or worries) can be useful in trying to prevent breathlessness episodes and is the first stage in empowering the individual to manage the anxiety that may cause or exacerbate the symptom (Powell, 2000).

Minimising the impact of breathlessness on people's lives

Numerous strategies can be utilised to help reduce the impact of breathlessness on people's ability to engage in valued activities. Energy conservation techniques such as task simplification can be of value in reducing the ventilatory requirements required to carry out an activity (Jantarakupt & Porock, 2005). Positioning objects, so as to avoid unnecessary walking or high or low reaching, offer simple examples as to how this can be achieved. The use of equipment to reduce energy consumption during activities such as showering or food preparation can also be considered. For some patients it may be beneficial for assistance to be arranged for these tasks (Cooper, 2006). Activity pacing has been found to be helpful in reducing the incidence and severity of breathlessness (Hochstetter *et al.*, 2005). This can be achieved by balancing activities, or components of activities, that require high use of energy with periods of rest and planning routines to ensure that tasks are spread throughout the day.

It is important that opportunities for breathless patients to lead fulfilled, meaningful lives are maximised at all stages of the cancer journey. Working with patients to establish rehabilitation priorities focused on goals that are important to them can help them to develop a sense of mastery over the symptom. Depending on individual patient's needs and wishes, therapists may be required to balance rehabilitative and compensatory approaches to promote the achievement of goals. For example rehabilitation to increase activity tolerance may assist some patients to achieve goals such as outdoors mobility or socialisation, whereas other patients with more advanced disease may be able to achieve similar goals through the provision of a wheelchair and O_2.

Conclusion

In recent years there have been significant advances in the treatment of the symptom of breathlessness in cancer and palliative care. Despite this, breathlessness remains a major source of morbidity for patients with progressive disease and a major cause of anxiety for their carers, representing a considerable challenge to the multidisciplinary team. Adapting to breathlessness is about coping with the frustration and distress caused by the loss of function, and setting a positive re-adaptation programme covering all domains of care, physical, social, occupational, spiritual and psychological. The skill of the therapist working with patients experiencing the very distressing symptom of breathlessness lies in walking the line between adapting to loss and positively readapting.

Case study

Mary, a 52-year-old woman, presented with locally advanced non-small-cell lung cancer following an episode of haemoptysis and a short history of weight loss, fatigue and feeling generally unwell. On diagnosis of lung cancer, she was also found to have widespread bony metastases and was short of breath on exertion. The lung tumour was irradiated to control the haemoptysis, but following this, her breathlessness symptoms became much more severe. Her performance status was poor and she opted to decline chemotherapy. On referral for breathlessness management, Mary was angry and shocked by her diagnosis, having been previously fit and well. Her main concern and goal was to attend her son's wedding, which was 2 months away. She was highly anxious about her life expectancy in relation to this event and felt profoundly unable to cope with the significant change in her physical status. A multidisciplinary approach was employed, in a step-by-step method, to accommodate her information needs and prevent overloading with too many strategies too quickly. The physiotherapist was appointed as her key worker and coordinated the care package that was delivered in a specialist cancer and palliative care community day unit.

Initially, Mary agreed to see the counsellor for help with coping with her diagnosis and her fears for the future. She was encouraged to redirect her anger towards more positive outcomes using cognitive–behavioural techniques that facilitated appropriate goal setting and enabled her to address unhelpful thoughts. Working with the counsellor, the physiotherapist and occupational therapist introduced practical skills to empower her to take control of her breathing. Breathing retraining, management of breathlessness on exertion and coping with fatigue were key elements. Task analysis, pacing and planning of activities were implemented and Mary began to realise that she could achieve the activities that were important to her by adjusting the methods she employed to do them.

A significant breakthrough in this adjustment process came after Mary attended the wedding rehearsal. At this time, she realised that she could not cope with all the excitement of the big day, with the distances needing to be covered from the car park to the church porch and then down the long isle inside the church, as well as maintain the social conversations required from the mother of the groom. The minister was extremely helpful, and simple problem solving was applied to the key issues. A sticking point for Mary had been the proposal of using a wheelchair for longer periods of activity. Her mobility was impaired only by her degree of breathlessness on exertion, so she reluctantly agreed to use a wheelchair to get from the car to the church porch, in her view a means to an end, in reality a significant step in her rehabilitation process. The minister opened the church on several occasions so that problem solving was applied to the real environment.

It was subsequently discovered that the aisle was too long for Mary to walk down and arrive at her seat in a non-distressed state. Despite the fact that she applied breathing control and pacing techniques very effectively, her condition was deteriorating steadily and her exercise tolerance was extremely poor. A compromise was reached by her entering the church through a side door, reducing the distance she would have to walk. Key friends and relatives were recruited to sit at specific locations along the aisle, so that Mary could stop by a friendly face as she employed her pacing and breathing control strategies as she walked to her seat on the arm of her husband, without being thought rude or having to explain herself. Her determination to appear as normal as possible in the church and to be in a fit state to enjoy the service was paramount to her emotional and psychological well-being. The minister was able to overcome her mistrust of religion and facilitate a profound shift in Mary's acknowledgement of her spiritual pain, which presented as anger and, at times, despair. Mary was observed to be far less anxious and agitated, with improved breathing, after a session with the minister.

All other symptom management issues were continually monitored and addressed by the palliative care team, e.g. pain, nausea and constipation. On the day of the wedding, Mary achieved her goals, following with military precision, the plans to enable her to walk to her seat. She participated fully in the service, singing the hymns and conversing without distress. She died 3 days later, supported at home by her family and the hospice at home team.

Key learning points

- A comprehensive understanding of the pathophysiology, causes and triggers of breathlessness and its impact on the patient's psychosocial functioning is essential to effective management.
- Skilled and comprehensive assessment is vital to holistic management, enabling the patient to develop the skills and coping strategies necessary for them to gain control of their breathlessness.
- Practical techniques such as breathing retraining, pacing and energy conservation as well as psychological management are intrinsic to supporting adaptation to a changed physical status resulting from breathlessness.
- A patient-centred multidisciplinary rehabilitative approach to addressing the many issues raised by the patient's experience of breathlessness is necessary for appropriate goal setting and attainment.

References

Bauldoff, G. S., Hoffman, L. A., Zullo, T. G. & Sciurba, F. C. (2002). Exercise maintenance following pulmonary rehabilitation: effect of distractive stimuli. *Chest, 122* (3), 948–954.

Beach, D. & Schwartzsein, R. M. (2006). The genesis of breathlessness. What do we understand? In: S. Booth & D. Dudgeon (Eds.), *Dyspnoea in advanced disease. A guide to clinical management.* Oxford: Oxford University Press.

Booth, S. & Dudgeon, D. (2006). A palliative approach to the breathless patient. In: S. Booth & D. Dudgeon (Eds.), *Dyspnoea in advanced disease. A guide to clinical management.* Oxford: Oxford University Press.

Boyd, K. J. & Kelly, M. (1997). Oral morphine as symptomatic treatment of dyspnoea in patients with advanced cancer. *Palliative Medicine, 11* (4), 277–281.

Bredin, M., Corner, J., Krishnasamy, M., Plant, H., Bailey, C. & A'Hern, R. (1999). Multicentre randomised controlled trial of nursing intervention for breathlessness in patients with lung cancer. *British Medical Journal, 318*, 901–906.

Bruera, E., Schmitz, B., Pither, J., Neumann, C. M. & Hanson, J. (2000). The frequency and correlates of dyspnoea in patients with advanced cancer. *Journal of Pain and Symptom Management, 19* (5), 357–362.

Carrieri-Kohlman, V. (2006). Non-pharmacological approaches. In: S. Booth & D. Dudgeon (Eds.), *Dyspnoea in advanced disease. A guide to clinical management.* Oxford: Oxford University Press.

Carrieri-Kohlman, V. & Dudgeon, D. (2006). Multidimensional assessment of dyspnoea. In: S. Booth & D. Dudgeon (Eds.), *Dyspnoea in advanced disease. A guide to clinical management.* Oxford: Oxford University Press.

Casaburi, R. (1992). Principles of exercise training. *Chest, 101*, 263S–275S.

Chan, C. W. H., Richardson, A. & Richardson, J. (2005). A study to assess the existence of the symptom cluster of breathlessness, fatigue and anxiety in patients with advanced lung cancer. *European Journal of Oncology Nursing, 9*, 325–333.

Chiu, T. Y., Hu, W. Y., Lue, B. H., Yao, C. A., Chen, C. Y. & Wakai, S. (2004). Dyspnoea and its correlates in Taiwanese patients with terminal cancer. *Journal of Pain and Symptom Management, 28* (2), 123–132.

Cooper, J. (Ed.) (2006). *Occupational therapy in oncology and palliative care* (2nd ed.). Chichester: John Wiley and Sons Ltd.

Corner, J. (1998). *The 4th Oxford Seminar in Palliative Care Therapeutics: Breathlessness,* CLIP Update Service March 1998. StOswald's Hospice, Newcastle, Hochland & Hochland Ltd, p. 31.

Corner, J. & O'Driscoll, M. (1999). Development of a breathlessness assessment guide for use in palliative care. *Palliative Medicine, 13,* 375–384.

Corner, J., Plant, H., A'Hern, R. & Bailey, C. (1996). Non-pharmacological intervention for breathlessness in lung cancer. *Palliative Medicine, 10,* 299–305.

Dudgeon, D. J., Kristjanson, L., Sloan, J. A., Lertzman, M. & Clement, K. (2001b). Dyspnoea in cancer patients: prevalence and associated factors. *Journal of Pain and Symptom Management, 21* (2), 95–102.

Dudgeon, D. J. & Lertzman, M. (1998). Dyspnoea in the advanced cancer patient. *Journal of Pain and Symptom Management, 16* (4), 212–219.

Dudgeon, D. J., Lertzman, M. & Askew, G. R. (2001a). Physiological changes and clinical correlations of dyspnoea in cancer outpatients. *Journal of Pain and Symptom Management, 21* (5), 373–379.

Edmonds, P., Karlsen, S. & Addington-Hall, J. (2001). A comparison of the palliative care needs of patients dying from chronic respiratory diseases and lung cancer. *Palliative Medicine, 15* (4), 287–295.

Ewer-Smith, C. (2002). *The Royal Marsden NHS Trust Breathlessness Management Programme.* London: The Royal Marsden NHS Trust Occupational Therapy Department. Unpublished. [Cited in: J. Cooper (Ed.), *Occupational therapy in oncology and palliative care* (2nd ed.). Chichester: John Wiley and Sons Ltd, 2006.]

Gosselink, R. (2003). Controlled breathing and dyspnoea in patients with chronic obstructive pulmonary disease (COPD). *Journal of Rehabilitation Research and Development, 40* (5), 25–34.

Hately, J., Laurence, V., Scott, A., Baker, R. & Thomas, P. (2003). Breathlessness clinics within specialist palliative care settings can improve the quality of life and functional capacity of patients with lung cancer. *Palliative Medicine, 17,* 410–417.

Hochstetter, J. K., Lewis, J. & Soares-Smith, L. (2005). An investigation into the immediate impact of breathlessness management on the breathless patient: a randomised controlled trial. *Physiotherapy, 91,* 178–185.

Hough, A. (1996). *Physiotherapy in respiratory care: a problem solving approach to respiratory and cardiac management* (2nd ed.). London: Chapman Hall.

Jantarakupt, P. & Porock, D. (2005). Dyspnoea management in lung cancer: applying the evidence from chronic obstructive pulmonary disease. *Oncology Nursing Forum, 32* (4), 785–797.

Johnson, M. & Moore, S. (2003). Research into practice: the reality of implementing a non-pharmacological breathlessness intervention into clinical practice. *European Journal of Oncology Nursing, 7* (1), 33–38.

Manning, H. L. & Schwartzstein, R. M. (1995). Pathophysiology of dyspnoea. *The New England Journal of Medicine, 333* (23), 1547–1553.

O'Driscoll, M., Corner, J. & Bailey, C. (1999). The experience of breathlessness in lung cancer. *European Journal of Cancer Care, 8,* 37–43.

Payne, R. A. (2000). *Relaxation techniques. A practical handbook for the health care professional.* Edinburgh: Churchill Livingstone.

Potter, J., Hami, F., Bryan, T. & Quigley, C. (2003). Symptoms in 400 patients referred to palliative care services: prevalence and patterns. *Palliative Medicine, 17,* 310–314.

Powell, T. (2000). *The mental health handbook* (revised ed.). Oxon: Speechmark Publishing Ltd.

Regnard, C. & Ahmedzai, S. (1990). Dyspnoea in advanced cancer – a flow diagram. *Palliative Medicine*, *4*, 311–315.

Reuben, D. B. & Mor, V. (1986). Dyspnea in terminally ill cancer patients. *Chest*, *89*, 234–236.

Souhami, R. & Tobias, J. (2003). *Cancer and its management* (4th ed.). Oxford: Blackwell Publishing.

Tanaka, K., Akechi, T., Okuyama, T., Nishiwaki, Y. & Uchitomi, Y. (2002). Factors correlated with dyspnoea in advanced lung cancer patients: organic causes and what else? *Journal of Pain and Symptom Management*, *23* (6), 490–500.

The American Thoracic Society (1999). Dyspnoea: mechanisms, assessment and management: a consensus statement. *American Journal of Respiratory Critical Care Medicine*, *159*, 321–340.

Thompson, E., Sola, I. & Subirana, M. (2005). Non-invasive interventions for improving well-being and quality of life in patients with lung cancer: a systematic review of the evidence. *Lung Cancer*, *50*, 163–176.

Contacts

See "Additional contacts" section at the end of the book.

Chapter 15
MAINTAINING MENTAL HEALTH

Professor Robin Davidson

Learning outcomes

Having read this chapter the reader should be able to:

- Relate psychological models which inform practice, including the health belief model and the transtheoretical model of change, to the emotional impact of cancer
- Understand psychological interventions which are used in the management of anxiety and depression in cancer patients and, in particular, cognitive–behavioural therapy
- Discuss the importance of good-quality communication between health care professionals and patients and the types of communication skills training which are available
- Understand the epidemiology of psychological morbidity among cancer patients

---

Introduction

This chapter will draw on psychological theory to help understand some of the issues associated with the management of cancer from initial diagnosis through to post-treatment rehabilitation. The concluding section will address specific sources of stress among allied health professional (AHPs) who work in an oncology setting and identify how these can be managed.

Supportive care refers to any intervention which optimises the impact of physical treatment and improves quality of life of the cancer patient. It is provided by all AHPs and includes self-help, provision of appropriate information, psychological support, social support, assistance with symptom control and rehabilitation. The National Institute for Clinical Excellence (NICE) (2004) guidance suggests that supportive care is an umbrella term for all of those services which may be required to support people with cancer and their carers. It is predicated on the view that holistic care of our patients requires treatment of the whole person rather than just the tumour. Supportive care is neither a particular speciality nor the domain of one group of health care professionals. It requires a range of skills which are central to good-quality, multi-professional care. This chapter focuses on those aspects of supportive care which have a particular psychological dimension.

Table 15.1 Factors associated with increased psychological morbidity among cancer patients.

History of mood disorder
History of alcohol/drug abuse
Cancer treatment associated with visible deformity
Younger age
An aversive experience of cancer in the family
Poor social support
Low expectation of effective treatment outcome
The presence of distressing side effects
Associated and concurrent stressful life events

The psychological impact of cancer

The psychological sequelae of cancer can occur at every stage of the disease trajectory. Emotional problems can range from worry to a depressive illness or a debilitating anxiety state. It is, however, important not to pathologise normal distress and most patients deal with the emotional impact of their illness with support from friends and family. The post-traumatic stress literature can help us here. Formal psychological intervention just after a trauma disempowers individuals and precludes them from mobilising their own social support network. Indeed, such intervention can increase, not decrease psychological morbidity, i.e. make people worse. It is likely that the same applies in cancer care (Edgar *et al.*, 1992). As is the case immediately post-trauma, just after a cancer diagnosis is not necessarily the optimum time for formal psychotherapy or counselling. Rather the patient should be encouraged to glean normal support from, for example, friends, family or ward staff. It is only for a minority of patients who have serious and persistent emotional adjustment problems that formal psychotherapy is required.

The presentation of serious depressive illness occurs in around 5–9% of newly diagnosed cancer patients. This is not much higher than that of the general population. However, the prevalence of clinically significant adjustment disorder with depressed mood is higher and estimates range from 16 to 25% (Sellick & Crooks, 1999). The predisposing factors associated with significant anxiety or depression are summarised in Table 15.1. It has been noted in the NICE (2004) guidance that patients and carers with significant psychopathology are likely to benefit from some form of professional psychological support. Such specialist services include counselling, psychotherapy and psychotropic drug therapy. A four-level model of psychological assessment and intervention is outlined in Table 15.2.

In summary, only a minority of cancer patients require the level 4 help of mental health specialists. However, most AHPs should be able to recognise psychological distress and be competent enough to perform at level 1 and, indeed, level 2. AHPs should therefore adopt the basic counselling principals of unconditional positive regard, empathy and congruence in their interaction with all patients and carers. *Unconditional positive regard* means genuinely caring and accepting the patient as a person, *empathy* is an ability to view the world through the patient's eyes and

Table 15.2 Levels of psychological assessment and support.

Level	Group	Assessment	Intervention
1	All health and social care professionals	Recognition of psychological needs	Effective information giving Compassionate communication and general psychological support
2	Health and social care professionals with additional expertise	Screening for psychological distress	Psychological techniques such as problem solving
3	Trained and accredited professionals	Assessed for psychological distress and diagnosis of some psychopathology	Counselling and specific psychological interventions such as anxiety management and solution-focused therapy, delivered according to an explicit theoretical framework
4	Mental health specialists	Diagnosis of psychopathology	Specialist psychological and psychiatric interventions such as psychotherapy, including cognitive–behavioural therapy

congruence refers to a consistency between the way the AHP feels and the way he or she behaves.

Psychological interventions

To date, five systematic reviews have been carried out on the impact of psychological assessment and intervention on patients with cancer. These are summarised in the NICE (2004) guidance and provide robust evidence that the benefits of such interventions include reduction in psychological distress, improvement in quality of life and greater compliance with cancer treatment. More specifically, psychological therapies, particularly cognitive–behavioural therapy, have been shown to produce positive outcomes for anxiety, depression and low self-esteem. There is some limited evidence that psychological interventions may convey survival advantage for particular illnesses, notably, melanoma and breast carcinoma. This latter evidence should, however, be treated with some caution at this stage pending further confirmatory studies (Fox, 1998).

Cognitive–behavioural psychotherapy is emerging as the most therapeutic and cost-effective intervention for cancer patients with significant psychopathology. Morrey *et al.* (1994) developed a cognitive intervention specifically tailored to the needs of cancer patients. This is a brief, problem-focused approach which helps to improve adjustment and enhance mood. The key components of this adjuvant psychological therapy (APT) are summarised in Table 15.3.

Table 15.3 Key components of adjuvant psychological therapy.

The promotion of emotional expression: This is the acknowledgement of negative emotions to help adjustment

Activity scheduling: Activities and daily structures are planned to promote mastery over one's personal environment, thereby promoting self-efficacy

Relaxation and visualisation: This helps patients deal with anxiety. Guided imagery of the host defences destroying cancer cells can be used in conjunction with hypnosis or relaxation

Cognitive restructuring: Monitoring thoughts and training in distraction, reality testing or reattribution of their meaning

---

Contemporary approaches to cancer rehabilitation adopted by AHPs include many of the elements of cognitive–behavioural therapy of which APT is an example. These include stress management programmes which commonly utilise relaxation and visualisation (see Chapter 3). Fatigue management groups conducted by physiotherapists and occupational therapists (OTs) will cover graded exercise and activity scheduling (Chapter 12). Problem-solving and behaviour modification techniques are key items in the dietitian's training. Cognitive–behavioural therapy essentially helps people reduce their distress through the process of modifying exaggerated or biased ways of thinking and behavioural experimentation.

Psychological adjustment to cancer

A number of common adjustment styles have emerged in factor analytic studies and these are summarised in Table 15.4.

Mental adjustment has been defined as 'cognitive and behavioural responses made by an individual' (Greer *et al.*, 1989). The most common measure of adjustment style is the mental adjustment to cancer (MAC) scale (Watson *et al.*, 1989). There is some evidence that the type of adjustment style is a determinant of psychological morbidity. It should be emphasised that encouraging 'fighting spirit' is not appropriate for everyone. Indeed, for some patients the beneficial effects of the 'denial' style have emerged so much so that this has been rechristened 'positive avoidance'. There is clear evidence that positive avoidance is an appropriate and helpful strategy for some patients. Such individuals may not search the internet for details of their cancer, they may not actively seek out information and they may not wish to be informed about the specific aspects of their illness by AHPs and medical staff.

It is also possible that adjustment style may enhance survival. Mystakidou *et al.* (2005) suggest that patients with 'fighting spirit' tend to live longer than those who

Table 15.4 Adjustment styles following a diagnosis of cancer.

Fighting spirit: 'I am not going to let this disease beat me'.
Positive avoidance: 'I don't really think that this is cancer'.
Stoic acceptance/fatalism: 'I am just going to have to learn to live with this'.
Helplessness/hopelessness: 'This is the end. There is nothing I can do'.
Anxious pre-occupation: 'I can't get the thought of this tumour out of my mind'.

---

adopt a 'helplessness' style. The link between adjustment style and longer survival has been discussed at length in the literature. While some studies have correlated 'fighting spirit' and 'positive avoidance' with longer survival, there have been other well-controlled studies which have found no such association (Osborne *et al.*, 2004). Nonetheless, the individual's personal MAC should inform the approach of all AHPs when treating their patients. Adjustment style will have some impact on motivation, which will in turn affect treatment compliance. Each person is an individual who will deal with the existential threat of cancer in his or her own way. The approach to each individual patient should be tailored to his or her particular adjustment style.

Brennan (2001) in his cognitive transition model of adjustment to cancer suggests that adjustment is an ongoing process of learning from and adapting to the changes which an individual faces as a result of living with and receiving treatment for cancer. He suggests that the degree of adjustment depends on the combined effects of coping responses, social support and cognitive appraisal of the cancer experience and the type of adjustment can change over time.

Communication

The importance of good-quality communication between cancer patients and AHPs has long been realised. In recent years there has been a great deal of research into professional–patient communication in a cancer environment. Fundamental qualities of the therapeutic relationship like open-ended questions, clarification, effective use of silence and empathy have been identified in a variety of studies (Butler *et al.*, 2005). AHPs should adopt a flexible approach to communication and through reflective practice should identify and deal with patients' concerns and emotions. The environment should be comfortable and the language appropriate to the patient's level of understanding.

There is a growing body of literature on the development of effective training programmes for cancer professionals in the area of communication. The NICE (2004) guidance states that training in communication skills can change health care professionals' attitudes and help elicit patients' concerns. The guidance details some evidence that intensive, skill-based training programmes can improve the communication behaviour of health care professionals. Generally, these training programmes consist of small groups with facilitators providing education and feedback.

There is normally also an experiential component to the training. The most effective approaches to communication skills training are quite intensive and employ patient models in simulated role-plays. Most of these programmes take the form of 3-day workshops.

The key question is whether or not any communication improvements are maintained after the training has been completed. Common areas addressed in most of the training programmes include breaking bad news, discussion of dying and bereavement, history taking, listening skills and recognition of patients' needs and emotional responses. In general, positive long-term outcomes for this type of communication training have been reported, and in a recent systematic review of 47 studies

Table 15.5 Breaking bad news: key steps.

See patients in a private setting.
Introduce yourself if you are not already known.
Find out what the patient knows and wants to know.
Start from the patient's starting point (aligning).
Give information in small chunks.
Use warning shot, 'I am afraid things aren't as straight forward as we thought'.
Use plain English.
Frequently monitor and acknowledge the patient's reaction: clarify accordingly.
If diagnosis is asked for start vaguely: move to more accurate predictions if the patient is able.
Warn that the interview is soon to close; e.g. 'I am afraid I am going to go in a minute, is there anything else you would like to know?'
Offer to speak to relatives.

Adapted from Buckman (1992).

Butler *et al.* (2005) concluded that relationships between health care professionals and patients do improve after these training programmes.

As noted above, the training is intensive and costly and there is a need for continuing research on cost-effective ways of providing good-quality communication skills training for all cancer care professionals. Almost all of the communication skills training programmes to date have been designed for doctors and nurses. There is clearly a need for a multidisciplinary approach to ensure that AHPs have access to such training.

A specific example of the importance of good communication skills is the breaking of bad news in a sensitive manner. Workers at the McMaster University in Canada have produced a body of research on training medical students to break bad news. Essentially the 1-day programme consists of video presentations, small group discussion and role-plays. This training has been shown to increase the student's sense of competency and the McMaster protocol is summarised in Table 15.5 (Buckman, 1992)

Rehabilitation

Behavioural and lifestyle factors contribute to almost half of cancer mortality. Smoking behaviour alone accounts for almost 30% of all new cancers. A number of cognitive models have been developed, which help us understand how people reduce carcinogenic behaviour and also adopt healthier lifestyles after diagnosis. Lifestyle management should be of interest to all AHPs.

The theory of planned behaviour (TPB) has been particularly influential and is arguably the most widely used model in this regard (Ajzen & Fishbein, 1980). This model demonstrates how individuals permanently acquire positive behaviours like breast and testicular self-examination, healthy eating habits, physical exercise and the like. It also enables us to understand how people reduce harmful behaviour like smoking and alcohol abuse. Essentially, it is a cognitive model which specifies the conditions of behaviour change which are under volitional control.

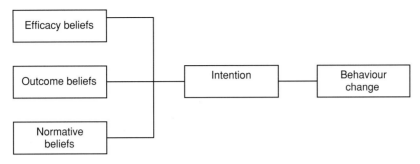

Figure 15.1 Theory of planned behaviour (Ajzen & Fishbein, 1980).

Figure 15.1 is a diagrammatic representation of the TPB. This indicates that the intention to change one's behaviour is determined by three cognitive variables, notably, beliefs about efficacy, outcome and the attitude of significant others to the proposed new behaviour. *Efficacy* refers to the belief in one's ability to engage successfully in the new behaviour. *Outcome* beliefs are expectations that the behavioural change will produce positive effects. *Normative* beliefs are about the importance which significant others in one's life attach to particular behavioural change.

Essentially, efficacy poses the question *can I succeed*? For outcome the question is, *will change be worthwhile*? For normative beliefs the question is, *do other people really want me to change*? Strong outcome and normative beliefs generally predict initiation of new positive health behaviours, while efficacy beliefs are better predictors of long-term maintenance of such behaviours. There is a very high correlation between these cognitive variables and permanent health behaviour outcome for a range of carcinogenic behaviour.

Andrykowski *et al.* (2006) examined the behavioural intentions of cancer patients towards *physical behaviours* such as eating a healthy diet and engaging in physical exercise. They also considered *psychosocial behaviours* such as reflecting on priorities in life, spending quality time with friends and loved ones, engaging in charitable or volunteer activities and spending time in religious and spiritual activities. These authors reported on 2-year outcomes for a large group of cancer patients and concluded that the TPB can serve as a comprehensive model for understanding long-term change in both physical and psychosocial behaviour after a cancer diagnosis. They demonstrate that the three cognitive variables are very strong predictors of the extent to which positive health behaviours are adopted and maintained.

The importance of cognitive predictors of post-treatment lifestyle management is more than just theoretically significant. The TPB can be used to inform the development and implementation of any practical rehabilitation intervention which involves conscious and permanent behavioural change. A key route to optimising the rehabilitation process would entail AHPs encouraging specific positive psychosocial behaviour, strengthening attitudes about outcome and helping people increase the sense of efficacy and behavioural control.

While rehabilitation interventions conducted by AHPs may have a primary physical focus, they will also carry significant psychological and social benefits. It has been noted that problems with mobility and daily activities arising from cancer can adversely affect the person's sense of control, self-esteem and quality of life. Good rehabilitation services promote a sense of empowerment and mastery which inoculate against emotional problems. General training in physical exercise and coping skills improves not only the physical but also the emotional well-being of cancer patients. Corner *et al.* (1996) found that a breathlessness intervention for lung cancer patients, which included breathing retraining, relaxation, coping skills training and adaption strategies, improved quality of life as well as functional ability. Holley and Borger (2001) explored group intervention for cancer-related fatigue. This included sessions on exercise, energy instruction and activity scheduling. The programme was found to improve quality of life and psychological distress. Lobrinzi *et al.* (1996) found that dietetic counselling aimed at weight maintenance had more general positive psychological effects. In all of this work, psychological theory can inform the AHP about psychological variables like choice, commitment, determination and behaviour change.

Motivation

Motivation to change one's behaviour is a key factor in producing permanent positive health behaviour outcomes either before or after a cancer diagnosis. A useful model which complements the theory of planned behaviour is the stages of change model. This model informs our thinking on motivational issues associated with behaviour change (Prochaska *et al.*, 1992) and is summarised in Figure 15.2.

Essentially, an individual does not change intentional behaviour instantaneously. Motivation evolves over time and there are a number of distinct motivational changes

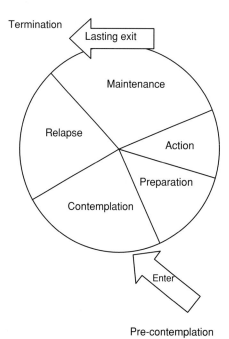

Figure 15.2 The stages model of motivational change. [Reproduced with permission from Prochaska *et al.*, 1992. Copyright © American Psychological Association.]

which the stage model has identified. In the *pre-contemplation stage* individuals are not aware of their difficulties, perhaps as a result of ambivalence, denial or selective exposure to information. As individuals become aware that their behaviour may be harmful they enter the *contemplation stage*. This involves thinking seriously about change and a specific evaluation of the pros and cons of changing behaviour. The next stage is the *preparation stage* when a commitment to the change plan is made. During the *action stage*, active coping is initiated and the behavioural change is made. Once this occurs, the individual enters the *maintenance stage* in which the new positive health behaviours are strengthened and integrated into one's overall lifestyle.

It takes some time to integrate new behaviours into an individual's lifestyle, but when this occurs one then exits the change system to *termination*. For many who are attempting to alter harmful behaviours, particularly smoking, alcohol use or poor diet, relapse is common, notably in the first 6 months or so. Relapse triggers can include negative self-evaluation, environmental pressures or inadequately prepared coping styles. It has been demonstrated that people do not progress in a linear fashion through the stages but rather exhibit a more cyclical pattern. It is said, for example, that an average successful ex-smoker makes three serious revolutions through the stages of change before becoming permanently free of the habit (Prochaska *et al.*, 1992).

This motivational model has not been free from criticism (Davidson, 1992 and West, 2005). It has, however, become ubiquitous in the health promotion literature and assists our understanding of motivational issues which promote positive behavioural change in cancer rehabilitation.

For individuals in the contemplation stage, *motivational interviewing* is the intervention of choice. Traditionally, AHPs may suggest lifestyle change. For example, physiotherapists may prescribe an exercise programme, SLTs may give instruction on homework or OTs may be clear about activities of daily living. However, these should take account of the motivational stage of the individual. Advice on diet is for life, not just a few weeks. Motivational interviewing is a skill which promotes decision making on the part of the patient, not the AHP. It is a strategy for enhancing motivation to embark on a permanent journey of lifestyle management. Increasingly, AHPs are opting for training in motivational interviewing as a supplement to the traditional methods of instruction and prescription. Motivational interviewing maximises the intention and determination of the individual patient to adopt permanent behavioural change (Miller & Rollnick, 2002).

The adoption of health behaviour in the context of a positive lifestyle is critical in cancer rehabilitation. The motivational stage model and the TPB help us understand the key motivational and cognitive variables which contribute to the initiation and permanent adoption of positive behaviour and elimination of negative behaviour.

Body image

Body image is in a state of constant flux throughout all of an individual's developmental stages. Price (1992) suggests that there are three related components to body image. *Body reality* is one's body as it really is, while *body ideal* is the body we would like to have. *Body presentation* is how we project ourselves through dress, grooming and posture. He notes that cancer does not intrude on a static body image, but rather on our ever-changing perception of how we think we appear to others.

There are many aspects of cancer and its treatment which can significantly alter body image. These can include stomas, mastectomies, lymphoedema, head-and-neck deformities or loss of hair through chemotherapy. Altered body image can also include other changes, which are not quite so visible, like incontinence, constipation, fatigue and impotence. Alteration of body image is one of the key areas in psychological management of cancer-related distress.

Issues about body image generally become manifest after the acute stage of coming to terms with the diagnosis and illness. Indeed, very often, body image problems will peak after the initial phase of active medical treatment has been completed. A key point in the cancer journey when psychopathology risks are high is just after discharge from active medical care. It is then that a patient is particularly vulnerable to distress and this is very often related to body image or fear of the future.

Body image is central to the work of many AHPs. There are a number of psychological theories which can help guide work in this area. Newell (1999) proposed a fear-avoidance model of psychological difficulty after disfigurement. This suggests that behavioural and cognitive avoidance associated with the disfigurement can lead to poor long-term psychological adjustment. Shearsmith-Farthing (2001) outlines the role for OT in the management of altered body image. She argues that, as in any intervention, it is essential to discuss the specific meaning and consequences of an altered body image with the patient. It may then be useful to employ the adaptation through occupation model, which is essentially a cognitive–behavioural approach. The patient is encouraged to express body image concerns in an accepting comfortable environment. This will set the scene for behavioural experiments aimed at helping the individual slowly adjust to body changes. This process of adjustment takes time and can be viewed rather like a bereavement reaction.

Another example would be speech and language training in oesophageal speech after a laryngectomy. Such work cannot be carried out in a vacuum and account should be taken of the motivational, cognitive and adjustment variables discussed in this chapter. Therapists must be careful not to minimise physical loss but rather encourage cancer survivors to reframe losses cognitively in ways which have meaning for them. When body image is conceptualised in such broad terms, it is something which all AHPs should address in their day-to-day work.

A variety of interventions based around emotional expression, grief work, cognitive–behavioural psychotherapy and family counselling can all play a significant role in dealing with alteration of body image associated with cancer or its treatment.

Group work

On occasions AHPs will be required to run support groups for people with cancer. The function of such groups could be for relaxation training, fatigue management, assertiveness work and activity scheduling or tumour-specific support. Since Spiegel *et al.* (1989) demonstrated that a support group could increase survival time for patients with metastatic breast cancer, there has been a great interest in the use of groups in a comprehensive approach to cancer care.

The effect of social support in itself can assist adjustment. However the results of a seminal early study on group work in cancer may help guide any AHPs who are designing group programmes for cancer patients (Evans & Connis, 1995). These authors randomly assigned cancer patients to a coping group, a support group and a control condition. The coping group was based on cognitive–behavioural principles and employed instruction in relaxation, cognitive reframing, assertiveness training, time management and goal setting. This group also had homework assignments and the use of role-play was extensive. The support group was more traditional in that people discussed their concerns and emotions relating to cancer adjustment. People in the control group did not receive any intervention. The results showed that the mental state of those in the control condition became worse; people in the support group reported reduction in anxiety and depression while those in the coping group not only improved in terms of anxiety and depression but also improved in a range of other areas including communication, assertiveness, ability to cope and empowerment. This finding on the efficacy of skill-based group interventions has been replicated over the years.

The Holley and Borger intervention referred to previously also explored group intervention for cancer-related fatigue. There were sessions on exercise, energy instruction and activity scheduling. The programme was found to improve quality of life and psychological distress. This is an example of a useful, evidence-based coping group approach which should be employed routinely in cancer treatment centres.

Looking after yourself

It is important that AHPs working within an oncology setting look after themselves. Burnout in a cancer care environment is not uncommon. The three components of burnout are emotional exhaustion, depersonalisation and reduced personal accomplishment (Maslach *et al.*, 1996). The characteristics of these components are outlined in Table 15.6.

Burnout among professional staff can lead to deterioration in the quality of care provided for the patient as well as low morale, absenteeism and poor physical and mental health. Job-related stresses specific to oncology have been identified (Davidson, 2006). These can include overinvolvement in highly personalised type of

Table 15.6 The characteristics of burnout.

Emotional exhaustion – Wearing out, depletion of emotional resources, loss of energy, debilitation and fatigue

Depersonalisation – Negative, callous, excessively detached towards other people, loss of idealism and irritability

Reduced personal accomplishment – Reduction in self-confidence, low productivity, poor morale and inability to cope

interaction with patients and families. Regularly confronting death can lead workers to question how a situation could have been managed better. There can be an incremental burnout effect due to what has been called accumulated grief.

Small informal staff support groups can be a useful antidote to burnout as can mentoring, effective teamwork and good-quality clinical supervision. It is also important that there is a mutually supportive atmosphere among colleagues. A recent survey of cancer professionals concluded that most people felt that the opportunity to simply talk things over with a colleague was the most useful coping strategy (Bruneau et al., 2004). It is important to identify sources of stress and put in place procedures for its identification and management.

A comprehensive approach to cancer care must emphasise the needs of the whole person. Thus multi-professional care is essential to improve the psychological as well as the physical health of our patients and AHPs are an integral part of the team. They are also just as prone to burnout as nursing and medical staff. Cancer work is emotionally demanding and all staff should ensure that they themselves are psychologically fit, which will in turn ensure best-quality care for our patients.

Key learning points

- Our understanding of evidence-based psychological interventions in cancer has increased considerably over the past two decades.
- Coping strategies adopted by cancer patients have a significant impact on an individual's adjustment to cancer and quality of life.
- There is robust literature on the training of effective communication skills for health care professionals, although most of the training has been piloted on doctors and nurses. There is a need for a multi-professional approach to communication skills training to include AHPs.
- When considering post-treatment lifestyle management the importance of cognitive variables cannot be overemphasised. Such variables like self-efficacy and perceived effectiveness are very good predictors of positive and permanent lifestyle change after a diagnosis of cancer.
- There is clear guidance in the literature as to which type of group interventions are most effective with cancer patients. Skill-based interventions are considerably more beneficial than traditional support groups.
- Burnout among professional staff caring for cancer patients is not uncommon. Key strategies for attenuating the effects of burnout include the identification of small groups offering peer support as well as effective teamwork and good-quality supervision.

References

Ajzen, I. & Fishbein, N. (1980). *Understanding attitudes and predicting behaviour.* Englewood Cliffs, NJ: Prentice Hall.

Andrykowski, M., Beacham, A., Schmidt, J. & Harper, F. (2006). Application of the theory of planned behaviour to understand intentions to engage in physical and psychosocial health behaviours after cancer diagnosis. *Psycho-Oncology, 15,* 759–771.

Brennan, J. (2001). Adjustment to cancer-coping or personal transition. *Psycho-Oncology*, *10*, 1–18.

Bruneau, B., Benjamin, M. & Ellison, G. (2004). Palliative care stress in a UK community hospital. *International Journal of Palliative Nursing*, *10*, 296–305.

Buckman, R. (1992). *How to break bad news; a guide for healthcare professionals*. London: Pan Books.

Butler, L., Degner, L., Baile, W. & Lany, M. (2005). Developing communication competency in the context of cancer: a critical interpretive analysis of provider training programmes. *Psycho-Oncology*, *14*, 861–872.

Corner, J., Plant, H., A'Hern, R. & Bailey, C. (1996). Non-pharmacological intervention for breathlessness in lung cancer. *Palliative Medicine*, *10*, 299–305.

Davidson, R. (1992). Prochaska and DeClemente's model of change; a case study. *British Journal of Addiction*, *87*, 821–822.

Davidson, R. (2006). Stress issues in palliative care. In: J. Cooper (Ed.), *Stepping into palliative care*. London: Routledge.

Edgar, L., Rossburger, Z. & Nowlis, D. (1992). Coping with cancer during the first year after diagnosis. *Cancer*, *69* (3), 817–828.

Evans, R. & Connis, R. (1995). Comparison of brief group therapy for depressed cancer patients who are receiving radiation treatment.*Public Health Report*, *110*, 306–311.

Fox, B. (1998). Hypotheses about Spiegel *et al.*'s paper on psychological intervention and breast cancer survival. *Psycho-Oncology*, *7* (5), 361–370.

Greer, S., Moorey, S. & Watson, M. (1989). Patient adjustment to cancer: the mental adjustment to cancer (MAC) scale vs clinical ratings. *Journal of Psychosomatic Research*, *33* (3), 373–377.

Holley, S. & Borger, D. (2001). Living with energy for lung cancer; preliminary findings of a cancer rehabilitation group intervention study. *Oncology Nursing Forum*, *28*, 1393–1396.

Lobrinzi, C., Athmannl, D., Kardinal, C. & O'Thallon, J. (1996). Randomized trial of dietitian counselling to try to prevent weight gain associated with breast cancer adjuvant chemotherapy. *Oncology*, *53*, 228–232.

Maslach, C., Jackson, S. & Leiter, M. (1996). *The Maslach Burnout Inventory* (3rd ed.). Palo Alto: Consulting Clinical Psychologists Press.

Miller, W. & Rollnick, S. (2002). *Motivational interviewing. Preparing people for change*. London: Guildford Press.

Morrey, S., Greer, S. & Watson, M. (1994). Adjuvant psychological therapy for patients with cancer: outcome at one year. *Psycho-Oncology*, *3*, 39–46.

Mystakidou, K., Watson, M., Tsilika, E., Parpa, E., Primikiri, A., Katsouda, E. & Viahos, L. (2005). Psychometric analysis of the mental adjustment to cancer scale (MAC) in a Greek palliative care unit. *Psycho-Oncology*, *14*, 16–24.

Newell, R. (1999). Altered body image: a fear avoidance model of psych-social difficulties following disfigurement. *Journal of Advanced Nursing*, *30*, 1230–1238.

National Institute for Clinical Excellence [NICE] (2004). *Improving supportive and palliative care for adults with cancer*. London: National Institute for Clinical Excellence.

Osborne, R., Sali, A., Aaronson, G., Elsworth, B., Medzewski, B. & Sinclair, A. (2004). Immune function and adjustment style: do they predict survival in breast cancer? *Psycho-Oncology*, *13*, 199–210.

Price, B. (1992). Living with altered body image; the cancer experience. *British Journal of Nursing*, *1*, 641–645.

Prochaska, J., DiClemente, C. & Norcross, J. (1992). In search of how people change: applications to addictive behaviour. *American Psychologist*, *7*, 1102–1104.

Sellick, S. & Crooks, D. (1999). Depression and cancer: an appraisal of the literature for prevalence, detection and practice guideline development for psychological intervention. *Psycho-oncology, 8* (4), 315–333.

Shearsmith-Farthing, K. (2001). The management of altered body image: a role for occupational therapy. *The British Journal of Occupational Therapy, 6*, 387–392.

Spiegel, D., Bloom, J., Cramer, H. & Gottheile, E. (1989) Effective psycho-social treatment on survival of patients with metastatic breast cancer. *Lancet, 2*, 888–891.

Watson, M., Greer, S. & Bliss, J. (1989). *Mental adjustment to cancer (MAC) scale users manual.* Sutton, Surrey, UK: CRC Psychological Medicine Research Group, Royal Marsden Hospital.

West, R. (2005). Time for a change: putting the transtheoretical (stages of change) model to rest. *Addiction, 100* (8), 1036.

ADDITIONAL CONTACTS

Macmillan Cancer Support
89 Albert Embankment, London, SE1 7UQ
Tel: 0808 808 2020
www.macmillan.org.uk

Roy Castle Lung Foundation
200 London Road, Liverpool, L3 9TA
Tel: 0800 358 7200
www.roycastle.org

Cancer BACUP
3 Bath Place, Rivington Street, London, EC2A 3JR
Tel: 020 7696 9003
Cancer info helpline: 0808 800 1234
www.cancerbacup.org.uk

British Lung Foundation
73–75 Goswell Road, London, EC1V 7ER
Tel: 08458 505020
www.britishlungfoundation.org

British Heart Foundation
14 Fitzhardinge Street, London, W1H 6DH
Tel: 020 7935 0185 or 0845 708070
www.bhf.org.uk

INDEX

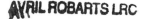